C000174152

Conquer the
PTEeXAM

Mary Peak

Conquer the PTEeXAM

Thomas M. Burch, MD

Assistant Professor
Department of Anesthesiology
University of Alabama at Birmingham
Birmingham, Alabama

Leanne Groban, MD

Associate Professor
Department of Anesthesiology
Cardiothoracic Section
Wake Forest University
Winston-Salem, North Carolina

David A. Zvara, MD

Jay J. Jacoby Professor and Chair
Department of Anesthesiology
The Ohio State University
Columbus, Ohio

SAUNDERS

ELSEVIER

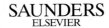

SAUNDERS
ELSEVIER

1600 John F. Kennedy Blvd.
Ste 1800
Philadelphia, PA 19103-2899

CONQUER THE PTEeXAM   ISBN: 978-1-4160-3833-7

Copyright © 2007, by Saunders, an imprint of Elsevier Inc.

All rights reserved. No part of this publication may be reproduced or transmitted in any form or by any means, electronic or mechanical, including photocopying, recording, or any information storage and retrieval system, without permission in writing from the publisher.
Permissions may be sought directly from Elsevier's Health Sciences Rights Department in Philadelphia, PA, USA: phone: (+1) 215 239 3804, fax: (+1) 215 239 3805, e-mail: healthpermissions@elsevier.com. You may also complete your request on-line via the Elsevier homepage (http://www.elsevier.com), by selecting 'Customer Support' and then 'Obtaining Permissions'.

NOTICE

Knowledge and best practice in this field are constantly changing. As new research and experience broaden our knowledge, changes in practice, treatment and drug therapy may become necessary or appropriate. Readers are advised to check the most current information provided (i) on procedures featured or (ii) by the manufacturer of each product to be administered, to verify the recommended dose or formula, the method and duration of administration, and contraindications. It is the responsibility of the practitioner, relying on their own experience and knowledge of the patient, to make diagnoses, to determine dosages and the best treatment for each individual patient, and to take all appropriate safety precautions. To the fullest extent of the law, neither the publisher nor the authors assumes any liability for any injury and/or damage to persons or property arising out of or related to any use of the material contained in this book

---

The Publisher

Library of Congress Cataloging-in-Publication Data
Conquer the PTEeXAM/editors, Thomas M. Burch, Leanne Groban, David A. Zvara. — 1st ed.
       p. ; cm.
ISBN 978-1-4160-3833-7
1. Transesophageal echocardiography — Examinations, questions, etc. 2.
Transesophageal echocardiography — Examinations — Study guides. I. Burch, Thomas M. 11. Groban, Leanne. 111. Zvara, David A.
[DNLM: 1. Anesthesia — Examination Questions. 2.
Anesthesiology — Examination Questions. 3. Anesthetics — Examination Questions. WO 18.2 C753 2007]

RD52.T73C667 2007
616.1'2075430076—dc22

                    2007000828

Executive Publisher: Natasha Andjelkovic
Editorial Assistant: Isabel Trudeau
Senior Production Manager: David Saltzberg
Design Direction: Steve Stave

Printed in China

Last digit is the print number: 9 8 7 6 5 4 3 2 1

Working together to grow
libraries in developing countries

www.elsevier.com | www.bookaid.org | www.sabre.org

ELSEVIER   BOOK AID International   Sabre Foundation

CONTENTS

Test 1, Part 1: Video Test Booklet 1

Test 1, Part 2: Written Test Booklet 31

Test 11, Part 1: Video Test Booklet 113

Test 11, Part 2: Written Test Booklet 145

Test 111, Part 1: Video Test Booklet 215

Test 111, Part 2: Written Test Booklet 243

Test 1V, Part 1: Video Test Booklet 313

Test 1V, Part 2: Written Test Booklet 343

Test V, Part 1: Video Test Booklet 419

Test V, Part 2: Written Test Booklet 451

Index 529

NOTE TO THE READER

Thanks for purchasing our product. Hopefully it will help you study for the **PTEeXAM**. We have invested a lot of time, energy and effort in preparing all the materials in this book and the accompanying CD-ROM as accurately as possible. However, nothing is ever perfect, and you should always look things up and consult other sources if anything looks questionable, especially before you make a clinical decision based on information contained in this book. To assist you with that we have listed references at the end of the explanations. Also, if you find a mistake please let us know so we can correct it. You can contact us via email with any questions, comments, criticisms or suggestions, at conquerthetest@yahoo.com

Take care, and good luck

The Authors

TEST I PART 1

Video Test Booklet

This product is designed to prepare people for the PTEeXAM. This booklet is to be used with the CD-ROM to practice for the video portion of the PTEeXAM.

Preface

As stated previously, this part of this product is designed to prepare people for the video component of the PTEeXAM. Please do not open this test booklet until you have read the instructions. During the PTEeXAM, instructions similar to these will be written on the back of the test booklet. You will be asked to read these instructions by a proctor at the exam. After you have read these instructions you will be asked to break the seal on the test booklet and to remove an answer sheet.

After you have filled out your name, test number, and other identifying information on the answer sheet you will be instructed to open the test booklet and begin. This test will involve video images shown on a computer monitor. You will share this monitor with three other examinees. This portion of the PTEeXAM has about 50 questions. It consists of about 17 cases, with 2 to 5 questions for each case. It is timed. Good luck!

Instructions

This test will consist of several cases, accompanied by 3 to 5 questions per case. Each case will show one or more images. For each case, you are to utilize the information written in this booklet and the information shown in the images to answer questions concerning each case. An audible chime or tone will assist in timing the exam. This tone alerts you when the test advances to the next step.

The order of the exam is as follows.

Tone/chime

> 1. Read the questions for case 1.

Tone/chime

> 2. View the images for case 1.

Tone/chime

> 3. Answer the questions for case 1.

Tone/chime

> 4. View the images for case 1 again.

Tone/chime

> 5. Check your answers to the questions for case 1.

Tone/chime

> 6. Read the questions for case 2.

Tone/chime

The process continues in this manner. In summary: tone, read, tone, view, tone, answer, tone, view, tone, check answers, tone.

Cases

Case 1

A 42-year-old male presents for kidney transplantation. Answer the following questions concerning his systolic function.

> 1. What is the best estimate of this patient's qualitative systolic function?

>> A. Normal systolic function LVEF >55%.

>> B. Mildly decreased systolic function LVEF = 45-50%.

>> C. Moderately decreased systolic function LVEF = 35-45%.

>> D. Severely decreased systolic function LVEF <20%.

>> E. It cannot be determined from the information given.

2. Which of the following is most likely to be true concerning this patient's segmental wall motion?

A. Severe global hypokinesis is present.

B. Severe anterior dyskinesis is present.

C. Severe inferior akinesis is present.

D. Severe septal akinesis is present.

3. This patient is at increased risk for which of the following?

A. Cerebral vascular accident due to thrombus in the left atrial appendage

B. Transplant failure due to inadequate renal perfusion

C. Fatal ventricular arrhythmias

D. All of the above

Case 2

4. Which of the following is the best estimate of this patient's fractional area change (FAC)?

A. 33%

B. 20%

C. 16%

D. 40%

E. None of the above

5. Which of the following best describes this patient's systolic function?

A. Normal

B. Hyperdynamic

C. Severely decreased

D. Slightly decreased

Case 3

6. What is the best estimate of this patient's fractional shortening (FS)?

    A. 8.8%

    B. 16.2%

    C. 11%

    D. 21%

    E. <5%

7. What wall is indicated by the arrow?

    A. Anterior

    B. Inferior

    C. Septal

    D. Anteroseptal

    E. Posterior

8. Which of the following statements concerning this patient is most likely true?

    A. Severe concentric left ventricular hypertrophy is present.

    B. Moderate left ventricular dilation is present.

    C. The inferior wall appears more robust (thickens more) than the other walls.

    D. The patient is hypovolemic.

Case 4

9. What mitral valve leaflet does the arrow in image 1 for case 4 indicate?

    A. Posterior

    B. Inferior

    C. Septal

    D. Anteroseptal

    E. Anterior

10. What view is shown in image I for case 4?

   A. Midesophageal four-chamber view

   B. Midesophageal two-chamber view

   C. Midesophageal long axis view

   D. Midesophageal mitral inflow view

   E. Transgastric mitral inflow view

11. What mitral valve leaflet does the arrow in image 2 for case 4 indicate?

   A. Posterior

   B. Inferior

   C. Septal

   D. Anteroseptal

   E. Anterior

12. What view is shown in image 2 for case 4?

   A. Transgastric mid papillary short axis view

   B. Transgastric left ventricular inflow view

   C. Transgastric basal short axis view

   D. Transgastric mitral valve commissural view

   E. Midesophageal mitral valve commissural view

13. The patient shown in image 3 for case 4 is scheduled to undergo mitral valve repair. For which post mitral valve repair complication is this patient at increased risk?

   A. Post repair mitral valve stenosis

   B. Mitral valve thrombus formation

   C. Ventricular fibrillation

   D. Complete heart block

   E. Systolic anterior motion of the anterior mitral valve leaflet

Case 5

14. What mitral valve scallop is indicated by the arrow?

    A. P1

    B. P2

    C. P3

    D. A1

    E. A2

15. What view is shown?

    A. Midesophageal four-chamber view

    B. Midesophageal two-chamber view

    C. Midesophageal long axis view

    D. Midesophageal mitral inflow view

    E. Transgastric mitral inflow view

Case 6

16. Which of the following best describes the severity of the mitral regurgitation seen in this patient?

    A. Trace

    B. Mild

    C. Moderate

    D. Severe

    E. Cannot be determined from the images shown

17. Which of the following measurements is most consistent with severe mitral regurgitation?

    A. Vena contracta at the base of the mitral regurgitant jet of 6.1 mm

    B. Color flow Doppler mitral regurgitant jet area of 5.5 cm^2

    C. Mitral regurgitant fraction of 50%

    D. Ratio of color flow Doppler jet area / left atrial area of 53%

    E. Systolic blunting of pulmonary vein inflow velocities by pulsed-wave Doppler

Case 7

18. In image 1 for case 7, which of the following is the best explanation for the difficulty in imaging the interventricular septum?

    A. Acoustic shadowing (echo dropout) artifact is present.

    B. The septum is not perpendicular to the ultrasound beam.

    C. The overall gain is set too low to image the septum.

    D. The time gain compensation is inadequate to allow imaging of the septum.

    E. Reverberation artifact is preventing imaging of the septum.

19. The angle between the mitral valve leaflets (α) is equal to 120 degrees and 120/180 = 0.67. Given this data and the information shown in the slides for case 4, what is the mitral valve area as determined by the proximal isovelocity surface area method?

    A. 0.62 cm^2

    B. 0.72 cm^2

    C. 0.82 cm^2

    D. 0.92 cm^2

    E. 1.2 cm^2

20. For the patient shown in case 7, a pulsed-wave Doppler interrogation of the left upper pulmonary vein is likely to show an enlargement of which of the following waves?

A. S wave

B. D wave

C. AR wave

D. E wave

E. F wave

Case 8

21. Which of the following best describes the chronic disease process illustrated in image 1 for case 8?

A. Severe aortic insufficiency

B. Severe aortic stenosis

C. Hypertrophic obstructive cardiomyopathy

D. Severe mitral stenosis

E. Severe mitral regurgitation

(*Note:* Use Figure A to answer the next 4 questions.)

22. Which of the flow volume loops shown in Figure A best describes the chronic disease process shown in image 1 for case 8?

A. A

B. B

C. C

D. D

E. E

23. Which of the flow volume loops shown in Figure A best describes the disease process shown in image 2 for case 8?

A. A

B. B

C. C

D. D

E. E

24. Which of the flow volume loops shown in Figure A best describes the disease process shown in images 3 and 4 for case 8?

A. A

B. B

C. C

D. D

E. E

25. Which of the flow volume loops shown in Figure A best describes the disease process shown in images 5 and 6 for case 8?

A. A

B. B

C. C

D. D

E. E

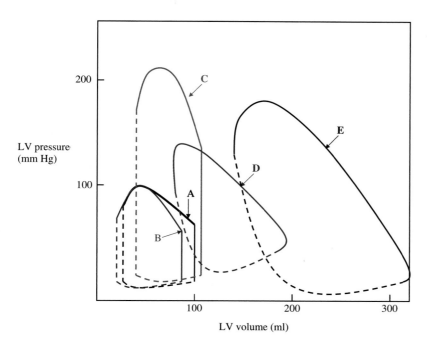

Figure A

Case 9

26. What is the diagnosis for the patient in case 9?

    A. Aortic stenosis

    B. Aortic regurgitation

    C. Pulmonic stenosis

    D. Kartagener's syndrome

    E. Pulmonic regurgitation

27. What view is illustrated in images 1 and 2 for case 9?

    A. Transgastric right ventricular outflow view

    B. Transgastric long axis view

    C. Deep transgastric long axis view

    D. Midesophageal long axis view

    E. Midesophageal right ventricular inflow/outflow view

Case 10

28. What tricuspid valve leaflets are shown in image 1 for case 10?

    A. Anterior and septal

    B. Posterior and septal

    C. Anterior and posterior

    D. Lateral and septal

    E. Left and right

29. What valve is being interrogated with color flow Doppler in image 2 for case 10?

   A. Aortic valve

   B. Pulmonic valve

   C. Tricuspid valve

   D. Mitral valve

   E. Eustachian valve

30. How would you grade the degree of regurgitation seen in image 2 for case 10?

   A. Trace

   B. Mild

   C. Moderate

   D. Severe

   E. Cannot be determined from the image shown

Case 11

31. Arrow 1 in image 2 for case 11 indicates which of the following?

   A. Right atrium

   B. Right ventricle

   C. Left atrium

   D. Left ventricle

   E. Inferior vena cava

32. Arrow 2 in image 2 for case 11 indicates which of the following?

   A. Tricuspid valve

   B. Mitral valve

   C. Eustachian valve

   D. Chiari network

   E. Christa terminalis

33. Arrow 3 in image 2 for case 11 indicates which of the following?

  A. Right ventricle

  B. Left ventricular outflow tract

  C. Right atrium

  D. Left atrium

  E. Main pulmonary artery

Case 12

34. What is the diagnosis?

  A. Constrictive pericarditis

  B. Pericardial tamponade

  C. Hemodynamically insignificant pericardial effusion

  D. Restrictive cardiomyopathy

  E. Acute myocardial infarction

35. What is the most appropriate definitive treatment for this patient?

  A. Heart transplantation

  B. Vasodilator therapy

  C. Inhaled nitric oxide

  D. Coronary revascularization

  E. Pericardial drainage

36. Which of the following transmitral flow velocity profiles would be expected in this patient?

  A. Normal

  B. Pseudonormal

  C. Impaired relaxation

  D. Restrictive

  E. Constrictive

37. Which of the following would be expected for this patient?

    A. Lateral mitral annular tissue Doppler E_M = 8.7 cm/sec

    B. Transmitral flow peak early filling velocity (E) = 62 cm/sec

    C. Transmitral flow velocity A wave velocity = 50 cm/sec

    D. Transmitral flow velocity E wave deceleration time = 215 milliseconds

    E. Isovolumic relaxation time = 110 milliseconds

38. Which of the following changes would be expected with spontaneous inspiration?

    A. Increased transmitral flow peak early filling velocity (E wave)

    B. Increased transmitral flow A-wave velocity

    C. Decreased lateral mitral annular tissue Doppler E_M

    D. Increased transmitral color M-mode Doppler flow propagation velocity

    E. Increased transtricuspid flow peak early filling velocity (E wave)

Case 13

39. Which of the following findings is/are seen in case 13?

    A. A pericardial effusion

    B. A right ventricular mass

    C. Right atrial inversion

    D. A lipomatous interatrial septum

    E. All of the above

40. Arrow 1 in image 2 for case 13 indicates which of the following?

    A. Right atrium

    B. Pericardial effusion

    C. Left atrium

    D. Left ventricle

    E. Right ventricle

41. Arrow 2 in image 2 for case 13 indicates which of the following?

    A. Right atrium

    B. Pericardial effusion

    C. Left atrium

    D. Left ventricle

    E. Right ventricle

42. Arrow 3 in image 5 for case 13 indicates which of the following?

    A. Left ventricular thrombus

    B. Lipomatous interventricular septum

    C. Normal ventricular wall

    D. Right ventricular hypertrophy

    E. Right ventricular mass

Case 14

43. Which of the following is the most likely diagnosis?

    A. Infiltrative amyloidosis

    B. Hemodynamically significant pericardial effusion

    C. Constrictive pericarditis

    D. Hodgkin's disease

    E. Carcinoid syndrome

44. Hypotension in this patient would likely be due to which of the following?

    A. Decreased left ventricular filling

    B. Impaired systolic function

    C. Constrictive diastolic dysfunction

    D. Severe mitral regurgitation

    E. Pulmonary hypertension

45. Arrow 1 in image 5 for case 14 indicates which of the following?

   A. Anterolateral papillary muscle

   B. Posteromedial papillary muscle

   C. Anterior papillary muscle

   D. Posterior papillary muscle

   E. Inferior papillary muscle

46. Arrow 2 in image 5 for case 14 indicates which of the following?

   A. Inferior wall

   B. Posterior wall

   C. Lateral wall

   D. Anterior wall

   E. Anteroseptal wall

Case 15

47. Which of the following best describes the degree of tricuspid regurgitation seen in case 15?

   A. Trace

   B. Mild

   C. Moderate

   D. Severe

   E. Cannot be determined from the data given

48. Arrow 1 indicates which of the following?

   A. Pulsed-wave Doppler hepatic vein S wave

   B. Pulsed-wave Doppler hepatic vein A wave

   C. Pulsed-wave Doppler hepatic vein D wave

   D. Pulsed-wave Doppler hepatic vein E wave

   E. Pulsed-wave Doppler hepatic vein V wave

49. Arrow 2 indicates which of the following?

    A. Pulsed-wave Doppler hepatic vein S wave

    B. Pulsed-wave Doppler hepatic vein A wave

    C. Pulsed-wave Doppler hepatic vein D wave

    D. Pulsed-wave Doppler hepatic vein E wave

    E. Pulsed-wave Doppler hepatic vein V wave

Case 16

50. How would you describe this patient's volume status as shown in images 1 and 2 for case 16?

    A. Normal (euvolemic)

    B. Mildly hypovolemic

    C. Severely hypovolemic

    D. Mildly volume overloaded

    E. Severely volume overloaded

51. How would you describe this patient's volume status as shown in image 3 for case 16?

    A. Normal (euvolemic)

    B. Mildly hypovolemic

    C. Severely hypovolemic

    D. Mildly volume overloaded

    E. Severely volume overloaded

52. What view is shown in image 2 for case 16?

    A. Transgastric deep long axis view

    B. Transgastric left ventricular inflow view

    C. Transgastric long axis view

    D. Transgastric two-chamber view

    E. Transgastric mitral valve commissural view

Case 17

53. Arrow 1 in image 2 for case 17 indicates which of the following?

    A. Anteroseptal wall

    B. Anterior wall

    C. Septal wall

    D. Lateral wall

    E. Posterior wall

54. Arrow 2 in image 2 for case 17 indicates which of the following?

    A. Coronary sinus

    B. Sinus of valsalva

    C. Left anterior descending coronary artery

    D. Circumflex coronary artery

    E. Right coronary artery

Case 18

55. Which of the following best describes the degree of regurgitation seen in case 18?

    A. Trace

    B. Mild

    C. Moderate

    D. Severe

    E. Cannot be determined from the given data

56. Which of the following measurements is labeled 1 in image 2 for case 18?

    A. Sinus of valsalva

    B. Aortic valve annulus

    C. Aortic root diameter

    D. Sinotubular ridge

    E. Aortic valve interspace

57. Which of the following measurements is labeled 2 in image 2 for case 18?

    A. Sinus of valsalva

    B. Aortic valve annulus

    C. Aortic root diameter

    D. Sinotubular ridge

    E. Aortic valve interspace

58. Which of the following measurements is labeled 3 in image 2 for case 18?

    A. Sinus of valsalva

    B. Aortic valve annulus

    C. Aortic root diameter

    D. Sinotubular ridge

    E. Aortic valve interspace

Case 19

59. Using the Carpentier classification of leaflet motion, which of the following describes the mitral valve leaflet motion seen in this patient?

    A. Type I leaflet motion

    B. Type II leaflet motion

    C. Type III leaflet motion

    D. Type IV leaflet motion

    E. Type V leaflet motion

60. Given the variance color flow Doppler map shown, which of the following colors indicates turbulent flow toward the transducer?

    A. Red

    B. Yellow

    C. Black

    D. Blue

    E. Green

61. Which of the following best describes the aortic valve shown?

   A. Bileaflet aortic valve prosthesis

   B. Sclerotic, calcified, and stenotic

   C. Myxomatous

   D. Bicuspid

   E. Infected bioprosthesis

Case 20

62. According to the American Society of Echocardiography 16-segment model, what numerical segment of the left ventricle is described by arrow 1?

   A. 3

   B. 4

   C. 5

   D. 6

   E. 7

63. According to the American Society of Echocardiography 16-segment model, what numerical segment of the left ventricle is described by arrow 2?

   A. 9

   B. 10

   C. 11

   D. 12

   E. 13

64. According to the American Society of Echocardiography 16-segment model, what numerical segment of the left ventricle is described by arrow 3?

   A. 7

   B. 8

   C. 9

   D. 10

   E. 11

65. According to the American Society of Echocardiography 16-segment model, what numerical segment of the left ventricle is described by arrow 4?

    A. 1

    B. 2

    C. 3

    D. 4

    E. 5

Case 21

66. What is the diagnosis?

    A. Ostium primum atrial septal defect

    B. Ostium secundum atrial septal defect

    C. Persistent left superior vena cava

    D. Sinus venosus atrial septal defect

    E. Perimembranous ventricular septal defect

67. Which of the following is associated with the disorder shown?

    A. Ostium primum atrial septal defect

    B. Ostium secundum atrial septal defect

    C. Coronary sinus atrial septal defect

    D. Sinus venosus atrial septal defect

    E. Patent foramen ovale

Case 22

68. What is the diagnosis?

    A. Bicuspid aortic valve

    B. Tricuspid aortic valve

    C. Quadracuspid aortic valve

    D. Normal aortic valve

    E. Clover leaf aortic valve

Answers:

1. D	24. C	47. D
2. A	25. A	48. A
3. D	26. C	49. C
4. B	27. A	50. C
5. C	28. A	51. A
6. A	29. B	52. D
7. B	30. A	53. B
8. B	31. C	54. D
9. E	32. A	55. A
10. A	33. A	56. B
11. E	34. B	57. A
12. C	35. E	58. D
13. E	36. D	59. C
14. B	37. A	60. B
15. C	38. E	61. B
16. D	39. E	62. B
17. A	40. B	63. B
18. A	41. C	64. A
19. D	42. E	65. A
20. C	43. D	66. C
21. A	44. A	67. C
22. E	45. B	68. C
23. B	46. D	

Explanations

Case 1

1. **Answer = D, Severely decreased systolic function LVEF <20%.** This patient has severely decreased systolic function with a qualitative ejection fraction of less than 20%.

2. **Answer = A, Severe global hypokinesis is present.**

3. **Answer = D, All of the above.** This patient is at increased risk for a cerebral vascular accident due to thrombus in the left atrial appendage (LAA), transplant failure due to inadequate renal perfusion, and fatal ventricular arrhythmias. There is a large thrombus in the LAA, shown in the midesophageal two-chamber view (case 1, image 4). The presence of this clot increases the risk of stroke or other untoward embolic phenomenon. This patient has decreased global perfusion and is therefore more likely to have decreased renal perfusion and graft failure. Patients with a left ventricular ejection fraction $\leq$ 35% have been shown to have a 28% lower risk of death with an automated internal cardiac defibrillator (AICD) when compared to Amiodarone.

Reference: Connolly SJ, Hallstrom AP, Cappato R, Schron EB, Kuck H, Zipes DP, et al. Meta-analysis of the implantable cardioverter defibrillator secondary prevention trials. AVID, CASH and CIDS studies. Antiarrhythmics vs Implantable Defibrillator study. Cardiac Arrest Study Hamburg. Canadian Implantable Defibrillator Study. *Eur Heart Journal* 2000;21:2071.

Case 2

4. **Answer = B, 20%.** The fractional areas change (FAC) calculation is as follows:

   FAC = (LVEDA - LVESA) / LVEDA
   - LVEDA = left ventricular end diastolic area
   - LVESA = left ventricular end diastolic area

Reference: Sidebotham D, Merry A, Legget M (eds.). *Practical Perioperative Transoesophageal Echocardiography.* Burlington, MA: Butterworth Heinemann 2003:103.

5. **Answer = C, Severe systolic dysfunction is present.** A normal fractional area change (FAC) = 50-70%. Therefore, FAC = 20% is severely depressed.

Reference: Perrino AC, Reeves S. *A Practical Approach to TEE.* Philadelphia: Lippincott Williams & Wilkins 2003:40.

Case 3

6. **Answer = A, 8.8% = the best estimate of this patient's fractional shortening (FS).** The calculation is as follows:

FS = LVEDd — LVESd / LVEDd.

- • LVEDd = left ventricular end diastolic dimension
- • LVESd = left ventricular end systolic dimension

Reference: Oh JK, Seward JB, Tajik AJ (eds.). *The Echo Manual*, Second Edition. Philadelphia: Lippincott Williams & Wilkins 1999:40.

7. **Answer = B, The inferior wall is indicated by the arrow.**

Reference: Sidebotham D, Merry A, Legget M (eds.). *Practical Perioperative Transoesophageal Echocardiography.* Burlington, MA: Butterworth Heinemann 2003:103.

8. **Answer = B, Moderate LV dilation is present.** The left ventricular end diastolic dimension is 60.5mm, which is consistent with moderate left ventricular dilation.

Reference: Gaasch W, Sundaram M, Meyer TE, et al. Managing asymptomatic patients with chronic aortic regurgitation. *Chest* 1997;111:1702-1709.

Case 4

9. **Answer = E, The arrow indicates the anterior mitral valve leaflet.** A four-chamber view is shown. In this view the anterior mitral valve leaflet lies on the septal side of the left ventricle. Sometimes the aorta can be seen near this location (five-chamber view), and this should remind the echocardiographer that anterior structures are located in this area.

Reference: Perrino AC, Reeves S. *A Practical Approach to TEE.* Philadelphia: Lippincott Williams & Wilkins 2003:146.

10. **Answer = A, The midesophageal four-chamber view is shown.**

11. **Answer = E, The arrow indicates the anterior mitral valve leaflet.** A transgastric basal short axis view is shown.

Reference: Sidebotham D, Merry A, Legget M (eds.). *Practical Perioperative Transoesophageal Echocardiography.* Burlington, MA: Butterworth Heinemann 2003:138.

12. **Answer = C, A transgastric basal short axis view is shown.** This view allows planimetry of the mitral valve, and assessment of the location of a mitral regurgitant jet with color flow Doppler. When utilizing this view to determine mitral valve area, care must be taken to find the smallest orifice because the mitral valve has a funnel shape.

Reference: Otto C. *Textbook of Clinical Echocardiography*, Third Edition. Philadelphia: Elsevier 2004:298.

13. **Answer = E, This patient is at increased risk for systolic anterior motion (SAM) of the anterior mitral valve leaflet with left ventricular outflow tract (LVOT) obstruction after mitral valve repair.** The distance from the coaptation point to the septum

(C-sept distance) can be used to help predict the risk of SAM with LVOT obstruction. C-sept ≤2.5 cm → increased risk, C-sept ≥ 3.0cm → decreased risk.

Reference: Perrino AC, Reeves S. *A Practical Approach to TEE.* Philadelphia: Lippincott Williams & Wilkins 2003:165-166.

Case 5

14. **Answer = B, The P2 scallop is shown.**

Reference: Perrino AC, Reeves S. *A Practical Approach to TEE.* Philadelphia: Lippincott Williams & Wilkins 2003:139-140.

15. **Answer = C, The midesophageal long axis view is shown.** This view is obtained between 110 and 150 degrees. The left ventricular outflow tract (LVOT) is shown. In this view, the A2 scallop lies adjacent to the LVOT and the P2 scallop is visualized attached to the posterior wall of the left ventricle.

Reference: Perrino AC, Reeves S. *A Practical Approach to TEE.* Philadelphia: Lippincott Williams & Wilkins 2003:139-140.

Case 6

16. **Answer = D, This patient has severe mitral regurgitation (MR).** The color flow Doppler jet area is 6.44 cm^2, which is consistent with severe mitral regurgitation. Note that the Nyquist limit for the color flow Doppler color map is 84 cm/sec. This is set very high and this makes the jet appear smaller, underestimating the degree of mitral regurgitation. A jet area of 6.44 cm^2 with such a high Nyquist limit certainly constitutes severe mitral regurgitation.

Reference: Perrino AC, Reeves S. *A Practical Approach to TEE.* Philadelphia: Lippincott Williams & Wilkins 2003:137.

17. **Answer = A, A vena contracta at the base of the mitral regurgitant jet of 6.1 mm is consistent with severe mitral regurgitation.** All other choices listed are consistent with mild or moderate mitral regurgitation.

Reference: Perrino AC, Reeves S. *A Practical Approach to TEE.* Philadelphia: Lippincott Williams & Wilkins 2003:137.

Case 7

18. **Answer = A, Acoustic shadowing from the heavily calcified rheumatic mitral valve prevents imaging of the intraventricular**

septum. Ultrasound cannot penetrate to reach this region, which appears as a dark area on the image.

Reference: Edelman SK. *Understanding Ultrasound Physics.* Woodlands, TX: ESP, Inc. 1994:207.

19. **Answer = D, The mitral valve area as determined by the proximal isovelocity surface area method (PISA) is 0.91cm².** PISA relies on the continuity of flow proximal to the valve and through the valve orifice.

- $Q_{pisa} = Q_{mv}$
- $Q_{pisa} = SV_{mv} * HR$
- $Q_{pisa} = MVA * TVI_{mv} * HR$
- $Q_{pisa} = MVA * V_{peak}$
- $MVA = Q_{pisa} / V_{peak}$ (Note: $TVI_{mv} {}^* HR = V_{peak}$)
- $MVA = (A_{pisa} * V_{alias}) / V_{peak}$ ($Q_{pisa} = A_{pisa} * V_{alias}$)
- $MVA = 2\pi r^2 (\alpha/180) * V_{alias} / V_{peak}$ $[A_{pisa} = 2\pi r^2 (\frac{\alpha}{180})]$

- $MVA = 2 (3.14)(1.2cm)^2 (0.67) (34cm/s) / (223cm/s)$
- $MVA = 0.92 \ cm^2$

Q_{pisa} = PISA flow, PISA = proximal isovelocity surface area, SV_{mv} = stroke volume through the mitral valve, HR = heart rate, TVI_{MV} = time velocity integral of flow through the mitral valve, V_{peak} = peak diastolic transmitral inflow velocity as measured by continuous wave Doppler, MVA = mitral valve area, V_{alias} = color flow Doppler aliasing velocity of blood flow through the mitral valve.

Reference: Perrino AC, Reeves S. *A Practical Approach to TEE.* Philadelphia: Lippincott Williams & Wilkins 2003:155.

20. **Answer = C, An enlarged AR wave would be expected in a patient with mitral stenosis.** The stenotic mitral valve increases left atrial pressure and inhibits forward flow. During atrial contraction, much of the blood will flow retrograde into the pulmonary vein (creating a large AR wave).

Reference: Perrino AC, Reeves S. *A Practical Approach to TEE.* Philadelphia: Lippincott Williams & Wilkins 2003:118.

Case 8

21. **Answer = A, Severe aortic insufficiency (AI) is seen in image I for case 8.** A color m-mode image of the left ventricular outflow tract (LVOT) is shown. A jet diameter / LVOT diameter ratio of greater than 65% is indicative of severe AI.

Degree of AI:	Trace (0-1+)	Mild (1-2+)	Moderate (2-3+)	Severe (3-4+)
AI jet d/ LVOT d:	1-24%	25-46%	47-64%	>65%

AI jet d = Aortic insufficiency jet diameter.
LVOT d = Left ventricular outflow tract diameter.

Reference: Perrino AC, Reeves S. *A Practical Approach to TEE.* Philadelphia: Lippincott Williams & Wilkins 2003:180.

22. **Answer = E, Severe aortic insufficiency (AI) is seen in image 1 for case 8.** A color m-mode image of the left ventricular outflow tract (LVOT) is shown. A jet diameter /LVOT diameter ratio of greater than 65% is indicative of severe AI. The question states that this is a chronic disease process. Flow volume loop E in Figure A (see page 9) indicates chronic AI.

Reference: Hensley HA, Martin DE, Gravlee GP. *A Practical Approach to Cardiac Anesthesia, Third Edition.* Philadelphia: Lippincott Williams & Wilkins 2002.

23. **Answer = B, Mitral stenosis MS is present.** Flow volume loop B in Figure A indicates mitral stenosis. Note that the left ventricular volume is decreased because of the narrow mitral orifice.

Reference: Hensley HA, Martin DE, Gravlee GP. *A Practical Approach to Cardiac Anesthesia, Third Edition.* Philadelphia: Lippincott Williams & Wilkins 2002.

24. **Answer = C, Aortic stenosis (AS) is shown.** Flow volume loop C in Figure A indicates AS. Note how high the left ventricular pressure is due to the narrow aortic orifice inhibiting systolic ejection.

Reference: Hensley HA, Martin DE, Gravlee GP. *A Practical Approach to Cardiac Anesthesia, Third Edition.* Philadelphia: Lippincott Williams & Wilkins 2002.

25. **Answer = A, Relatively normal valvular function is present.** A normal flow volume loop is shown in Figure A, loop A.

Reference: Hensley HA, Martin DE, Gravlee GP. *A Practical Approach to Cardiac Anesthesia, Third Edition.* Philadelphia: Lippincott Williams & Wilkins 2002.

Case 9

26. **Answer = C, Pulmonic stenosis is present.** The patient is an infant with congenital pulmonic stenosis and right ventricular hypertrophy. The pressure gradient across the pulmonic valve is 109 mmHg.

27. **Answer = A, The transgastric right ventricular outflow view is shown.** This is also sometimes called the transgastric right ventricular inflow outflow view.

Reference: Perrino AC, Reeves S. *A Practical Approach to TEE.* Philadelphia: Lippincott Williams & Wilkins 2003:334.

Case 10

28. **Answer = A, The anterior and septal tricuspid valve leaflets are shown.**

Reference: Sidebotham D, Merry A, Legget M (eds.). *Practical Perioperative Transoesophageal Echocardiography.* Burlington, MA: Butterworth Heinemann 2003:203.

29. **Answer = B, The pulmonic valve is shown.**

30. **Answer = A, Trace pulmonic regurgitation is shown.**

Reference: Perrino AC, Reeves S. *A Practical Approach to TEE.* Philadelphia: Lippincott Williams & Wilkins 2003:227.

Case 11

31. **Answer = C, Arrow 1 indicates the left atrium.**

32. **Answer = A, Arrow 2 indicates the tricuspid valve.**

33. **Answer = A, Arrow 3 indicates the right ventricle.**

Case 12

34. **Answer = B, Cardiac tamponade is present.** Systolic right atrial inversion and late diastolic right ventricular collapse are characteristics of a hemodynamically significant pericardial effusion.

35. **Answer = E, Pericardial drainage is the treatment of choice for a hemodynamically significant pericardial effusion.**

36. **Answer = D, Restrictive diastolic function is expected.**

Reference: Perrino AC, Reeves S. *A Practical Approach to TEE.* Philadelphia: Lippincott Williams & Wilkins 2003:125.

37. **Answer = A, A normal lateral mitral annular tissue Doppler E_M (8.7 cm/sec) would be expected in a patient with pericardial tamponade.** The myocardial tissue itself is normal, and the restrictive filling pattern results from compression by the effusion.

Reference: Perrino AC, Reeves S. *A Practical Approach to TEE.* Philadelphia: Lippincott Williams & Wilkins 2003:125.

38. **Answer = E, An increased transtricuspid early peak flow velocity profile (E wave) is expected.** With spontaneous inspiration, intrathoracic pressure is decreased (resulting in dilation of the thin-walled right ventricle and thus increased right ventricular forward flow). This increased right ventricular inflow dilates the RV and causes the interventricular septum to bulge into the left ventricle, impeding LV filling. Thus, right-sided filling is increased and left-sided filling is decreased. The increased right ventricular filling will increase the transtricuspid peak E-wave velocity as early diastolic transtricuspid flow is increased. The decreased left-sided filling results in a decreased transmitral E-wave peak velocity and a decreased pulmonary vein D-wave peak velocity.

References: Otto C. *Textbook of Clinical Echocardiography, Third Edition.* Philadelphia: Elsevier 2004:179; Groban L, Dolinski SY. Transesophageal echocardiographic evaluation of diastolic function. *Chest* 2005;128;3652-3663.

Case 13

39. **Answer = E, This patient has a right ventricular mass, a lipomatous interatrial septum, atrial inversion, and a pericardial effusion.**

40. **Answer = B, Arrow 1 indicates a pericardial effusion.**

41. Answer = **C, Arrow 2 indicates the left atrium.**

42. Answer = **E, Arrow 3 indicates a right ventricular mass.**

Case 14

43. Answer = **D, An anterior mediastinal mass compressing the anterolateral aspect of the left ventricle is seen.** The only choice consistent with an anterior mediastinal mass is Hodgkin's disease. Biopsy confirmed the diagnosis in this pregnant 24-year-old female.

44. Answer = **A, The mass is compressing the left ventricle and decreasing left ventricular filling.** Constrictive diastolic dysfunction does not exist. With normal left atrial size, and normal right ventricular size and function, severe mitral regurgitation and/or pulmonary hypertension are unlikely.

45. Answer = **B, The posteromedial papillary muscle is indicated by arrow 1.**

46. Answer = **D, The anterior left ventricular wall is shown by arrow 2.**

Case 15

47. Answer = **D, Severe tricuspid regurgitation (TR) is present.** Retrograde systolic hepatic vein flow is indicative of severe TR.

48. Answer = **A, Arrow 1 indicates the pulsed-wave Doppler hepatic vein S wave.**

49. Answer = **C, Arrow 2 indicates the pulsed-wave Doppler hepatic vein D wave.**

Case 16

50. Answer = **C, Severe hypovolemia is present.**

51. Answer = **A, This patient's volume status is best described as normal or euvolemic.**

52. Answer = **D, The transgastric two chamber view is shown.**

Case 17

53. Answer = **B, The anterior wall is shown.**

54. Answer = **D, The circumflex coronary artery is shown.**

Case 18

55. Answer = **A, Trace AI is seen.**

56. Answer = **B, The aortic valve annulus is measured.**

57. Answer = **A, The sinus of valsalva is measured.**

58. Answer = **D, The sinotubular ridge is measured.**

Case 19

59. Answer = **C, Type III mitral valve leaflet motion is present.** Using the Carpentier system of classification, restrictive leaflet motion is referred to as type III. The Carpentier classification system of leaflet motion for mitral regurgitation is as follows.

Carpentier class	Leaflet motion
Type I:	Normal
Type II:	Excessive
Type III:	Restrictive

Reference: Perrino AC, Reeves S. *A Practical Approach to TEE.* Philadelphia: Lippincott Williams & Wilkins 2003:162-163.

60. Answer = **B, Yellow indicates turbulent flow toward the transducer. A variance color flow map (bar) is shown.**

Reference: Edelman SK. *Understanding Ultrasound Physics.* Woodlands, TX: ESP, Inc. 1994:155.

61. Answer = **B, A sclerotic calcified stenotic aortic valve is shown.**

Case 20

62. Answer = **B, Segment 4 (the basal posterior wall segment) is indicated by arrow 1.**

Reference: ASE/SCA. ASE/SCA Guidelines for Performing a Comprehensive Intraoperative Multiplane Transesophageal Echocardiography Examination. *J Am Soc Echo* 1999;12:884-900.

63. Answer = **B, Segment 10 (the mid posterior wall segment) is indicated by arrow 2.**

Reference: ASE/SCA. ASE/SCA Guidelines for Performing a Comprehensive Intraoperative Multiplane Transesophageal Echocardiography Examination. *J Am Soc Echo* 1999;12:884-900.

64. Answer = **A, Segment 7 (the mid anteroseptal segment) is indicated by arrow 3.**

Reference: ASE/SCA. ASE/SCA Guidelines for Performing a Comprehensive Intraoperative Multiplane Transesophageal Echocardiography Examination. *J Am Soc Echo* 1999;12:884-900.

65. Answer = **A, Segment 1 (the basal anteroseptal segment) is indicated by arrow 4.**

Reference: ASE/SCA. ASE/SCA Guidelines for Performing a Comprehensive Intraoperative Multiplane Transesophageal Echocardiography Examination. *J Am Soc Echo* 1999;12:884-900.

Case 21

66. **Answer = C, A dilated coronary sinus with a persistent left superior vena cava is shown.** Agitated saline injected into a left-arm intravenous line shows the flow of blood into the coronary sinus from the left upper extremity via a left superior vena cava.

67. **Answer = C, A coronary sinus atrial septal defect is associated with this disorder.**

Case 22

68. **Answer = C, A quadracuspid aortic valve is shown.**

TEST I PART 2
Written Test Booklet

1. Which of the following best describes the frequencies at which echocardiography machines commonly operate?

   A. < 2 MHz

   B. 2–10 MHz

   C. 5–18 MHz

   D. 10–20 MHz

   E. > 20 MHz

2. Which of the following best approximates the speed of ultrasound through soft tissue?

   A. 0.154 mm/μs

   B. 1.54 mm/μs

   C. 15.4 mm/μs

   D. 154 mm/μs

   E. 1540 mm/μs

3. Which of the following media will have the highest ultrasound propagation velocity?

   A. Blood

   B. Liver

   C. Myocardium

   D. Lung

   E. Bone

4. Which of the following is the correct formula for acoustic impedance (Z)?

    A. Z = density * velocity

    B. Z = density / velocity

    C. Z = resonant frequency * velocity

    D. Z = resonant frequency / velocity

    E. Z = resonant frequency / bandwidth

5. Which of the following is an advantage of low-frequency transducers?

    A. Improved spatial resolution

    B. Improved lateral resolution

    C. Improved axial resolution

    D. Improved temporal resolution

    E. Decreased attenuation

6. Which of the following correctly matches the coronary blood supply to the numerical myocardial segment as described by the 16-segment model found in the ASE/SCA guidelines for perioperative TEE?

    A. Right coronary artery → segment 11

    B. Left anterior descending coronary artery → segment 10

    C. Left anterior descending coronary artery → segment 4

    D. Circumflex coronary artery → segment 5

    E. Right coronary artery → segment 1

7. Which of the following correctly matches the coronary blood supply to the numerical myocardial segment as described by the 16-segment model found in the ASE/SCA guidelines for perioperative TEE?

    A. Left anterior descending coronary artery → segment 5

    B. Circumflex coronary artery → segment 4

    C. Left anterior descending coronary artery → segment 11

    D. Right coronary artery → segment 2

    E. Posterior descending coronary artery → segment 3

8. Which of the following correctly matches the coronary blood supply to the numerical myocardial segment as described by the 16-segment model found in the ASE/SCA guidelines for perioperative TEE?

   A. Left coronary artery → segment 5

   B. Right coronary artery → segment 1

   C. Circumflex coronary artery → segment 11

   D. Left anterior descending coronary artery → segment 2

   E. Circumflex coronary artery → segment 7

9. Which of the following correctly matches the coronary blood supply to the numerical myocardial segment as described by the 16-segment model found in the ASE/SCA guidelines for perioperative TEE?

   A. Right coronary artery → segment 9

   B. Left anterior descending coronary artery → segment 1

   C. Circumflex coronary artery → segment 6

   D. Circumflex coronary artery → segment 11

   E. Left anterior descending coronary artery → segment 5

10. Which of the following correctly matches the coronary blood supply to the numerical myocardial segment as described by the 16-segment model found in the ASE/SCA guidelines for perioperative TEE?

   A. Left anterior descending coronary artery → segment 13

   B. Left anterior descending coronary artery → segment 15

   C. Circumflex coronary artery → segment 16

   D. Right coronary artery → segment 14

   E. Right coronary artery → segment 2

11. Which of the following correctly describes the three cusps of the pulmonic valve?

   A. Right, left, and posterior

   B. Right, left, and middle

   C. Anterior, posterior, and inferior

   D. Lateral, medial, and anterior

   E. Right, left, and anterior

12. Which of the following mitral valve chordae tendinae arise from the ventricular wall (not the papillary muscles) and are present on the posterior mitral valve leaflet where they attach to the base of the mitral valve leaflet?

A. First-order chordae

B. Second-order chordae

C. Third-order chordae

D. Fourth-order chordae

E. None of the above

13. Which of the following views passes through the "high" (more basal) axis of the mitral valve annulus and is therefore the appropriate view in which to assess leaflet prolapse?

A. Midesophageal four-chamber view

B. Midesophageal mitral valve commissural view

C. Midesophageal two-chamber view

D. Midesophageal long axis view

E. Transgastric basal short axis view

14. The intensity of the transmitral regurgitant jet relative to the intensity of the transmitral diastolic inflow by continuous wave Doppler reflects which of the following?

A. Mitral valve regurgitant volume

B. The pressure gradient between the left ventricle and the left atrium

C. The left atrial compliance

D. The mean velocity of the mitral valve regurgitant jet

E. The degree to which the blood flow and the ultrasound beam are parallel (how close the angle of incidence is to 0 degrees).

15. An increase in which of the following is **not** associated with an increase in the severity of mitral regurgitation?

A. The intensity of the regurgitant jet relative to the intensity of the transmitral diastolic inflow by continuous wave Doppler

B. Mitral valve regurgitant orifice area

C. Mitral valve regurgitant volume

D. Color flow Doppler mitral regurgitant jet area

E. Peak velocity of the mitral valve regurgitant jet

16. A patient scheduled for lung transplantation has a tricuspid regurgitant jet area to right atrial area ratio of 18%. Which of the following best describes the severity of tricuspid regurgitation in this patient?

A. Trace (grade I)

B. Mild (grade II)

C. Moderate (grade III)

D. Severe (grade IV)

E. It cannot be determined from the given information

NOTE: Use Table 1.2A to answer the next eight (8) questions.

Table 1.2A.

PISA aliasing velocity = 34 cm/sec	TVI_{MRjet} = 85 cm	LA diameter = 51 mm
PISA radius = 10 mm	$V_{MVpeakinflow}$ = 240 cm/sec	LVOT diameter = 2 cm
$TVI_{MV\ inflow}$ = 50 cm	BSA = 2 m^2	TVI_{LVOT} = 8 cm
PISA angle correction (α) = 130°	BP = 180/30	TVI_{AV} = 7.5 cm

PISA = proximal isovelocity surface area, LA = left atrial, BSA = body surface area, LVOT = left ventricular outflow tract, TVI_{MRjet} = time velocity integral of the mitral regurgitant jet, BP = blood pressure, $V_{MVpeak\ inflow}$ = peak mitral valve inflow velocity, $TVI_{MVinflow}$ = time velocity integral of mitral valve inflow, TVI_{LVOT} = time velocity integral of blood flow through the left ventricular outflow tract, TVI_{AV} = time velocity integral of blood flow through the aortic valve.

17. What is the mitral valve area?

    A. 0.64 cm^2

    B. 0.84 cm^2

    C. 1.04 cm^2

    D. 1.24 cm^2

    E. 1.44 cm^2

18. What is the mitral valve stroke volume?

    A. 32 ml

    B. 42 ml

    C. 67 ml

    D. 78 ml

    E. 84 ml

19. What additional information is needed to calculate the right ventricular systolic pressure?

    A. Peak early pulmonic insufficiency jet velocity

    B. Peak late pulmonic insufficiency jet velocity

    C. Peak mitral insufficiency jet velocity

    D. Peak velocity of left – to – right flow across a patent foramen ovale

    E. Peak left-to-right flow across a patent ductus arteriosus

20. What is the mitral valve regurgitant volume?

    A. 5 ml

    B. 7 ml

    C. 11 ml

    D. 21 ml

    E. 31 ml

21. What is the mitral valve regurgitant orifice area?

    A. 0.8 mm^2

    B. 8.2 mm^2

    C. 18 mm^2

    D. 28 mm^2

    E. 83 mm^2

22. What is the mitral valve regurgitant fraction?

    A. 2%

    B. 22%

    C. 32%

    D. 42%

    E. 52%

23. Which of the following best describes the degree of mitral regurgitation?

    A. Mild

    B. Moderate

    C. Severe

    D. It cannot be determined without the mitral valve pressure half time

    E. It cannot be determined without the peak velocity of the MR jet

24. Which of the following best describes the degree of mitral stenosis?

    A. None (normal valve area)

    B. Mild

    C. Moderate

    D. Severe

    E. It cannot be determined from the given data

25. Which of the following correctly describes the pulse repetition period?

    A. It is the distance from the start of one pulse to the start of the next pulse.

    B. It is the reciprocal of the pulse repetition frequency.

    C. It is determined by the medium through which the ultrasound beam travels.

    D. It cannot be altered by the echocardiographer.

26. The output is decreased such that the power of an ultrasound system is 1/10 the original power. This can be represented as:

    A. −3 dB

    B. −6 dB

    C. −9 dB

    D. −10 dB

    E. −12 dB

27. Which of the following is the correct formula for power?

    A. For power: $dB = Log\ P_2\ /\ P_1$

    B. For power: $dB = 10\ Log\ P_2\ /\ P_1$

    C. For power: $dB = 20\ Log\ P_2\ /\ P_1$

    D. For power: $dB = 30\ Log\ P_2\ /\ P_1$

    E. None of the above

28. A 20-MHz TEE probe with initial amplitude of 1 mm is utilized. What would the amplitude be at a depth of 8 cm?

    A. 1×10^{-2} mm

    B. 1×10^{-3} mm

    C. 1×10^{-4} mm

    D. 1×10^{-5} mm

    E. None of the above

29. A 16-MHz TEE probe is used to image at a depth of 0.375 cm. If the initial power is 20 mWatts, which of the following most closely estimates the power at 0.375 cm?

    A. 5 mWatts

    B. 10 mWatts

    C. 15 mWatts

    D. 18 mWatts

    E. 20 mWatts

NOTE: Use Table 1.2B for the next five (5) questions.

Table 1.2B.			
Medium 1	**Medium 2**	**Medium 3**	**Medium 4**
Density = 0.5	Density = 0.5	Density = 1	Density = 2
Elasticity = 0.5	Elasticity = 2	Elasticity = 1	Elasticity =1

30. In which of the media in Table 1.2B is the *velocity* of the ultrasound beam *most* likely to be the *highest?*

    A. Medium 1

    B. Medium 2

    C. Medium 3

    D. Medium 4

31. An ultrasound beam travels from left to right through all of the media: medium 1 →medium 2 →medium 3 →medium 4. If this beam has an orthogonal angle of incidence, at which interface between the media is refraction *most* likely to be the *greatest?*

    A. Between medium 1 and medium 2

    B. Between medium 2 and medium 3

    C. Between medium 3 and medium 4

    D. None of the above

32. Which of the following properties of the media influence(s) the acoustic impedance?

    A. Density

    B. Elasticity

    C. Velocity

    D. All of the above

33. Given the data concerning medium 1 and medium 2 in Table 1.2B, which of these two media will *most* likely have the higher acoustic impedance?

    A. Medium 2.

    B. Medium 1.

    C. They are equal.

    D. It cannot be determined from the given data.

34. If an ultrasound beam travels from medium1 to medium 2 with a perpendicular angle of incidence, what will occur at the interface between the two media?

    A. Transmission only

    B. Transmission, reflection, and refraction

    C. Transmission and reflection

    D. Reflection only

NOTE: Use the following data and Table 1.2C to answer the next four (4) questions.

A TEE ultrasound beam travels from left to right through:

medium 1 → medium 2 →medium 3 →medium 4.

Table 1.2C.

	Medium 1	Medium 2	Medium 3	Medium 4
Acoustic Impedance (Z):	Z = 1 rayls	Z = 1 rayls	Z = 1 rayls	Z = 2 rayls
Attenuation coefficient (AC):	AC = 3 dB/cm	AC =3 dB/cm	AC = 3 dB/cm	AC = 3 dB/cm
Velocity (V):	V = 1540 m/s	V = 1600 m/s	V = 1540 m/s	V = 1540 m/s

35. If the incident angle between medium 2 and medium 3 is 73 degrees, which statement is correct concerning the angle of transmission?

   A. It is greater than 73 degrees.

   B. It is 73 degrees.

   C. It is less than 73 degrees.

   D. Transmission will not occur.

36. If the incident angle between medium 1 and medium 2 is 80 degrees, which statement is correct concerning the angle of transmission?

   A. It is greater than 80 degrees.

   B. It is less than 80 degrees.

   C. It is equal to 80 degrees.

   D. Transmission will not occur.

   E. None of the above.

37. If the incident angle between medium 2 and medium 3 is 76 degrees, what can be said of the reflection angle between medium 3 and medium 4?

   A. Reflection will not occur between media 3 and 4.

   B. It is less than 76 degrees.

   C. It is greater than 76 degrees.

   D. It is 76 degrees.

38. If the incident angle between medium 3 and medium 4 is 72 degrees, what is most likely true concerning the reflection angle at this interface?

   A. It is greater than 72 degrees.

   B. It is less than 72 degrees.

   C. It is 72 degrees.

   D. Reflection will not occur.

39. Which of the following most likely has the highest acoustic impedance?

    A. Skin

    B. Matching layer

    C. Fat

    D. Piezoelectric crystal

    E. Ultrasound gel

NOTE: Use the data in Table 1.2D for the next question.

Table 1.2D.

Crystal Property	Crystal A	Crystal B	Crystal C	Crystal D
Crystal density	2	1	2	0.6
Crystal diameter	1	0.75	2	2
Acoustic impedance	0.5	1	0.5	1.2
Crystal thickness	0.2	0.25	0.10	0.11

40. Which of the crystals described in Table 1.2D is most likely to produce the highest beam divergence in the far field?

    A. Crystal A

    B. Crystal B

    C. Crystal C

    D. Crystal D

41. The ability to accurately identify structures that lie close together when one is in front of the other (one is deeper than the other) is called:

    A. Longitudinal resolution

    B. Angular resolution

    C. Transverse resolution

    D. Lateral resolution

42. An unfocused continuous wave ultrasound beam has a near zone length of 10 cm. At the focus the beam is 3 mm wide. What is the diameter of the piezoelectric crystal in this transducer?

   A. 2 mm

   B. 3 mm

   C. 6 mm

   D. 10 mm

43. Which of the following is true concerning *line density?*

   A. As it increases temporal resolution decreases.

   B. It is the number of pulses per scan line.

   C. As it increases frame rate increases.

   D. It increases as imaging depth increases.

44. An increase in which of the following is *most* likely to increase *temporal resolution?*

   A. Heart rate

   B. Line density

   C. Imaging depth

   D. Frame rate

   E. Number of foci per scan line (number of pulses per scan line)

NOTE: Using Figure 1.2A, which shows an ultrasound probe and six red blood cells all traveling at a speed of 4 m/s in the direction indicated by the arrows. Answer the following five (5) questions concerning Doppler ultrasound.

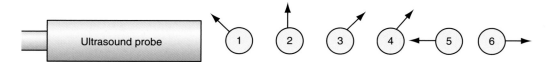

Fig. 1-2A

45. Which red blood cells will produce a positive Doppler shift?

    A. 2

    B. 1, 5

    C. 5

    D. 3, 4, 6

    E. 6

46. Which red cells will produce a negative Doppler shift?

    A. 2

    B. 1, 5

    C. 5

    D. 3, 4, 6

    E. 6

47. Which red cells will not produce a Doppler shift?

    A. 2

    B. 1, 5

    C. 5

    D. 3, 4, 6

    E. 6

48. Which red blood cell will produce the maximum positive Doppler shift?

    A. 2

    B. 1, 5

    C. 5

    D. 3, 4, 6

    E. 6

49. Which red blood cell will produce the maximum negative Doppler shift?

   A. 2

   B. 1, 5

   C. 5

   D. 3, 4, 6

   E. 6

NOTE: Use Table 1.2E to answer question 50.

Table 1.2E.

Transducer:	A	B	C	D	E
Blood Velocity: (cm/s)	58 cm/s	22 cm/s	30 cm/s	62 cm/s	30 cm/s
Angle of incidence: (degrees)	0 degrees	30 degrees	60 degrees	90 degrees	0 degrees
Transmitted frequency: (MHz)	10 MHz	8 MHz	10 MHz	8 MHz	9 MHz
Sample volume size: (mm)	2 mm	4 mm	5 mm	4 mm	2 mm

50. Given the information listed in Table 1.2E, which transducer will observe the largest Doppler shift (ΔF)? Note that the angle of incidence is the angle between the direction of blood flow and the ultrasound beam.

   A. Transducer A

   B. Transducer B

   C. Transducer C

   D. Transducer D

   E. Transducer E

51. Blood flow is perpendicular to a TEE ultrasound beam (the angle of incidence is 90 degrees). What color would be expected on a color flow Doppler exam?

   A. Blue

   B. Black

   C. Red

   D. Green

   E. It depends on the colors on the color flow map (color bar)

52. Which of the following atrial septal defects (ASDs) is located in the fossa ovalis?

    A. Ostium secundum

    B. Ostium primum

    C. Sinus venosus

    D. Coronary sinus

    E. Perimembranous

53. Which of the following is the *most* common congenital heart defect observed in adult patients?

    A. Perimembranous ventricular septal defect

    B. Ostium secundum atrial septal defect

    C. Aortic coarctation

    D. Ostium primum atrial septal defect

    E. Bicuspid aortic valve

54. Which of the following is the *most* common type of atrial septal defect?

    A. Ostium secundum

    B. Ostium primum

    C. Sinus venosus

    D. Coronary sinus

    E. Perimembranous

55. Which of the following atrial septal defects is associated with a cleft mitral valve?

    A. Ostium secundum

    B. Ostium primum

    C. Sinus venosus

    D. Coronary sinus

    E. Perimembranous

56. Which of the following atrial septal defects is associated with anomalous drainage of the pulmonary veins?

A. Ostium secundum

B. Ostium primum

C. Sinus venosus

D. Coronary sinus

E. Perimembranous

57. Which of the following best describes a right-to-left reversal of the thoracic and abdominal viscera?

A. Dextroversion

B. Situs inversus

C. Dextrocardia

D. Dextroinversus

E. Dextrotransposition

58. Which of the following best describes a rightward shift of the cardiac apex without mirror-image inversion?

A. Dextroversion

B. Situs inversus

C. Dextrocardia

D. Dextroinversus

E. Dextrotransposition

NOTE: Use Table 1.2F to answer the next five (5) questions.

Table 1.2F.

TVI_{LVOT} = 12 cm	HR = 100 beats/min	LVOT diameter = 20 mm
$\text{TVI}_{\text{AIjet}}$ = 30 cm	BP = 130/80	Sinus of valsalva diameter = 32 mm
TVI_{AV} = 20 cm	BSA = 2.0 m^2	Sinotubular ridge diameter = 22 mm
TVI_{MV} = 25 cm	CVP = 10 mmHg	Mitral valve annulus diameter = 34 mm

TVI_{LVOT} = time velocity integral of flow through the left ventricular outflow tract by pulsed-wave Doppler,
$\text{TVI}_{\text{AIjet}}$ = time velocity integral of the aortic insufficiency jet (regurgitant aortic valve flow TVI),
TVI_{AV} = time velocity integral of flow through the aortic valve (TVI of systolic flow through the AV),
TVI_{MV} = time velocity integral of flow through the mitral valve (diastolic mitral inflow TVI),
HR = heart rate, BP = blood pressure, BSA = body surface area, CVP = central venous pressure,
LVOT = left ventricular outflow tract.

59. Given the data in Table 1.2F, what is the left ventricular outflow tract stroke volume?

   A. 38 cm^3

   B. 48 cm^3

   C. 58 cm^3

   D. 68 cm^3

   E. 78 cm^3

60. Given the information in Table 1.2F, which of the following is the best estimate of the cardiac output through the left ventricular outflow tract?

   A. 3800 cm^3/min

   B. 4800 cm^3/min

   C. 5800 cm^3/min

   D. 6800 cm^3/min

   E. 7800 cm^3/min

61. Given the information in Table 1.2F, which of the following is the best estimate of the cardiac index?

   A. 1.9 L/min/m^2

   B. 2.4 L/min/m^2

   C. 2.9 L/min/m^2

   D. 3.4 L/min/m^2

   E. 3.9 L/min/m^2

62. What is the aortic valve area?

   A. < 1 cm^2

   B. 1.9 cm^2

   C. 2.4 cm^2

   D. 2.8 cm^2

   E. It cannot be determined due to this patient's mitral regurgitation.

63. What is the stroke volume of flow through the aortic valve?

   A. 38 cm^3

   B. 48 cm^3

   C. 58 cm^3

   D. 68 cm^3

   E. 78 cm^3

NOTE: Use Table 1.2G to answer the next five (5) questions.

Table 1.2G.

V_{MRpeak} = 600 cm/sec	BP = 150/80 mmHg	TVI_{MR} = 180 cm
PISA radius = 0.9 cm	BSA = 2.0 m^2	LVOT diameter = 22 mm
PISA alias velocity = 34 cm/sec	CVP = 10 mmHg	TVI_{LVOT} = 13 cm
PISA angle correction (α) = 150°	HR = 100 beats/min	$V_{LVOTpeak}$ = 90 cm/sec

V_{MRpeak} = peak velocity of the mitral valve regurgitant jet, HR = heart rate, BP = blood pressure, PISA radius = distance from the mitral valve leaflet tips to the first aliasing velocity, PISA alias velocity = the color flow Doppler aliasing velocity on the color flow map (Nyquist limit), PISA angle correction (α) = the correction angle required to account for the PISA hemisphere shape (it is not a perfect hemisphere), BSA = body surface area, TVI_{MR} = time velocity integral of the mitral regurgitant jet, $V_{LVOTpeak}$ = peak velocity of flow through the left ventricular outflow tract.

64. Which of the following is the best estimate of the left atrial pressure (LAP) as calculated from the data in Table 1.2G?

   A. 4 mmHg

   B. 6 mmHg

   C. 8 mmHg

   D. 10 mmHg

   E. 12 mmHg

65. Which of the following is the best estimate of the MV regurgitant orifice area?

   A. 0.12 cm^2

   B. 0.15 cm^2

   C. 0.17 cm^2

   D. 0.20 cm^2

   E. 0.24 cm^2

66. Which of the following is the best estimate of the mitral valve regurgitant volume as calculated from the data in Table 1.2G?

    A. 23 cm^3

    B. 33 cm^3

    C. 43 cm^3

    D. 53 cm^3

    E. 63 cm^3

67. Which of the following is the best estimate of the mitral valve stroke volume?

    A. 52.6 cm^3

    B. 62.6 cm^3

    C. 72.6 cm^3

    D. 82.6 cm^3

    E. 92.6 cm^3

68. Which of the following is the best estimate of the MV regurgitant fraction?

    A. 27%

    B. 37%

    C. 47%

    D. 57%

    E. 67%

69. An aortic aneurysm extends from 1 cm below the left subclavian artery to the celiac trunk. How would this aneurysm be best described according to the Crawford classification system?

    A. Crawford type I

    B. Crawford type II

    C. Crawford type III

    D. Crawford type IV

    E. Crawford type V

NOTE: Use Figure 1.2B to answer the next three (3) questions.

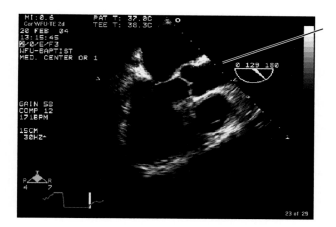

No evidence of root involvement

Fig. 1-2B1

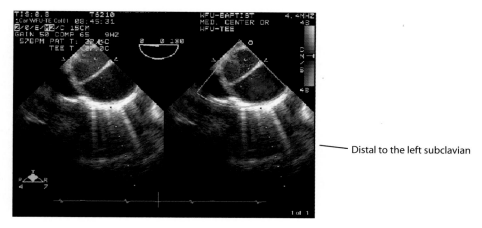

Distal to the left subclavian

Fig. 1-2B2

70. Which of the following is true concerning the disorder shown in Figure 1.2B?

   A. A Stanford type B dissection is shown.

   B. Stanford type A dissections occur more frequently than Stanford type B.

   C. Medical and surgical treatments for this patient have similar mortality rates.

   D. A DeBakey type III dissection is shown.

   E. All of the above are true.

71. Which of the following is true concerning the sensitivity of tests for aortic dissection?

    A. TEE is less sensitive than aortography.

    B. CT is more sensitive than MRI.

    C. MRI is the most sensitive test for aortic dissection.

    D. CT is more sensitive than TEE.

    E. CT is less sensitive than aortography.

       (TEE = Transesophageal echocardiography, CT = computed tomography, MRI = magnetic resonance imaging, aortography = angiography)

72. Which of the following is true concerning the differentiation of the true lumen (TL) from the false lumen (FL) in an aortic dissection?

    A. The TL is often round in the short axis view.

    B. The TL typically expands during systole.

    C. The TL has laminar flow on color flow Doppler exam.

    D. The FL is usually larger.

    E. All of the above are true.

73. Which of the following disorders is most likely to produce a restrictive transmitral pulsed-wave Doppler flow velocity profile?

    A. Myocardial ischemia

    B. Left ventricular hypertrophy

    C. Hypertrophic cardiomyopathy

    D. Constrictive pericarditis

    E. All of the above

74. A patient with normal diastolic function preoperatively is undergoing an off pump coronary artery bypass graft procedure. What type of diastolic function would you expect during an ischemic period following temporary occlusion of the left anterior descending artery?

    A. Constrictive

    B. Restrictive

    C. Impaired relaxation

    D. Normal

    E. Pseudonormal

75. Which of the following describes how a patient with normal diastolic function responds to a decrease in preload?

    A. Lateral mitral annular tissue Doppler E_M decreases

    B. Transmitral color M-mode Doppler flow propagation velocity (V_P) increases

    C. Transmitral pulsed-wave Doppler E/A ratio remains unchanged

    D. Transmitral pulsed-wave Doppler E wave increases

    E. Transmitral A wave increases and the E wave decreases

76. Which of the following would suggest that a patient with normal-appearing transmitral pulsed-wave Doppler E and A waves has pseudonormal diastolic dysfunction?

    A. Transmitral color M-mode Doppler flow propagation velocity (V_P) = 50 cm/sec

    B. Lateral mitral annular tissue Doppler E_M = 8.4 cm/sec

    C. Pulmonary vein S wave > D wave

    D. Transmitral E/A ratio increases with nitroglycerin administration

    E. Pulmonary vein A-wave (PV_{AR}) = 37 cm/sec

NOTE: Use the information in Table 1.2H to answer the next question.

Table 1.2H.

Transmitral E = 80 cm/sec	ET = 240 msec
Transmitral A = 50 cm/sec	Tissue Doppler E_M = 8.6
IVRT = 80 msec	Dp/dt = 1200
IVCT = 80 msec	V_p = 57 cm/sec

IVCT = ICT = isovolumic contraction time, IVRT = IRT = isovolumic relaxation time, ET = ejection time,
V_p = transmitral color M-mode Doppler flow propagation velocity,
Dp/dt = change in pressure with respect to time during isovolumetric LV contraction.

77. Given the data in Table 1.2H, what is this patient's index of myocardial performance?

    A. 0.33

    B. 0.42

    C. 0.5

    D. 0.67

    E. 0.75

78. Which of the following changes in diastolic function would be expected with normal aging?

    A. Transmitral E wave increases as age increases

    B. Transmitral A wave increases as age increases

    C. Lateral mitral annular tissue Doppler E_M increases as age increases

    D. Isovolumic relaxation time (IVRT) decreases as age increases

    E. Transmitral E-wave deceleration time (DT) decreases as age increases

79. In a patient with delayed relaxation (impaired relaxation), increasing preload would be expected to cause which of the following?

    A. Decreased lateral mitral annular tissue Doppler E_M

    B. Decreased transmitral tissue Doppler E wave peak velocity

    C. Prolonged isovolumic relaxation time (IVRT)

    D. Decreased deceleration time (DT)

    E. Decreased transmitral color M-mode Doppler flow propagation velocity (V_p)

NOTE: Use Figure 1.2C to answer the next four (4) questions.

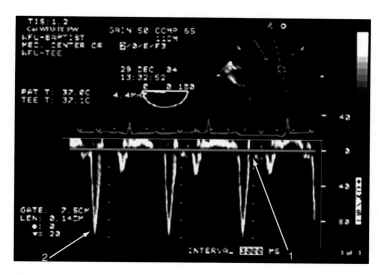

Fig. 1-2C

80. Given the transmitral flow velocities in Figure 1.2C, which of the following best describes this patient's diastolic function?

   A. Impaired relaxation

   B. Constrictive diastolic dysfunction

   C. Restrictive diastolic dysfunction

   D. Normal diastolic function

   E. Pseudonormal

81. Given the transmitral flow velocities shown, which of the following would be expected?

   A. Pulmonary vein S-wave peak velocity > D-wave peak velocity

   B. Transmitral color M-mode Doppler flow propagation velocity (V_P) > 50 cm/sec

   C. Lateral mitral annular tissue Doppler E_M > 8 cm/sec

   D. Left atrial catheter pressure > 13 mmHg

   E. E/E_M ratio less than 15

   (E = pulsed-wave Doppler transmitral early filling velocity, E_M = lateral mitral annular tissue Doppler E wave (E_M = E' = E prime), S wave = pulmonary vein systolic flow wave, D wave = pulmonary vein diastolic flow wave)

82. The arrow labeled 1 in Figure 1.2C indicates the beginning of which of the following phases of diastole?

   A. Isovolumic relaxation

   B. Atrial contraction

   C. Early filling

   D. Diastasis

   E. Late ventricular filling

83. What name best describes the wave illustrated by the arrow labeled 2 in Figure 1.2C?

   A. Transmitral pulsed-wave Doppler E wave

   B. Transmitral pulsed-wave Doppler A wave

   C. Transmitral pulsed-wave Doppler S wave

   D. Transmitral pulsed-wave Doppler D wave

   E. Transmitral pulsed-wave Doppler V wave

NOTE: Use Figure 1.2D to answer the next question.

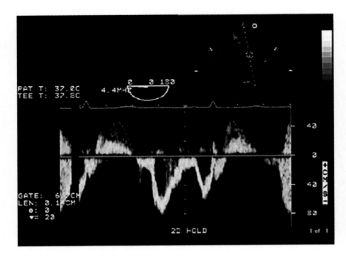
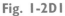

Fig. 1-2D1

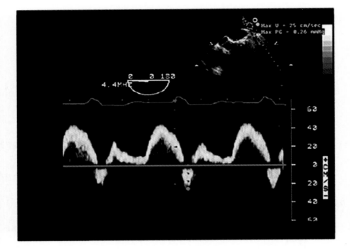

Fig. 1-2D2

84. Given the transmitral pulsed-wave Doppler flow velocities and the pulmonary vein flow velocity profile shown in Figure 1.2D, which of the following best describes this patient's diastolic function?

    A. Normal

    B. Pseudonormal

    C. Impaired relaxation

    D. Constrictive

    E. Restrictive

NOTE: Use the transmitral flow velocity profile shown in Figure 1.2E to answer the next three (3) questions.

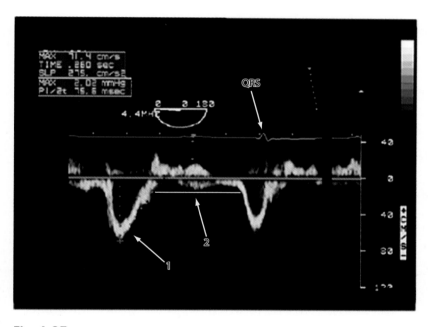

   Fig. 1-2E

85. Which of the following statements concerning the transmitral pulsed-wave Doppler profiles shown in Figure 1.2E is true?

    A. The E-wave deceleration time is prolonged.

    B. The E/A ratio will increase with nitroglycerin administration.

    C. Restrictive diastolic dysfunction is present.

    D. The pulmonary vein (PV) pulsed-wave Doppler profile likely shows S < D.

    E. The PV pulsed-wave Doppler profile likely shows PV_{AR} > 35 cm/sec.

86. Which of the following best describes the wave labeled 1 in Figure 1.2E?

    A. PV_{AR} wave

    B. S wave

    C. D wave

    D. E wave

    E. A wave

87. Which of the following best describes the phase of diastole indicated by arrow 2 in Figure 1.2E?

    A. Isovolumic relaxation

    B. Atrial contraction

    C. Diastasis

    D. Late filling

    E. Early filling

NOTE: Use Table 1.2I to answer the next five (5) questions.

Table 1.2I.

LVED diameter = 52 mm	LA diameter = 40 mm	LV free wall thickness = 12 mm
LVES diameter = 33 mm	RA diameter = 30 mm	BP = 110/62 mmHg
V_{Allate} = 350 cm/sec	LVOT diameter = 2 cm	CVP = 10 mmHg
$V_{Alearly}$ = 280 cm/sec	TVI_{LVOT} = 15 cm	V_{TRjet} = 200 cm/sec

$V_{Alearly}$ = early peak aortic regurgitant velocity, V_{Allate} = late peak aortic regurgitant velocity, LVED = left ventricular end diastolic, LVES = left ventricular end systolic, RA = right atrial, LVOT = left ventricular outflow tract, TVI = time velocity integral, CVP = central venous pressure, BP = blood pressure, LV = left ventricular, V_{TRjet} = peak tricuspid regurgitant velocity.

88. Given the data in Table 1.2I, which of the following is the best estimate of the left ventricular end diastolic pressure (LVEDP)?

    A. 5 mmHg

    B. 8 mmHg

    C. 13 mmHg

    D. 14 mmHg

    E. 16 mmHg

89. Which of the following is the best estimate of the wall tension?

    A. 238 mmHg mm

    B. 338 mmHg mm

    C. 438 mmHg mm

    D. 538 mmHg mm

    E. 638 mmHg mm

90. Which of the following is the best estimate of the wall stress?

    A. 5 mmHg

    B. 8 mmHg

    C. 13 mmHg

    D. 14 mmHg

    E. 16 mmHg

91. Which of the following is the best estimate of the right ventricular systolic pressure?

    A. 16 mmHg

    B. 26 mmHg

    C. 36 mmHg

    D. 46 mmHg

    E. 56 mmHg

92. Which of the following is the best estimate of the fractional shortening?

    A. 26.5%

    B. 36.5%

    C. 46.5%

    D. 56.5%

    E. 66.5%

93. Which of the following Doppler changes would most likely be consistent with acute rejection in a heart transplant patient?

   A. Decreased transmitral E-wave peak velocity

   B. Prolonged transmitral E-wave deceleration time (DT)

   C. Decreased isovolumic relaxation time (IVRT)

   D. Increased transmitral E-wave pressure half time

   E. Increased lateral mitral annular tissue Doppler E_M

94. Which of the following would be expected in right ventricular pressure overload?

   A. Paradoxical septal motion occurring in systole

   B. Paradoxical septal motion occurring in late diastole

   C. Paradoxical septal motion occurring in both systole and diastole

   D. None of the above

95. Which of the following would be expected in constrictive pericarditis?

   A. Decreased transmitral peak E-wave velocity

   B. Dilated left atrium

   C. Fractional area change (FAC) = 30%

   D. Left ventricular free wall thickness = 15 mm

   E. Left ventricular end diastolic diameter (LVEDd) = 70 mm

96. Which of the following would be expected to increase with spontaneous inspiration in constrictive pericarditis?

   A. Lateral mitral annular tissue Doppler E_M wave

   B. Hepatic venous S-wave peak velocity

   C. Hepatic venous D-wave peak velocity

   D. Transtricuspid E-wave peak velocity

   E. Pulmonary venous D-wave peak velocity

97. Which of the following is **not** a relative contraindication to TEE probe placement?

   A. History of dysphagia or odynophagia

   B. Cervical arthritis

   C. History of mediastinal radiation treatment

   D. Deformities of the oral pharynx

   E. All of the above are relative contraindications

NOTE: Use Figure 1.2F to answer the following question.

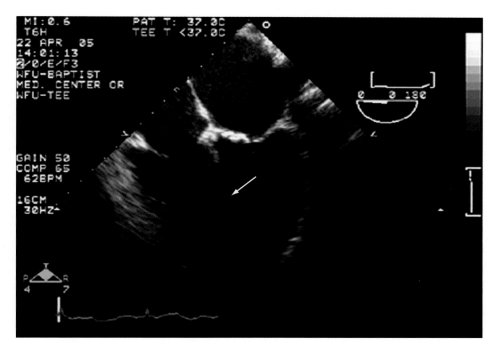

Fig. 1-2F

98. What type of artifact results in this difficulty in visualizing the wall shown in Figure 1.2F?

   A. Mirroring

   B. Acoustic speckle

   C. Beam width artifact

   D. Acoustic shadowing

   E. Reverberation artifact

99. Which of the following can result in artifact formation?

    A. Violation of the assumptions that are incorporated into the design of ultrasound systems.

    B. Violation of the assumptions of the viewer.

    C. Violation of the assumption that ultrasound travels in a straight line.

    D. Violation of the assumption that ultrasound travels at 1540 m/s.

    E. All of the above can result in artifact formation.

100. Which of the following artifacts is best described as equally spaced "objects" that have the appearance of a ladder? This artifact results when two or more strong reflectors lie in the path of an ultrasound beam and sound ricochets back and forth between the two reflectors before returning to the transducer.

    A. Mirroring

    B. Acoustic resonance

    C. Beam width artifact

    D. Acoustic shadowing

    E. Reverberation artifact

101. Which of the following is an embryologic remnant of the sinus venosus?

    A. Cor triatriatum

    B. Moderator band

    C. Eustachian valve

    D. Coumadin ridge

    E. Transverse sinus

102. Which of the following is associated with a patent foramen ovale?

    A. Moderator band

    B. Coumadin ridge

    C. Chiari network

    D. Lipomatous interatrial septum

    E. Crista terminalis

103. Which of the following is associated with an interatrial septal aneurysm?

A. Moderator band

B. Coumadin ridge

C. Chiari network

D. Lipomatous interatrial septum

E. Crista terminalis

104. Which of the following is a muscular ridge that extends anteriorly from the superior vena cava (SVC) to the inferior vena cava (IVC) and divides the trabeculated portion of the right atrium from the posterior smooth-walled sinus venarum segment?

A. Transverse sinus

B. Moderator band

C. Crista terminalis

D. Coumadin ridge

E. Cor triatriatum

105. Which of the following is true concerning the Nyquist limit?

A. It is infinite with pulsed-wave Doppler.

B. It is the max Doppler shift that can be measured.

C. It is equal to 1/3 the pulse repetition frequency.

D. It is the max velocity that can be measured.

E. None of the above are correct.

106. Which of the following will decrease aliasing artifact?

A. Decreasing the Nyquist limit

B. Decreasing the size of the sample gate

C. Decreasing the depth of the sample volume

D. Decreasing the pulse repetition frequency

E. Increasing the velocity of blood flow in the sample gate

107. Which of the following views can be used to estimate the right ventricular stroke volume?

   A. Upper esophageal aortic arch short axis view

   B. Upper esophageal aortic arch long axis view

   C. Midesophageal right ventricular inflow/outflow view

   D. Transgastric right ventricular inflow view

   E. Midesophageal bicaval view

108. Which of the following views can be used for visualization of the pulmonary artery bifurcation?

   A. Midesophageal ascending aortic short axis view

   B. Upper esophageal aortic arch long axis

   C. Upper esophageal aortic arch short axis

   D. Midesophageal aortic arch long axis

   E. Midesophageal aortic arch short axis

109. In which of the following views is it possible to see a cross-sectional (short axis) view of the superior vena cava?

   A. Bicaval view

   B. Midesophageal ascending aortic short axis view

   C. Midesophageal ascending aortic long axis view

   D. Upper esophageal aortic arch long axis view

   E. Midesophageal aortic arch short axis view

NOTE: Use Table 1.2J to answer the next five (5) questions.

Table 1.2J.

TVI_{TV} = 12 cm	HR = 100 beats/min	PA diameter = 2.4 cm
TVI_{TRjet} = 180 cm	CVP = 18 mmHg	LVOT diameter = 20 mm
TVI_{PA} = 13 cm	BSA = 2.0 M^2	Tricuspid valve area = 6 cm^2
TVI_{AV} = 22 cm	BP = 120/80 mmHg	IVC diameter = 21 mm

TVI_{TV} = time velocity integral of diastolic transtricuspid inflow,
TVI_{TRjet} = time velocity integral of the tricuspid valve regurgitant jet,
TVI_{PA} = time velocity integral of flow through the pulmonary artery,
TVI_{AV} = time velocity integral of flow through the aortic valve, HR = heart rate, CVP = central venous pressure,
BSA = body surface area, BP = systemic blood pressure, PA = pulmonary artery,
LVOT = left ventricular outflow tract, IVC = inferior vena cava, SV = stroke volume.

110. Which of the following is the best estimate of the SV of flow through the tricuspid valve?

A. 32 ml

B. 42 ml

C. 52 ml

D. 62 ml

E. 72 ml

111. What is the best estimate of the stroke volume of flow through the pulmonic valve?

A. 38.8 ml

B. 48.8 ml

C. 58.8 ml

D. 68.8 ml

E. 78.8 ml

112. What is the best estimate of tricuspid valve regurgitant volume?

A. 8.2 ml

B. 10.2 ml

C. 11.2 ml

D. 13.2 ml

E. 14.2 ml

113. What is the best estimate of the tricuspid valve regurgitant fraction?

A. 6.3%

B. 8.3%

C. 12.3%

D. 15.3%

E. 18.3%

114. What is the best estimate of the tricuspid valve regurgitant orifice area?

    A. 0.053 cm^2

    B. 0.063 cm^2

    C. 0.073 cm^2

    D. 0.083 cm^2

    E. 0.093 cm^2

115. An increase in which of the following will create more shades of dark black and bright white, with fewer shades of gray on the image?

    A. Gain

    B. Focus

    C. Time gain compensation

    D. Power

    E. Dynamic range

116. Which of the following is best defined as fully reversible myocardial dysfunction that persists up to 24 hours after reperfusion despite restoration of normal or near-normal coronary blood flow?

    A. Ischemic myocardium

    B. Stunned myocardium

    C. Hibernating myocardium

    D. Somnolent myocardium

    E. Inhibited myocardium

117. Which of the following is best defined as reversible left ventricular dysfunction due to chronic coronary artery disease with normal or slightly reduced myocardial blood flow and limited coronary reserve?

    A. Ischemic myocardium

    B. Stunned myocardium

    C. Hibernating myocardium

    D. Somnolent myocardium

    E. Inhibited myocardium

118. Which of the following post-revascularization findings can be predicted by dobutamine stress echocardiography?

   A. Left ventricular remodeling

   B. Survival

   C. Regional improvements in wall motion

   D. Left ventricular ejection fraction improvements

   E. All of the above

119. Which of the following can be used to distinguish acutely ischemic myocardium from stunned myocardium in the operating room?

   A. Dobutamine stress echocardiography

   B. ST-segment analysis

   C. Perioperative transesophageal echocardiography

   D. Myocardial contrast echocardiography

   E. Positron emission tomography (PET) scanning

120. Which of the following is regarded as the gold standard and the final arbiter in decisions regarding myocardial viability?

   A. Dobutamine stress echocardiography

   B. Positron emission tomography (PET) imaging

   C. Technetium-99m sestamibi assessment

   D. Thallium scintigraphy

   E. Single photon emission computerized tomography (SPECT) imaging

121. Which of the following left ventricular wall thickness measurements is consistent with moderate left ventricular hypertrophy in an adult?

   A. 4 mm

   B. 11 mm

   C. 12 mm

   D. 16 mm

   E. 20 mm

122. The right atrial pressure tracing X-descent corresponds with which of the following pulsed-wave Doppler hepatic venous flow waves?

    A. S wave

    B. A wave

    C. D wave

    D. V wave

    E. E wave

123. Which of the following echocardiographic features is **not** consistent with restrictive cardiomyopathy?

    A. Left ventricular ejection fraction = 60%.

    B. Right ventricular free wall thickness = 6 mm.

    C. Left ventricular free wall thickness = 15 mm.

    D. Superior vena cava diameter = 25 mm.

    E. All of the above are consistent with restrictive cardiomyopathy.

124. Which of the following would be expected with chronic hypertension?

    A. Concentric left ventricular hypertrophy

    B. Aortic valve sclerosis

    C. Mitral annular calcification

    D. Aortic root dilation

    E. All of the above

125. Which of the following would be expected with chronic hypertension?

    A. Left ventricular free wall thickness = 11 mm

    B. Aortic root diameter = 32 mm

    C. Pulsed-wave Doppler transmitral E/A < 1

    D. Lateral mitral annular tissue Doppler E_M = 8.2 cm/sec

    E. Color M-mode transmitral propagation velocity (V_P) = 63 cm/sec

126. Which of the following transducers is capable of creating multiple focal zones per scan line?

    A. Vector array transducers

    B. Annular array transducers

    C. Phased array transducers

    D. Convex switch array transducers

127. Which of the following is true concerning an increase in line density at a given imaging depth?

    A. As line density increases the number of sound pulses per image decreases.

    B. As line density increases the temporal resolution is increased.

    C. As line density increases frame rate decreases.

    D. As line density increases propagation velocity increases.

128. Which of the following is an indication for a dobutamine stress echo (DSE)?

    A. Diagnosis of myocardial ischemia

    B. Risk stratification after an acute myocardial infarction

    C. Preoperative evaluation for a major noncardiac surgical procedure

    D. Identification of severe coronary artery disease

    E. All of the above

NOTE: Use Figure 1.2G to answer the following two (2) questions.

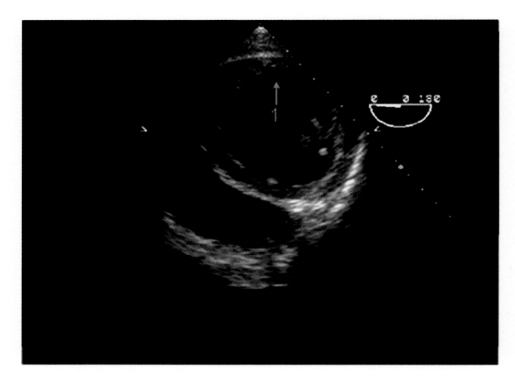

Fig. 1-2G

129. During a dobutamine stress echo (DSE) the left ventricular wall becomes hyperdynamic except for the region indicated by the arrow in Figure 1.2G. What is the diagnosis?

    A. Left anterior descending artery ischemia.

    B. Circumflex coronary artery ischemia.

    C. Right coronary artery ischemia.

    D. Left main coronary artery ischemia.

    E. It cannot be determined from the given information.

130. Which of the following is the most sensitive sign of myocardial ischemia during a dobutamine stress echo (DSE)?

    A. Left ventricular cavity dilation

    B. Globally decreased left ventricular systolic function

    C. New onset mitral regurgitation

    D. Worsening mitral regurgitation

    E. New regional wall motion abnormality

131. Which of the following valves is least likely to be affected by endocarditis?

    A. Pulmonic valve

    B. Tricuspid valve

    C. Aortic valve

    D. Mitral valve

    E. All valves are equally likely to have vegetations with endocarditis

132. A patient has normal aortic and mitral valve function, with both tricuspid and pulmonic valve disease. What is the most likely cause of this valvular pathology?

    A. Rheumatic heart disease

    B. Myxomatous valve disease

    C. Carcinoid syndrome

    D. Marfans syndrome

    E. Ebstein's anomaly

133. Which of the following is the most likely complication of mitral valve repair?

    A. Left anterior descending coronary artery damage

    B. Damage to the right coronary cusp of the aortic valve

    C. Shortening of the P-R interval with creation of an accessory conduction pathway

    D. Ventricular rupture

    E. Left ventricular outflow tract obstruction due to systolic anterior motion of the posterior mitral valve leaflet

134. A patient has aortic insufficiency (AI), mitral regurgitation (MR), and mitral stenosis (MS). Which of the following methods of determining mitral valve area is *not* influenced by aortic insufficiency and mitral regurgitation?

    A. Pressure half time method.

    B. Proximal isovelocity surface area method (PISA).

    C. Deceleration time method.

    D. Continuity equation method.

    E. All of the listed methods are influenced by AI and MR.

135. What is the most common cause of mitral stenosis in adult patients?

   A. Cor triatriatum

   B. Rheumatic heart disease

   C. Degenerative calcific mitral stenosis

   D. Carcinoid syndrome

   E. Ebstein's anomaly

136. Which of the following mitral valve disorders is most amenable to surgical repair (most likely to result in a good long term repair)?

   A. Mitral regurgitation due to P_2 prolapse

   B. Mitral regurgitation due a flail A_2 scallop

   C. Mitral regurgitation due to a ruptured cord attached to the P_1 scallop

   D. Mitral regurgitation due to restricted leaflet motion secondary to rheumatic mitral valve disease

   E. Mitral regurgitation due to A_2 prolapse

Answers:

1. B	31. D	61. A
2. B	32. D	62. B
3. E	33. B	63. A
4. A	34. C	64. B
5. E	35. C	65. E
6. A	36. A	66. C
7. B	37. B	67. E
8. D	38. C	68. C
9. B	39. D	69. A
10. A	40. C	70. E
11. E	41. A	71. C
12. C	42. C	72. E
13. D	43. A	73. D
14. A	44. D	74. C
15. E	45. B	75. C
16. B	46. D	76. E
17. A	47. A	77. D
18. A	48. C	78. B
19. E	49. E	79. D
20. B	50. A	80. C
21. B	51. B	81. D
22. B	52. A	82. D
23. A	53. E	83. A
24. D	54. A	84. B
25. B	55. B	85. A
26. D	56. C	86. D
27. B	57. B	87. C
28. C	58. A	88. C
29. B	59. A	89. B
30. A	60. A	90. D

Answers:—continued

91. B	107. A	123. E
92. B	108. A	124. E
93. C	109. B	125. C
94. A	110. E	126. C
95. B	111. C	127. C
96. C	112. D	128. E
97. E	113. E	129. C
98. D	114. C	130. E
99. E	115. E	131. A
100. E	116. B	132. C
101. C	117. C	133. D
102. C	118. E	134. B
103. C	119. D	135. B
104. C	120. B	136. A
105. B	121. D	
106. C	122. A	

Explanations

1. **Answer = B, 2 to 10 MHz is the frequency range within which most echocardiography machines operate.**

Reference: Sidebotham D, Merry A, Legget M (eds.). *Practical Perioperative Transoesophageal Echocardiography.* Burlington, MA: Butterworth Heinemann 2003:13.

2. **Answer = B, 1.54 mm/μs (1540 m/s) is the speed of ultrasound in soft tissue.**

Reference: Sidebotham D, Merry A, Legget M (eds.). *Practical Perioperative Transoesophageal Echocardiography.* Burlington, MA: Butterworth Heinemann 2003:14.

3. **Answer = E, Bone will have the highest propagation velocity.** The velocity of ultrasound depends on the properties of the media through which it travels. Propagation speed is inversely related to density, and directly related to stiffness. Assuming all other properties of the medium are held constant, as density increases velocity decreases, and as stiffness increases velocity increases. Paradoxically, propagation velocity is usually

higher in denser materials because they tend to be stiffer and because stiffness differences among materials are usually larger than density differences.

Reference: Sidebotham D, Merry A, Legget M (eds.). *Practical Perioperative Transoesophageal Echocardiography.* Burlington, MA: Butterworth Heinemann 2003:14.

4. Answer = A, Acoustic impedance (Z) = density * velocity.

Reference: Sidebotham D, Merry A, Legget M (eds.). *Practical Perioperative Transoesophageal Echocardiography.* Burlington, MA: Butterworth Heinemann 2003:17.

5. Answer = E, Decreased attenuation is an advantage of low-frequency transducers.

Reference: Sidebotham D, Merry A, Legget M (eds.). *Practical Perioperative Transoesophageal Echocardiography.* Burlington, MA: Butterworth Heinemann 2003:18.

6. Answer = A, The right coronary artery supplies segment 11, the mid inferior wall.

References: Shanewise JS, Cheung AT, Aronson S, Stewart WJ, Weiss RL, Mark JB, et al. ASE/SCA guidelines for performing a comprehensive intraoperative multiplane transesophageal echocardiography examination. *J Am Soc Echocardiog* 1999;12:884-900; Konstadt SN, Shernon S, Oka Y (eds). *Clinical Transesophageal Echocardiography: A Problem-Oriented Approach, Second Edition.* Philadelphia: Lippincott Williams & Wilkins 2003:45.

7. Answer = B, The circumflex coronary artery supplies segment 4, the basal posterior wall.

References: Shanewise JS, Cheung AT, Aronson S, Stewart WJ, Weiss RL, Mark JB, et al. ASE/SCA guidelines for performing a comprehensive intraoperative multiplane transesophageal echocardiography examination. *J Am Soc Echocardiog* 1999;12:884–900; Konstadt SN, Shernon S, Oka Y (eds). *Clinical Transesophageal Echocardiography: A Problem-Oriented Approach, Second Edition.* Philadelphia: Lippincott Williams & Wilkins 2003:45.

8. Answer = D, The left anterior descending coronary artery supplies segment 2, the basal anterior wall.

References: Shanewise JS, Cheung AT, Aronson S, Stewart WJ, Weiss RL, Mark JB, et al. ASE/SCA guidelines for performing a comprehensive intraoperative multiplane transesophageal echocardiography examination. *J Am Soc Echocardiog* 1999;12:884-900; Konstadt SN, Shernon S, Oka Y (eds). *Clinical Transesophageal Echocardiography: A Problem-Oriented Approach, Second Edition.* Philadelphia: Lippincott Williams & Wilkins 2003:45.

9. Answer = B, The left anterior descending coronary artery supplies segment 1, the basal anteroseptal wall.

References: Shanewise JS, Cheung AT, Aronson S, Stewart WJ, Weiss RL, Mark JB, et al. ASE/SCA guidelines for performing a comprehensive intraoperative multiplane transesophageal echocardiography examination. *J Am Soc Echocardiog* 1999;12:884-900; Konstadt SN, Shernon S, Oka Y (eds). *Clinical Transesophageal Echocardiography: A Problem-Oriented Approach, Second Edition.* Philadelphia: Lippincott Williams & Wilkins 2003:45.

10. **Answer = A, The left anterior descending coronary artery supplies segment 13, the apical anterior wall.**

References: Shanewise JS, Cheung AT, Aronson S, Stewart WJ, Weiss RL, Mark JB, et al. ASE/SCA guidelines for performing a comprehensive intraoperative multiplane transesophageal echocardiography examination. *J Am Soc Echocardiog* 1999;12:884-900; Konstadt SN, Shernon S, Oka Y (eds). *Clinical Transesophageal Echocardiography: A Problem-Oriented Approach, Second Edition.* Philadelphia: Lippincott Williams & Wilkins 2003:45.

11. **Answer = E, The pulmonic valve has 3 cusps: anterior, left, and right.**

Reference: Netter FH (ed.). *Atlas of Human Anatomy*, Second Edition. Summit, NJ: Novartis 2003: plate 210.

12. **Answer = C, Third-order chordae tendinae arise from the ventricular wall (not the papillary muscles) and are present only on the posterior mitral valve leaflet, where they attach to the base of the mitral leaflet.** First and second-order chordae tendinae arise from the papillary muscles. First-order chordae tendinae attach to the mitral valve leaflet tips, and second-order chordae tendinae attach to the undersurface of the mitral valve leaflets.

Reference: Sidebotham D, Merry A, Legget M (eds.). *Practical Perioperative Transoesophageal Echocardiography.* Burlington, MA: Butterworth Heinemann 2003:133.

13. **Answer = D, The midesophageal long axis view passes through the "high" (more basal) axis of the mitral annular and is therefore the appropriate view in which to assess leaflet prolapse.**

Reference: Sidebotham D, Merry A, Legget M (eds.). *Practical Perioperative Transoesophageal Echocardiography.* Burlington, MA: Butterworth Heinemann 2003:138.

14. **Answer = A, The intensity of the transmitral regurgitant jet relative to the intensity of the transmitral diastolic inflow by continuous wave Doppler reflects the severity of mitral regurgitation or the mitral valve regurgitant volume.**

Reference: Sidebotham D, Merry A, Legget M (eds.). *Practical Perioperative Transoesophageal Echocardiography.* Burlington, MA: Butterworth Heinemann 2003:145.

15. **Answer = E, An increase in the peak velocity of the mitral regurgitant jet is not associated with an increase in the severity of the mitral regurgitant jet.** The velocity of the mitral regurgitant jet reflects the pressure gradient between the left atrium and the left ventricle and is not directly related to the degree of mitral regurgitation. In fact, the velocity may be lower with the elevated left atrial pressures seen in significant mitral regurgitation.

Reference: Sidebotham D, Merry A, Legget M (eds.). *Practical Perioperative Transoesophageal Echocardiography.* Burlington, MA: Butterworth Heinemann 2003:146.

16. **Answer = B, A TR jet area to RA area of 18% is indicative of mild (grade II) tricuspid regurgitation** (see Table 1.2K).

Reference: Konstadt SN, Shernon S, Oka Y, et. al. *Clinical Transesophageal Echocardiography: A Problem-Oriented Approach, Second Edition.*Philadelphia: Lippincott Williams & Wilkins 2003:429.

Table 1.2K.

Degree of TR	Trace (grade I)	Mild (grade II)	Moderate (grade III)	Severe (grade IV)
TR jet area / RA area	< 15%	16–30%	31–60%	> 60%

17. **Answer = A, 0.64 cm² is the mitral valve area.** The calculation is as follows.

$Q_{MV} = Q_{PISA}$

$A_{MV} * V_{peak\ MVinflow} = A_{PISA} * V_{alias}$

$A_{MV} = A_{PISA} * V_{alias} / V_{peak\ MVinflow}$

$A_{MV} = [(2\pi r^2 * \alpha / 180°) * V_{alias}]/ V_{peak\ MVinflow}$

$A_{MV} = [(2\pi\ cm^2 * 130°/180°) * 34\ cm/sec] / 240\ cm/sec$

$A_{MV} = 0.64\ cm^2$

Where:

Q_{MV} = flow through the mitral valve

Q_{PISA} = PISA flow

A_{MV} = mitral valve area

V_{alias} = PISA aliasing velocity

$V_{peak\ MVinflow}$ = peak mitral valve inflow velocity

PISA = proximal isovelocity surface area

Reference: SCA/ASE Annual Comprehensive Review and Update of Perioperative Hemodynamics Workshop. Feb. 17, 2005, San Diego, CA; discussion led by Stanton Shernon, et al.

18. **Answer = A, 32 ml is the stroke volume of blood flow through the mitral valve.** The calculation is as follows.

$$SV_{MV} = A_{MV} \, {}^*TVI_{MVinflow}$$

$$SV_{MV} = 0.64 \text{ cm}^2 \, {}^* \, 50 \text{ cm} = 32 \text{ ml}$$

$$Q_{MV} = Q_{PISA}$$

$$A_{MV} \, {}^*V_{peak \, MVinflow} = A_{PISA} \, {}^* \, V_{alias}$$

$$A_{MV} = A_{PISA} \, {}^* \, V_{alias} / V_{peak \, MVinflow}$$

$$A_{MV} = [(2\pi r^2 \, {}^*\alpha/180°) {}^* \, V_{alias}] / V_{peak \, MVinflow}$$

$$A_{MV} = [(2\pi \text{ cm}^2 \, {}^* \, 130°/180°) \, {}^* \, 34 \text{ cm/sec}] \, /240 \text{ cm/sec}$$

$$A_{MV} = 0.64 \text{ cm}^2$$

Where:

Q_{MV} = flow through the mitral valve

Q_{PISA} = PISA flow

A_{MV} = mitral valve area

V_{alias} = PISA aliasing velocity

$V_{peak \, MVinflow}$ = peak mitral valve inflow velocity

PISA = proximal isovelocity surface area

$TVI_{MV \, inflow}$ = time velocity integral of blood flow through the mitral valve

Reference: SCA/ASE Annual Comprehensive Review and Update of Perioperative Hemodynamics Workshop. 17 Feb. 2005, San Diego, CA; discussion led by Stanton Shernon, et al.

19. **Answer = E, The peak left to right flow across a patent ductus arteriosus could be used with the systolic blood pressure to calculate the right ventricular systolic pressure, which is equal to the pulmonary artery systolic pressure assuming no pulmonic stenosis is present.** The calculation is as follows.

$$\Delta P = 4V^2$$

$$SBP - PASP = 4(V_{PDA})^2$$

$$RVSP = PASP = SBP - 4(V_{PDA})^2$$

Where:

ΔP = the change in pressure

SBP = systolic blood pressure

PASP = pulmonary artery systolic pressure

V_{PDA} = peak left to right flow velocity across a PDA

PDA = patent ductus arteriosus

RVSP = right ventricular systolic pressure

Reference: SCA/ASE Annual Comprehensive Review and Update of Perioperative Hemodynamics Workshop. 17 Feb. 2005, San Diego, CA; discussion led by Stanton Shernon, et al.

20. **Answer = B, 7 ml is the mitral valve regurgitant volume.** The calculation is as follows.

$$\text{MV regurgitant volume} = SV_{MV} - SV_{LVOT}$$

$$\text{MV regurgitant volume} = 32 \text{ ml} - \{A_{LVOT} * TVI_{LVOT}\}$$

$$\text{MV regurgitant volume} = 32 \text{ ml} - \{\pi r^2 * 8 \text{ cm}\}$$

$$\text{MV regurgitant volume} = 32 \text{ ml} - 25 \text{ ml} = \underline{\textbf{7 ml}}$$

$$SV_{MV} = A_{MV} * TVI_{MVinflow}$$

$$SV_{MV} = 0.64 \text{ cm}^2 * 50 \text{ cm} = 32 \text{ ml}$$

$$Q_{MV} = Q_{PISA}$$

$$A_{MV} * V_{peak\ MVinflow} = A_{PISA} * V_{alias}$$

$$A_{MV} = A_{PISA} * V_{alias} / V_{peak\ MVinflow}$$

$$A_{MV} = [(2\pi r^2 * \alpha/180°) * V_{alias}] / V_{peak\ MVinflow}$$

$$A_{MV} = [(2\pi \text{ cm}^2 * 130°/180°) * 34 \text{cm/sec}] / 240 \text{ cm/sec}$$

$$A_{MV} = 0.64 \text{ cm}^2$$

Where:

Q_{MV} = flow through the mitral valve

Q_{PISA} = PISA flow

A_{MV} = mitral valve area

V_{alias} = PISA aliasing velocity

$V_{peak\ MVinflow}$ = peak mitral valve inflow velocity

PISA = proximal isovelocity surface area

$TVI_{MV\ inflow}$ = time velocity integral of blood flow through the mitral valve

SV_{LVOT} = stroke volume of blood flow through the left ventricular outflow tract

TVI_{LVOT} = time velocity integral of blood flow through the left ventricular outflow tract

A_{LVOT} = area of the left ventricular outflow tract

MV = mitral valve

SV_{MV} = stroke volume of blood flow through the mitral valve

Reference: SCA/ASE Annual Comprehensive Review and Update of Perioperative Hemodynamics Workshop. 17 Feb. 2005, San Diego, CA; discussion led by Stanton Shernon, et al.

21. **Answer = B, 8.2 mm^2 (0.082 cm^2) is the mitral valve regurgitant orifice area.** The calculation is as follows.

$$MV_{ROA} = MV \text{ regurgitant volume} / TVI_{MRjet} = 7 \text{ cm}^3 / 85 \text{cm} = \underline{\textbf{0.082 cm}^2}$$

$$MV \text{ regurgitant volume} = SV_{MV} - SV_{LVOT}$$

$$MV \text{ regurgitant volume} = 32 \text{ ml} - \{A_{LVOT} * TVI_{LVOT}\}$$

$$MV \text{ regurgitant volume} = 32 \text{ ml} - \{\pi r^2 * 8 \text{ cm}\}$$

$$MV \text{ regurgitant volume} = 32 \text{ ml} - 25 \text{ ml} = \underline{7 \text{ ml}}$$

$$SV_{MV} = A_{MV} * TVI_{MVinflow}$$

$$SV_{MV} = 0.64 \text{ cm}^2 * 50 \text{ cm} = 32 \text{ ml}$$

$$Q_{MV} = Q_{PISA}$$

$$A_{MV} * V_{peak\ MVinflow} = A_{PISA} * V_{alias}$$

$$A_{MV} = A_{PISA} * V_{alias} / V_{peak\ MVinflow}$$

$$A_{MV} = [(2\pi r^2 * \alpha/180°) * V_{alias}] / V_{peak\ MVinflow}$$

$$A_{MV} = [(2\pi \text{ cm}^2 * 130°/180°) * 34 \text{ cm/sec}] / 240 \text{ cm/sec}$$

$$A_{MV} = 0.64 \text{ cm}^2$$

Where:

Q_{MV} = flow through the mitral valve

Q_{PISA} = PISA flow

A_{MV} = mitral valve area

V_{alias} = PISA aliasing velocity

$V_{peak\ MVinflow}$ = peak mitral valve inflow velocity

PISA = proximal isovelocity surface area

$TVI_{MV\ inflow}$ = time velocity integral of blood flow through the mitral valve

SV_{LVOT} = stroke volume of blood flow through the left ventricular outflow tract

TVI_{LVOT} = time velocity integral of blood flow through the left ventricular outflow tract

A_{LVOT} = area of the left ventricular outflow tract

SV_{MV} = stroke volume of blood flow through the mitral valve

MV = mitral valve

TVI_{MRjet} = time velocity integral of the mitral valve regurgitant jet

Reference: SCA/ASE Annual Comprehensive Review and Update of Perioperative Hemodynamics Workshop. 17 Feb. 2005, San Diego, CA; discussion led by Stanton Shernon, et al.

22. **Answer = B, 22% is the mitral valve regurgitant fraction.** The calculation is as follows.

MV regurgitant fraction = MV RVol / SV_{MV} = 7 ml / 32 ml = 22%

Where:

MV RVol = mitral valve regurgitant volume

SV_{MV} = mitral valve stroke volume

Reference: SCA/ASE Annual Comprehensive Review and Update of Perioperative Hemodynamics Workshop. 17 Feb. 2005, San Diego, CA; discussion led by Stanton Shernon, et al.

23. **Answer = A, Mild mitral valve regurgitation is present** (see Table 1.2L).

Reference: Perrino AC, Reeves S. *A Practical Approach to TEE.* Philadelphia: Lippincott Williams & Wilkins 2003:137.

Table 1.2L.

Degree of MR	Mild	Moderate	Severe
Regurgitant orifice area (PISA)	< 10 mm^2	10–25 mm^2	> 25 mm^2
Regurgitant fraction	20–30%	30–50%	> 55%

24. **Answer = D, Severe mitral stenosis is present** (see Table 1.2M).

Reference: Perrino AC, Reeves S. *A Practical Approach to TEE.* Philadelphia: Lippincott Williams & Wilkins 2003:137.

Table 1.2M.

Degree of Mitral Stenosis	Mild	Moderate	Severe
Mitral valve area	1.6–2.0 cm^2	1–1.5 cm^2	< 1.0 cm^2
Pressure half time	100 msec	200 msec	> 300 msec

25. **Answer = B, The pulse repetition period (PRP) is the reciprocal of the pulse repetition frequency.** It is the time from the start of one pulse to the start of the next pulse. It is determined by the ultrasound source, not the medium. The echocardiographer can alter the PRP by altering the imaging depth, which changes the listening time and thereby changes the pulse repetition period.

Reference: Edelman SK. *Understanding Ultrasound Physics.* Woodlands, TX: ESP, Inc. 1994:30.

26. **Answer = D, –10 dB represents a decrease of the power to 1/10 of the original power.** For power: dB = 10 log P_2 / P_1, where P_2 is the new power and P_1 is the initial or reference power. In this case, 10 log P_2 / P_1 = ? If the power is decreased by 1/10, then P_2/P_1 is equal to 1/10 and this substitution yields: 10 Log 0.1 = X →X = 10 (log 0.1) = 10 (−1) = −10. Remember that the log of a numeral is defined as the number of times 10 must be multiplied by itself to get that numeral. $\log_{10} Z = Y$ →$10^y = Z$ (for example, $\log_{10} 1 = 0$ →$10^0 = 1$).

Reference: http://www.phys.unsw.edu.au/~jw/dB.html.

27. **Answer = B, Power: dB = 10 Log P_2 / P_1.** The following are the correct formulas.

    - Pressure: dB = 20 Log p_2 / p_1
    - Intensity: dB = 10 Log I_2 / I_1
    - Amplitude: dB = 20 Log A_2 / A_1
    - Power: dB = 10 Log P_2 / P_1

Reference: http://www.phys.unsw.edu.aul/~jw/dB.html.

28. **Answer = C, 1×10^{-4} mm.** For ultrasound in soft tissue, the attenuation coefficient (AC) = 1/2 Frequency = 10 dB/cm. The total amount of attenuation is the AC times the path length = $-10 * 8 = -80$ dB. Therefore: $20\, LogA_2 / A_1 = -80 \rightarrow LogA_2 / A_1 = -4 \rightarrow A_2 = A_1 \times 10^{-4} \rightarrow A_2 = 1 \times 10^4$. Note that the arrow ($\rightarrow$) means/symbolizes "implies." Note that the symbol * refers to "times." For example: $(2 * 2) = (2 \times 2) = 4$.

Reference: Edelman SK. *Understanding Ultrasound Physics.* Woodlands, TX: ESP, Inc. 1994:55.

29. **Answer = B, 10 mWatts = power at 0.375 cm.** For ultrasound in soft tissue: Attenuation Coefficient (AC) = 1/2 * 16 = 8 dB/cm, path length = 0.375 cm, total amount of attenuation = (0.375 cm) * 8 dB/cm = 3 dB. Therefore:

    $10\, LogP_2 / P_1 = -3 \rightarrow LogP_2/P_1 = -0.3 \rightarrow P_2 / P_1 = 10^{-0.3} \rightarrow$

    $P_2 = 10^{-0.3}\, P_1 \rightarrow P_2 = 1/10^{0.3}\, P_1 = 1/2\, P_1 = 10$ mWatts.

    Note that the arrow ($\rightarrow$) means/symbolizes "implies." Note that the symbol * refers to "times." For example: $(2 * 2) = (2 \times 2) = 4$.

Reference: Edelman SK. *Understanding Ultrasound Physics.* Woodlands, TX: ESP, Inc. 1994:55.

30. **Answer = A, Medium 1 will have the highest velocity because it has the lowest density and elasticity.** Velocity will be the highest where density is the lowest and stiffness is the greatest. Elasticity is the reciprocal of stiffness, and thus velocity and elasticity are inversely related. As elasticity increases stiffness decreases and velocity decreases.

Reference: Edelman SK. *Understanding Ultrasound Physics.* Woodlands, TX: ESP, Inc. 1994:19.

31. **Answer = D, None of the above.** Refraction will not occur with an orthogonal angle. Orthogonal = right = normal = perpendicular.

Reference: Kremkau FW. *Diagnostic Ultrasound: Principles Instruments and Exercises, Third Edition.* Philadelphia: Saunders 1989:45.

32. **Answer = D, All of the above.** Impedance = density * velocity. Velocity is determined by the density and the elasticity. Therefore, the elasticity, by virtue of its effect on velocity, has influence on the impedance.

Reference: Kremkau FW. *Diagnostic Ultrasound: Principles Instruments and Exercises, Third Edition.* Philadelphia: Saunders 1989:293.

33. **Answer = B, Medium 1 will have a higher impedance.** For ultrasound: Impedance = density * velocity. Velocity is determined by the density and the elasticity. Therefore, medium 1 with its lower elasticity will have a higher velocity and higher impedance.

References: Kremkau FW. *Diagnostic Ultrasound: Principles Instruments and Exercises, Third Edition.* Philadelphia: Saunders 1989:293; Edelman SK. *Understanding Ultrasound Physics.* Woodlands, TX: ESP, Inc. 1994:19.

34. **Answer = C, Transmission and reflection.** With a normal incidence and different acoustic impedances between the media, transmission and reflection will occur. Refraction cannot occur with a perpendicular incidence.

Reference: Edelman SK. *Understanding Ultrasound Physics.* Woodlands, TX: ESP, Inc. 1994:62, 67.

35. **Answer = C, It is less than 73 degrees.** The velocity of medium 2 is greater than the velocity of medium 3, and thus the transmission angle will be less than the incident angle. Snell's law determines the physics of refraction by the following relationship (see Figure 1.2H).

$$\sin \theta_t / \sin \theta_i = V_2 / V_3$$

Where:

θ_t = Transmitted angle

θ_i = Incident angle

V_2 = Velocity of sound in medium 2

V_3 = Velocity of sound in medium 3

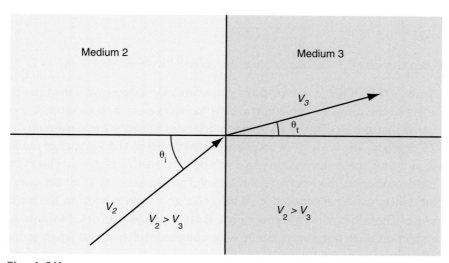

Fig. 1-2H

Reference: Kremkau FW. *Diagnostic Ultrasound: Principles Instruments and Exercises, Third Edition.* Philadelphia: Saunders 1989:46.

36. **Answer = B, It is less than 80 degrees.** The velocity of medium 1 is less than the velocity of medium 2, and thus the transmission angle will be less than the incident angle. Snell's law determines the physics of refraction by the following relationship

1994:68.

$$Sin\ \theta_t\ /\ Sin\ \theta_i = V_1 / V_2$$

Where:

θ_i = Incident angle

θ_t = Transmitted angle

V_1 = Velocity of sound in medium 1

V_2 = Velocity of sound in medium 2

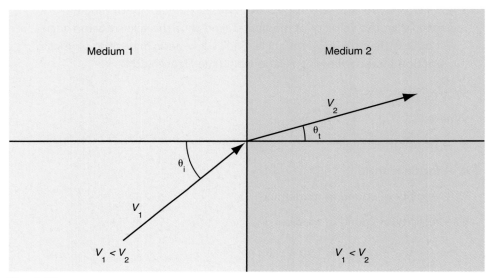

Fig. 1-21

Reference: Edelman SK. *Understanding Ultrasound Physics.* Woodlands, TX: ESP, Inc.

37. **Answer = B, This is a two-part question.** First determine the incident angle of the ultrasound beam traveling from medium 3 to medium 4. We know that the incident angle at the interface of medium 2 and medium 3 is 76 degrees. The velocity of medium 2 is greater than the velocity of medium 3, and thus the transmission angle will be less than 76 degrees. This is the incident angle at the interface of medium 3 and medium 4. With oblique incidence, when reflection occurs the reflection angle is equal to the incident angle. Therefore, the reflection angle is less than 76 degrees. Note that reflection does not always occur with oblique incidence, but when it does the reflection angle is equal to the incident angle. The reflection angle equals the angle between the reflected sound and the interface between the tissue. We cannot easily predict if reflection will occur when the incident angle is oblique, but if it does occur the incident angle equals the reflection angle.

Reference: Edelman SK. *Understanding Ultrasound Physics.* Woodlands, TX: ESP, Inc. 1994:66–68.

38. **Answer = C, With oblique incidence, when reflection occurs the reflection angle is equal to the incident angle and therefore the reflection angle is 72 degrees.** Note that reflection does not always occur with oblique incidence, but when it does the reflection angle is equal to the incident angle. The reflection angle equals the angle between the reflected sound and the interface between the tissue. We cannot easily predict if reflection will occur when the incident angle is oblique, but if it does occur the incident angle equals the reflection angle.

Reference: Edelman SK. *Understanding Ultrasound Physics.* Woodlands, TX: ESP, Inc. 1994:66–68.

39. **Answer = D, The piezoelectric crystal (PZT) has the highest acoustic impedance of the items listed.**
    • Acoustic impedance = Z = density * velocity.
    Acoustic impedance: PZT > matching layer > Gel > Skin

Reference: Edelman SK. *Understanding Ultrasound Physics.* Woodlands, TX: ESP, Inc. 1994:66–74.

40. **Answer = C, Crystal C will produce the highest beam divergence in the far field because it has the most shallow focal depth.** Focal depth is dependent on crystal diameter and frequency. Of the crystals shown, crystal C will have the shallowest focal depth because it has the largest diameter, and the lowest frequency. The frequency of the crystal is dependent on the thickness of the crystal and on the velocity of sound through the crystal. Velocity increases as acoustic impedance increases and density decreases. Therefore, the crystal with the most shallow focal length will have the following properties: highest density, lowest acoustic impedance, thinnest crystal, and largest diameter.

Reference: Edelman SK. *Understanding Ultrasound Physics.* Woodlands, TX: ESP, Inc. 1994:85.

41. **Answer = A, Longitudinal resolution is defined as the ability to accurately identify structures that lie close together when one is in front of the other (one is deeper than the other).** *Angular, transverse,* and *lateral* resolutions are synonyms defined as the ability to identify/discern two structures that lie side by side.

Reference: Edelman SK. *Understanding Ultrasound Physics.* Woodlands, TX: ESP, Inc. 1994:90.

42. **Answer = C, 6 mm is the diameter of the piezoelectric crystal.** With an unfocused transducer operating in the continuous mode, the beam diameter at the focus is one-half the transducer diameter.

Reference: Edelman SK. *Understanding Ultrasound Physics.* Woodlands, TX: ESP, Inc. 1994:81–83.

43. **Answer = A, As line density increases temporal resolution decreases.** Line density = number of lines per image. An increase in line density (number of scan lines per image) will decrease the frame rate (number of images per second) and thereby decrease the temporal

resolution. Increasing imaging depth does not necessarily change the line density.

Reference: Edelman SK. *Understanding Ultrasound Physics.* Woodlands, TX: ESP, Inc. 1994: 122–123.

44. **Answer = D, An increase in frame rate (number of images per second) will increase temporal resolution.** Temporal resolution depends on the following two main factors.

    • How much the object being imaged moves
    • The frame rate = number of frames per second = number of images per second

   The frame rate depends on the following factors.

    • Line density = number of scan lines per image
    • Number of foci (focal points) per line = pulses per scan line
    • Imaging depth (listening time)

   Decreasing the imaging depth decreases the time the machine has to wait for echoes to return to the transducer (listening time) and thereby allows the machine to increase the number of images per second (frame rate). This improves the temporal resolution, which is the ability to accurately locate the position of moving structures at a particular instance in time. An increase in heart rate will increase the movement of the heart and decrease temporal resolution. An increase in line density (number of scan lines per image) will decrease the frame rate (number of images per second) and thereby decrease the temporal resolution. Increasing the number of foci per scan line increases the time required to image each scan line. This will decrease the frame rate and thereby decrease temporal resolution.

Reference: Edelman SK. *Understanding Ultrasound Physics.* Woodlands, TX: ESP, Inc. 1994: 122–124.

45. **Answer = B, Red cells 1 and 5 are moving toward the transducer and will therefore produce a positive Doppler shift.** Note that this concept is a little difficult because if $\Delta F = Ft - Fr$ it seems that ΔF would be negative for cells 1 and 5 because $Ft < Fr$. This is not the standard. A Doppler shift is considered positive if $Ft < Fr$ and negative if $Ft > Fr$. The direction of blood flow is what determines if the Doppler shift is positive. The velocity of red cells moving away from the transducer will be negative, and the velocity of red cells moving toward the transducer will be positive by convention.

    • Ft = transmitted frequency
    • Fr = reflected frequency

Reference: Edelman SK. *Understanding Ultrasound Physics.* Woodlands, TX: ESP, Inc. 1994:144.

46. **Answer = D, Red cells 3, 4, and 6 are moving away from the transducer and will therefore produce a negative Doppler shift.** Note that this concept is a little difficult because if $\Delta F = Ft - Fr$ it seems that ΔF would be positive for cells 3, 4, and 6 because $Ft > Fr$. This is not

the standard. A Doppler shift is considered positive if Ft < Fr and negative if Ft > Fr. The direction of blood flow is what determines if the Doppler shift is positive. The velocity of red cells moving away from the transducer will be negative, and the velocity of red cells moving toward the transducer will be positive by convention.

Reference: Edelman SK. *Understanding Ultrasound Physics.* Woodlands, TX: ESP, Inc. 1994:144.

47. **Answer = A, Red cell 2 will not produce a Doppler shift because the direction of blood flow is perpendicular to the ultrasound beam.** The incident angle is 90 degrees and cos 90 = 0.

Reference: Edelman SK. *Understanding Ultrasound Physics.* Woodlands, TX: ESP, Inc. 1994:144.

48. **Answer = C, Red cell 5 will produce the largest positive Doppler shift.** Although both cell 1 and cell 5 will produce a positive Doppler shift, cell 5 has a lower angle of incidence.

Reference: Edelman SK. *Understanding Ultrasound Physics.* Woodlands, TX: ESP, Inc. 1994:144.

49. **Answer = E, Red cell 6 will produce the largest negative Doppler shift.** Red cells 3, 4, and 6 will produce negative Doppler shifts because they are moving away from the ultrasound transducer. Red cell 6 has the lowest angle of incidence and will therefore have the largest negative Doppler shift.

Reference: Edelman SK. *Understanding Ultrasound Physics.* Woodlands, TX: ESP, Inc. 1994:144.

50. **Answer = A, Transducer A will have the highest observed Doppler shift (ΔF).**

$\Delta F = V \cos \theta \, 2 \, (F_t) / C$

Where:

ΔF = Doppler shift = (Ft −Fr)

Ft = transmitted frequency

Fr = reflected frequency

V = blood flow velocity

θ = incident angle

C = 1540 m/s (speed of ultrasound in soft tissue)

Given this formula and the data in the table, the Doppler shift (ΔF) is greatest for transducer A. Note that things that increase the Doppler shift include increasing the velocity of blood flow, increasing the transmitted frequency (Ft), and decreasing the angle of incidence (cos 0 = 1, cos 90 = 0). The sample volume size does not affect the Doppler shift.

Reference: Perrino AC, Reeves S. *A Practical Approach to TEE.* Philadelphia: Lippincott Williams & Wilkins 2003:79.

51. **Answer = B, Black = the color indicated by blood flow perpendicular to the ultrasound beam.** Flow perpendicular to the ultrasound beam does not cause a Doppler shift. This means that no blood flow is detected. This is coded on the color bar as black.

Reference: Edelman SK. *Understanding Ultrasound Physics.* Woodlands, TX: ESP, Inc. 1994:155.

52. **Answer = A, Ostium secundum atrial septal defects (ASDs) are located in the fossa ovalis.**

Reference: Sidebotham D, Merry A, Legget M (eds.). *Practical Perioperative Transoesophageal Echocardiography.* Burlington, MA: Butterworth Heinemann 2003:222.

53. **Answer = E, A bicupsid aortic valve is the most common congenital heart defect seen in adults, occurring in 1 to 2% of the population.** It is the most common cause of symptomatic aortic stenosis in patients under the age of 65. Planimetry of a bicuspid valve is not accurate and valve area should be determined by the continuity equation. The bicuspid valve is often functional until age 50 to 60 years, when aortic stenosis from fibrocalcific changes occurs. Patients with a bicuspid aortic valve are at increased risk for aortic stenosis, aortic aneurysms, and ventricular septal defects (VSDs). Although VSDs are common congenital heart defects, they are generally noticed early if they are large and close spontaneously prior to adulthood if they are small.

Reference: Otto C. *Textbook of Clinical Echocardiography, Third Edition.* Philadelphia: Elsevier 2004:461.

54. **Answer = A, Ostium secundum atrial septal defects are the most common type accounting for 70% of all atrial septal defects (ASDs).**

Reference: Perrino AC, Reeves S. *A Practical Approach to TEE.* Philadelphia: Lippincott Williams & Wilkins 2003:287.

55. **Answer = B, Ostium primum atrial septal defects are frequently associated with a cleft anterior mitral valve leaflet.** These occur in the lower portion of the interatrial septum and may occur in conjunction with an inlet ventricular septal defect, creating an AV canal defect (AV septal defect). AV canal defects are more frequent in patients with Down's syndrome.

Reference: Otto C. *Textbook of Clinical Echocardiography, Third Edition.* Philadelphia: Elsevier 2004:466.

56. **Answer = C, Sinus venosus atrial septal defects are associated with anomalous pulmonary venous return.** These defects occur adjacent to the entrance of the vena cava, most commonly the superior vena cava.

Reference: Otto C. *Textbook of Clinical Echocardiography, Third Edition.* Philadelphia: Elsevier 2004:466.

57. **Answer = B, Situs inversus describes a right-to-left reversal of the thoracic and abdominal viscera.**

Reference: Otto C. *Textbook of Clinical Echocardiography, Third Edition.* Philadelphia: Elsevier 2004:457.

58. **Answer = A, Dextroversion dexbribes a rightward shift in the cardiac apex without mirror-image inversion.**

Reference: Otto C. *Textbook of Clinical Echocardiography, Third Edition.* Philadelphia: Elsevier 2004:457.

59. **Answer = A, SV_{LVOT} = 38 cm³.** The calculation is as follows.

$$SV_{LVOT} = A_{LVOT} * TVI_{LVOT}$$

$$SV_{LVOT} = \pi r^2 * TVI_{LVOT}$$

$$SV_{LVOT} = \pi (1)^2 * 12 = 38 \text{ cm}^3$$

Reference: Perrino AC, Reeves S. *A Practical Approach to TEE.* Philadelphia: Lippincott Williams & Wilkins 2003:99.

60. **Answer = A, CO_{LVOT} = 3.8 L/min.** The calculation is as follows.

$$CO_{LVOT} = SV_{LVOT} * HR$$

$$CO_{LVOT} = 38 \text{ cm}^3 * 100 \text{ beats/min} = 3.8 \text{ L/min}$$

$$SV_{LVOT} = A_{LVOT} * TVI_{LVOT}$$

$$SV_{LVOT} = \pi r^2 * TVI_{LVOT}$$

$$SV_{LVOT} = \pi (1)^2 * 12 = 38 \text{ cm}^3$$

Reference: Perrino AC, Reeves S. *A Practical Approach to TEE.* Philadelphia: Lippincott Williams & Wilkins 2003:99.

61. **Answer = A, CI = 1.9 L/min/m².** The calculation is as follows.

$$CI = CO/BSA$$

$$CI = (3.8 \text{ L/min}) / 2.0 \text{ m}^2$$

$$CI = 1.9 \text{ L/min/m}^2$$

$$CO_{LVOT} = SV_{LVOT} \ast HR$$

$$CO_{LVOT} = 38 \text{ cm}^3 \ast 100 \text{ beats/min} = 3.8 \text{ L/min}$$

$$SV_{LVOT} = A_{LVOT} \ast TVI_{LVOT}$$

$$SV_{LVOT} = \pi r^2 \ast TVI_{LVOT}$$

$$SV_{LVOT} = \pi (1)^2 \ast 12 = 38 \text{ cm}^3$$

Reference: Perrino AC, Reeves S. *A Practical Approach to TEE.* Philadelphia: Lippincott Williams & Wilkins 2003:99.

62. **Answer = B, 1.9 cm² = the aortic valve area (AVA) (A$_{AV}$).** The calculation is based on the continuity principle and the equation is as follows.

$Q_{AV} = Q_{LVOT}$

$SV_{AV} = SV_{LVOT}$

$A_{AV} \ast TVI_{AV} = A_{LVOT} \ast TVI_{LVOT}$

$A_{AV} = A_{LVOT} \ast TVI_{LVOT} / TVI_{AV}$

$A_{AV} = \pi r^2 \ast TVI_{LVOT} / TVI_{AV}$

$A_{AV} = \pi (1 \text{ cm})^2 \ast 12 \text{ cm} / 20 \text{ cm}$

$A_{AV} = 1.9 \text{ cm}^2$

Reference: Perrino AC, Reeves S. *A Practical Approach to TEE.* Philadelphia: Lippincott Williams & Wilkins 2003:100.

63. **Answer = A, SV$_{AV}$ = SV$_{LVOT}$ = 38 cm³.** This is the basis for the continuity equation used to calculate the aortic valve area.

$SV_{LVOT} = A_{LVOT} \ast TVI_{LVOT}$

$SV_{LVOT} = \pi r^2 \ast TVI_{LVOT}$

$SV_{LVOT} = \pi (1 \text{ cm})^2 \ast 12 \text{ cm} = 38 \text{ cm}^3$

Reference: Perrino AC, Reeves S. *A Practical Approach to TEE.* Philadelphia: Lippincott Williams & Wilkins 2003:99.

64. **Answer = B, 6 mmHg is the left atrial pressure as determined from the data in the table.** The calculation is as follows.

$\Delta P = 4V^2$

$\Delta P_{MV} = 4(V_{MR})^2$

$(LVSP - LAP) = 4(V_{MR})^2$

$(SBP - LAP) = 4(V_{MR})^2$

$LAP = SBP - 4(V_{MR})^2$

$LAP = 150 - 4(6)^2$

$LAP = 6 \text{ mmHg}$

Reference: Perrino AC, Reeves S. *A Practical Approach to TEE.* Philadelphia: Lippincott Williams & Wilkins 2003:105.

65. **Answer = E, 0.24 cm^2 is the mitral valve regurgitant orifice area (MVROA).** The calculation is essentially a form of the continuity principle. Flow just proximal to the hole in the mitral valve is the same as flow through the hole in the valve.

$Q_{hole} = Q_{PISA}$

$SV_{hole} = Q_{PISA}$

$A_{hole} * V_{MRpeak} = A_{PISA} * V_{alias}$

$MVROA * V_{MRpeak} = A_{PISA} * V_{alias}$

$MVROA = A_{PISA} * V_{alias} / V_{MRpeak}$

$MVROA = (2\pi r^2 * \alpha / 180) \text{ cm}^2 * 34 \text{ cm/sec} \div (600 \text{ cm/sec})$

$MVROA = 0.24 \text{ cm}^2$

Reference: SCA/ASE Annual Comprehensive Review and Update of Perioperative Hemodynamics Workshop. 17 Feb. 2005, San Diego, CA; discussion led by Stanton Shernon, et al.

66. **Answer = C, 43 cm^3 is the mitral valve regurgitant volume (MVRVOL).** The calculation is as follows.

$$MVRVOL = MVROA * TVI_{MR}$$

$$MVRVOL = (0.24 \text{ cm}^2) * (180 \text{ cm})$$

$$MVRVOL = 43.2 \text{ cm}^3$$

$$Q_{hole} = Q_{PISA}$$

$$Sv_{hole} = SV_{PISA}$$

$$A_{hole} * V_{MRpeak} = A_{PISA} * V_{alias}$$

$$MVROA * V_{MRpeak} = A_{PISA} * V_{alias}$$

$$MVROA = A_{PISA} * V_{alias} / V_{MRpeak}$$

$$MVROA = (2\pi r^2 * \alpha/180) \text{ cm}^2 * 34 \text{ cm/sec} \div (600 \text{ cm/sec})$$

$$MVROA = 0.24 \text{ cm}^2$$

Where:

Q_{hole} = flow through the mitral valve regurgitant orifice area (MVROA)

SV_{hole} = stroke volume through the MVROA

A_{hole} = MVROA (get your mind out of the gutter)

V_{MRpeak}= peak velocity of the mitral regurgitant jet as measure with continuous wave Doppler

A_{PISA} = area PISA (proximal isovelocity surface area)

V_{alias} = aliasing velocity

V_{MRpeak} = peak mitral diastolic inflow velocity

Reference: SCA/ASE Annual Comprehensive Review and Update of Perioperative Hemodynamics Workshop. 17 Feb. 2005, San Diego, CA; discussion led by Stanton Shernon, et al.

67. **Answer = E, 92.6 cm³ is the mitral valve stroke volume.** The calculation is as follows.

$$SV_{MV} - SV_{LVOT} = RVol \rightarrow SV_{MV} = RVol + SV_{LVOT}$$

$$SV_{MV} = RVol + (\pi r^2 * TVI_{LVOT})$$

$$SV_{MV} = 43.2 \text{ cm}^3 + (49.4 \text{ cm}^3)$$

$$SV_{MV} = 92.6 \text{ cm}^3$$

$$MVRVOL = MVROA * TVI_{MR}$$

$$MVRVOL = (0.240 \text{ cm}^2) * (180 \text{ cm})$$

$$MVRVOL = 43.2 \text{ cm}^3$$

$$Q_{hole} = Q_{PISA}$$

$$A_{hole} * V_{MRpeak} = A_{PISA} * V_{alias}$$

$$MVROA * V_{MRpeak} = A_{PISA} * V_{alias}$$

$$MVROA = A_{PISA} * V_{alias} / V_{MRpeak}$$

$$MVROA = (2\pi r^2 * \alpha/180) \text{ cm}^2 * 34 \text{ cm/sec} \div (600 \text{ cm/sec})$$

$$MVROA = 0.24 \text{ cm}^2$$

Where:

SV_{LVOT} = stroke volume through the left ventricular outflow tract

SV_{MV} = stroke volume of blood flow through the mitral valve

RVol = MVRVOL = mitral valve regurgitant volume

Q_{hole} = flow through the mitral valve regurgitant orifice area (MVROA)

SV_{hole} = stroke volume through the MVROA

A_{hole} = MVROA (get your mind out of the gutter)

V_{MRpeak}= peak velocity of the mitral regurgitant jet as measure with continuous wave Doppler

A_{PISA} = area PISA (proximal isovelocity surface area)

V_{alias} = aliasing velocity

V_{MRpeak} = peak mitral diastolic inflow velocity

Reference: SCA/ASE Annual Comprehensive Review and Update of Perioperative Hemodynamics Workshop. 17 Feb. 2005, San Diego, CA; discussion led by Stanton Shernon, et al.

68. **Answer = C, 46.6% is the mitral valve regurgitant fraction (Reg Fx).** The calculation is as follows.

Reg Fx = MVRVol / SV_{MV}

Reg Fx = 43.2 cm^3 / 92.7 cm^3

Reg Fx = 46.6%

Reference: SCA/ASE Annual Comprehensive Review and Update of Perioperative Hemodynamics Workshop. 17 Feb. 2005, San Diego, CA; discussion led by Stanton Shernon, et al.

69. **Answer = A, A Crawford type I aortic aneurysm is described.** This thoracoabdominal aneurysm begins near the left subclavian artery and extends distally to a location above the renal arteries (see Table 1.2N).

Reference: Perrino AC, Reeves S. *A Practical Approach to TEE.* Philadelphia: Lippincott Williams & Wilkins 2003:252.

Table 1.2N. CRAWFORD CLASSIFICATION FOR THORACOABDOMINAL ANEURYSMS

Type	Origin	Extends Distally:
I	Near left subclavian artery	Above renal arteries
II	Near left subclavian artery	Below renal arteries
III	More distal than types I or II but above the diaphragm	Below renal arteries
IV	Below the diaphragm (abdominal)	Below renal arteries

70. **Answer = E, all of the above.** A Stanford type B dissection is shown. This dissection originates distal to the left subclavian artery and does not involve the aortic arch. Stanford type A dissections involve the ascending aorta regardless of the location of the intimal tear. Type A dissections occur more frequently than type B dissections, comprising about 70%. Medical and surgical management of type B dissections have similar mortality rates. The dissection shown is also consistent with a DeBakey type III dissection because it involves an intimal tear distal to the aortic arch (near the left subclavian artery) without arch involvement (see Table 1.2O).

Reference: Hensley HA, Martin DE, Gravlee GP. *A Practical Approach to Cardiac Anesthesia, Third Edition.* Philadelphia: Lippincott Williams & Wilkins 2002:621.

Table 1.2O. DEBAKEY CLASSIFICATION FOR AORTIC DISSECTIONS

Type	Origin	Extends Distally:	Stanford classification
I	Ascending thoracic aorta	To aortic bifurcation	A
II	Ascending thoracic aorta	To brachiocephalic trunk (ends before the arch)	A
IIIa	Near the left subclavian artery	Above the diaphragm	B
IIIb	Near the left subclavian artery	Aortic bifurcation	B

71. **Answer = C, MRI is the most sensitive test for aortic dissection.** Sensitivity: MRI > TEE = CT > Aortography. TEE has the advantage of allowing rapid bedside assessment with high sensitivity and specificity. TEE

also allows for identification of valvular abnormalities (aortic insufficiency), pericardial effusions, coronary artery involvement, and segmental wall motion abnormalities. Aortography and TEE are the only modalities listed that allow coronary artery assessment. TEE is not as good at identifying branch vessel involvement, and a "blind spot" exists where the trachea and left main bronchus occlude a portion of the distal ascending aorta and proximal aortic arch.

Reference: Perrino AC, Reeves S. *A Practical Approach to TEE.* Philadelphia: Lippincott Williams & Wilkins 2003:254.

72. **Answer = E, All of the above are true statements concerning the differentiation of the true lumen from the false lumen.** The true lumen (TL) is often round in the short axis and the false lumen (FL) is typically crescent shaped in short axis. The TL expands during systole, and has laminar flow on color flow Doppler. The FL is typically larger than the TL, and may have spontaneous echo contrast suggestive of sluggish flow.

Reference: Perrino AC, Reeves S. *A Practical Approach to TEE.* Philadelphia: Lippincott Williams & Wilkins 2003:179.

73. **Answer = D, Constrictive pericarditis is most likely to produce a restrictive transmitral pulsed wave Doppler flow velocity profile.** The other disorders listed are more likely to produce impaired left ventricular relaxation.

Reference: Oh JK, Seward JB, Tajik AJ (eds). *The Echo Manual, Second Edition.* Philadelphia: Lippincott Williams & Wilkins 1999:52.

74. **Answer = C, Impaired relaxation (delayed relaxation) is the most likely diastolic function to observe during an episode of acute ischemia in a patient who previously had normal diastolic function.**

Reference: Oh JK, Seward JB, Tajik AJ (eds). *The Echo Manual, Second Edition.* Philadelphia: Lippincott Williams & Wilkins 1999:52.

75. **Answer = C, The transmitral E/A ratio remains unchanged.** As preload is decreased in patients with normal diastolic function both E and A will decrease to the same extent and the E/A ratio will remain constant. E_M and V_P are not altered by decreases in loading conditions, and this is one of their advantages over transmitral pulsed-wave Doppler flow velocities. Note that the response of E and A waves to decreases in preload depends on the degree of diastolic dysfunction. As indicated in Table 1.2P, restrictive diastolic dysfunction will pseudonormalize if the diastolic dysfunction is reversible. Pseudonormal diastolic dysfunction will revert to an impaired relaxation waveform pattern with preload reduction. Also note that in impaired relaxation E and A will both decrease, but E will decrease more than A (resulting in a decrease in the E/A ratio). The decrease in early diastolic filling results from a decrease in the pressure gradient between

the left atrium and the left ventricle in response to preload reduction (see Table 1.2P).

Reference: Perrino AC, Reeves S. *A Practical Approach to TEE*. Philadelphia: Lippincott Williams & Wilkins 2003:117.

Table 1.2P.   RESPONSE OF TRANSMITRAL FLOW VELOCITIES TO PRELOAD REDUCTION

Flow Pattern	E	A	E/A Ratio
Normal	Decreased	Decreased	No change
Impaired relaxation	Decreased	Decreased	Decreased
Pseudonormal	Decreased	Decreased	Decreased
Restrictive (reversible)	Decreased	Increased	Decreased
Restrictive (irreversible, end stage)	No change	No change	No change

76. **Answer = E, An elevated pulmonary vein atrial reversal wave (PV$_{AR}$) suggests pseudonormal diastolic dysfunction in the presence of normal appearing transmitral E and A waves.** Normally the PV$_{AR}$ wave is less than 25 cm/sec. Pseudonormal diastolic function can be distinguished from normal diastolic function by the following:

    - Decreased transmitral color M-mode Doppler flow propagation velocity (VP) < 45 cm/sec
    - Tissue Doppler E$_M$ < 8 cm/sec
    - Pulm Vein S < D
    - PVAR duration > E-wave duration
    - PVAR > 25 cm/sec
    - E/A ratio decreases with decrease in preload

References: Perrino AC, Reeves S. *A Practical Approach to TEE*. Philadelphia: Lippincott Williams & Wilkins 2003:126; Groban L, Dolinski SY. Transesophageal echocardiographic evaluation of diastolic function. *Chest* 2005;128;3652–3663.

77. **Answer = D, 0.67 is the index of myocardial performance (IMP). The calculation is as follows.**

    IMP = (IVCT + IVRT) / ET = 160 / 240 = 2 / 3 = 0.67

    Where:

    IVCT = ICT = isovolumic contraction time

    IVRT = IRT = isovolumic relaxation time

    ET = ejection time

Reference: Oh JK, Seward JB, Tajik AJ (eds). *The Echo Manual, Second Edition*. Philadelphia: Lippincott Williams & Wilkins 1999:56.

78. **Answer = B, The transmitral pulsed wave Doppler A wave increases as age increases.** As patients age, relaxation becomes impaired or delayed. With normal aging, the transmitral flow velocities approach an impaired relaxation pattern with the following findings.

E wave decreased, A wave increased, E/A decreased, DT increased (prolonged), E_M decreased, V_P decreased, S/D increased (S > D), IVRT increased

Where:

V_P = transmitral color M-mode Doppler flow propagation velocity

E = pulsed-wave Doppler transmitral early filling velocity

A = pulsed-wave Doppler transmitral peak A-wave velocity

E_M = lateral mitral annular tissue Doppler E wave (E_M = E′ = E prime)

IVRT = isovolumic relaxation time

DT = deceleration time

References: Perrino AC, Reeves S. *A Practical Approach to TEE.* Philadelphia: Lippincott Williams & Wilkins 2003:126; Groban L, Dolinski SY. Transesophageal echocardiographic evaluation of diastolic function. *Chest* 2005;128;3652–3663.

79. **Answer = D, A decrease in deceleration time (steeper deceleration slope) would be expected with an increase in preload in patients with delayed (impaired) relaxation.** Other changes that might be expected include the following: increased transmitral E-wave peak velocity, decreased isovolumic relaxation time (IVRT), and decreased A-wave peak velocity. Lateral mitral annular tissue Doppler E_M and transmitral color M-mode Doppler flow propagation velocity (V_P) are not influenced by changes in preload.

References: Otto C. *Textbook of Clinical Echocardiography, Third Edition.* Philadelphia: Elsevier 2004:179; Groban L, Sylvia Y. Transesophageal echocardiographic evaluation of diastolic function. *Chest* 2005;128;3652–3663.

80. **Answer = C, Restrictive diastolic dysfunction is shown.**

Reference: Groban L, Dolinski SY. Transesophageal echocardiographic evaluation of diastolic function. *Chest* 2005;128;3652–3663.

81. **Answer = D, A left atrial catheter pressure should be greater than 13 mmHg, given the high early peak transmitral filling velocities shown.** In the restrictive pattern shown, the following findings would be expected.

S<D, E_M < 8 cm/sec, V_P < 45 cm/sec, E/E_M > 15

Where:

E = pulsed-wave Doppler transmitral early filling velocity

E_M = lateral mitral annular tissue Doppler E wave (E_M = E′ = E prime)

S wave = pulmonary vein systolic flow wave, D wave = pulmonary vein diastolic flow wave

Reference: Groban L, Dolinski SY. Transesophageal echocardiographic evaluation of diastolic function. *Chest* 2005;128;3652–3663.

82. **Answer = D, The arrow indicates the beginning of diastasis.** The four phases of diastole are isovolumic left ventricular relaxation, early filling, diastasis, and atrial contraction. Early filling is associated with the transmitral pulsed-wave Doppler E wave, diastasis is the period between early filling and atrial contraction when flow is negligible, and late filling/atrial contraction is associated with the A wave.

Reference: Groban L, Sylvia Y. Transesophageal echocardiographic evaluation of diastolic function. *Chest* 2005;128;3652–3663.

83. **Answer = A, The transmitral early filling (E wave) is indicated by the arrow.**

Reference: Konstadt SN, Shernon S, Oka Y (eds). *Clinical Transesophageal Echocardiography: A Problem-Oriented Approach, Second Edition.* Philadelphia: Lippincott Williams & Wilkins 2003: 74–77.

84. **Answer = B, Pseudonormal diastolic dysfunction is present.** A normal transmitral pulsed-wave Doppler diastolic velocity profile is shown. This normal E- and A-wave profile could result from normal or pseudonormal diastolic function. The pulmonary vein pattern shown is classic for pseudonormal diastolic function: S < D, enlarged PV_{AR} wave. The S wave is decreased because the elevated left atrial pressure decreases systolic inflow. The D wave is preserved or increased because the left atrial pressure decreases rapidly upon opening of the mitral valve and pulmonary vein flow increases in diastole. The PV_{AR} wave duration and peak velocity increase because the decreased left ventricular compliance inhibits forward flow through the mitral valve and favors retrograde flow into the pulmonary veins.

Reference: Groban L, Dolinski SY. Transesophageal echocardiographic evaluation of diastolic function. *Chest* 2005;128;3652–3663.

85. **Answer = A, The deceleration time is prolonged.** The image shows a transmitral pulsed-wave Doppler velocity profile. The profile shown has characteristics of impaired relaxation and of normal diastolic function. The transmitral E-wave deceleration time (DT) is prolonged (normal DT = 150 to 220), but the E/A ratio is greater than 1. To determine this patient's diastolic function, another modality needs to be investigated, such as the lateral mitral annular tissue Doppler E_M peak velocity. The E/A ratio will never increase with nitroglycerin administration, regardless of the diastolic function. Restrictive diastolic dysfunction is characterized by E >> A. This is not present. In both impaired relaxation and normal diastolic function, the pulmonary vein S wave is greater than the D wave, and the PV_{AR} wave peak velocity is less than 25 cm/sec.

Reference: Groban L, Dolinski SY. Transesophageal echocardiographic evaluation of diastolic function. *Chest* 2005;128;3652-3663.

86. **Answer = D, The arrow indicates the transmitral pulsed-wave Doppler early filling velocity profile (E wave).**

Reference: Groban L, Dolinski SY. Transesophageal echocardiographic evaluation of diastolic function. *Chest* 2005;128;3652–3663.

87. **Answer = C, The yellow arrow 2 indicates diastasis.** The four phases of diastole are isovolumic left ventricular relaxation, early filling, diastasis, and atrial contraction. Early filling is associated with the transmitral pulsed-wave Doppler E wave, diastasis is the period between early filling and atrial contraction when flow is negligible, and late filling/atrial contraction is associated with the A wave.

Reference: Groban L, Dolinski SY. Transesophageal echocardiographic evaluation of diastolic function. *Chest* 2005;128;3652–3663.

88. **Answer = C, LVEDP = 13.** The calculation is as follows.

$\Delta P = 4V^2$

$(DBP - LVEDP) = 4\,(V_{Allate})^2$

$LVEDP = DBP - 4\,(3.5)^2$

$LVEDP = 62 - 49$

$LVEDP = 13$ mmHg

Where:

V_{Allate} = late peak aortic regurgitant velocity

LVEDP = left ventricular end diastolic pressure

DBP = diastolic blood pressure

Reference: Sidebotham D, Merry A, Legget M (eds.). *Practical Perioperative Transoesophageal Echocardiography.* Burlington, MA: Butterworth Heinemann 2003:241.

89. **Answer = B, 338 mmHg mm = the wall tension.** The calculation is as follows.

Wall Tension = (P * R)

Wall Tension = 13 mmHg * 26 mm

Wall Tension = 338 mmHg mm

$\Delta P = 4V^2$

$(DBP - LVEDP) = 4\,(V_{Allate})^2$

$LVEDP = DBP - 4\,(3.5)^2$

$LVEDP = 62 - 49$

$LVEDP = 13$ mmHg

Where:

V_{Allate} = late peak aortic regurgitant velocity

P = LVEDP = left ventricular end diastolic pressure

DBP = diastolic blood pressure

R = left ventricular end diastolic radius

Reference: Otto C. *Textbook of Clinical Echocardiography, Third Edition.* Philadelphia: Elsevier 2004:133.

90. **Answer = D, 14 mmHg = left ventricular wall stress.** The law of LaPlace determines wall stress.

    Wall stress = Wall Tension / 2(wall thickness)

    Wall stress = P * R / 2 T

    Wall stress = (13 mmHg * 26 mm)/2(12 mm)

    Wall stress = 14 mmHg

    $\Delta P = 4V^2$

    $(DBP - LVEDP) = 4(V_{Allate})^2$

    $LVEDP = DBP - 4 (3.5)^2$

    LVEDP = 62 − 49

    LVEDP = 13 mmHg

Where:

P = left ventricular end diastolic pressure, R = left ventricular internal radius, T = free wall thickness

NOTE: Wall Tension = P * R and is a component of wall stress

Reference: Otto C. *Textbook of Clinical Echocardiography, Third Edition.* Philadelphia: Elsevier 2004:133.

91. **Answer = B, 26 mmHg = the right ventricular systolic pressure (RVSP).** The calculation is as follows.

    $\Delta P = 4V^2$

    $(RVSP - RAP) = 4V_{TR}^2$

    $(RVSP - CVP) = 4V_{TR}^2$

    $RVSP = 4V^2 + CVP$

    $RVSP = 4(2 \text{ m/s})^2 + 10$

    RVSP = 26 mmHg

Where:

RVSP = right ventricular systolic pressure

CVP = central venous pressure

V_{TR} = peak tricuspid regurgitant velocity as measured by CWD

92. **Answer = B, 36.5% is the fractional shortening (FS).** The calculation is as follows.

FS = (LVEDd − LVESd) / LVEDd

FS = (52 − 33) / 52

FS = 36.5%

Where:

LVEDd = left ventricular end diastolic diameter

LVESd = left ventricular end systolic diameter

Reference: Perrino AC, Reeves S. *A Practical Approach to TEE.* Philadelphia: Lippincott Williams & Wilkins 2003:38.

93. **Answer = C, Decreased isovolumic relaxation time would be expected in a patient with acute transplant rejection.** Other expected findings include the following: increased transmitral E-wave peak velocity, shortened transmitral E-wave deceleration time, decreased transmitral E-wave pressure half time, and decreased lateral mitral annular tissue Doppler E_M.

Reference: Otto C. *Textbook of Clinical Echocardiography, Third Edition.* Philadelphia: Elsevier 2004:250.

94. **Answer = A, Paradoxical septal motion occurring in systole is indicative of right ventricular pressure overload.** The interventricular septum usually moves toward the left ventricle during systole as the left ventricle contracts. With right ventricular pressure overload, the septum paradoxically flattens and becomes concave toward the right ventricle during systole when right ventricular pressure is highest. One explanation for the paradoxical motion seen with pressure overload is as follows: the septum moves toward the center of mass of the heart during systole and with right ventricular hypertrophy the center of mass of the heart is shifted toward the right ventricle, causing the septum to move in that direction. In contrast to pressure overload, with right ventricular volume overload the paradoxical septal motion occurs during late diastole when right ventricular volume is highest. During this right ventricular volume overload, the septum is flattened and becomes concave toward the right ventricle in late diastole.

Reference: Otto C. *Textbook of Clinical Echocardiography, Third Edition.* Philadelphia: Elsevier 2004:252.

95. **Answer = B, A dilated left atrium would be expected in constrictive pericarditis due to chronically elevated left atrial pressures.** Other expected findings include normal systolic function (FAC > 50%), restrictive diastolic dysfunction (elevated transmitral peak E velocity), normal left ventricular free wall thickness, and normal left ventricular dimensions.

Reference: Otto C. *Textbook of Clinical Echocardiography, Third Edition.* Philadelphia: Elsevier 2004:270.

96. **Answer = C, An increase in the hepatic venous D wave on pulsed-wave Doppler would be expected during spontaneous inspiration in a patient with constrictive pericarditis.** With spontaneous inspiration, the negative intrathoracic pressure dilates the thin-walled right ventricle and favors RV filling at the expense of LV filling and LV stroke volume (a reciprocal respiratory filling pattern). Lateral mitral annular tissue Doppler E_M is not affected by changes in loading conditions.

Reference: Otto C. *Textbook of Clinical Echocardiography, Third Edition.* Philadelphia: Elsevier 2004:270–272.

97. **Answer = E, All of the above are relative contraindications to TEE.** Relative contraindications to TEE include the following: esophageal diverticulum, large hiatal hernia, recent esophageal or gastric surgery, esophageal varices, history of dysphagia or odynophagia, cervical arthritis, history of radiation to the mediastinum, deformities of the oral pharynx, and severe coagulopathy.

Reference: Savage RM, Aronson S, Thomas JD, Shanewise JS, Shernan SK. *Comprehensive Textbook of Intraoperative Transesophageal Echocardiography.* Philadelphia: Lippincott Williams & Wilkins 2004:108.

98. **Answer = D, Acoustic shadowing results from inability of the ultrasound beam to penetrate the heavily calcified mitral valve annulus.**

Reference: Savage RM, Aronson S, Thomas JD, Shanewise JS, Shernan SK. *Comprehensive Textbook of Intraoperative Transesophageal Echocardiography.* Philadelphia: Lippincott Williams & Wilkins 2004:39.

99. **Answer = E, All of the above can result in artifact formation.**

100. **Answer = E, Reverberation artifact is best described as equally spaced "objects" that have the appearance of a ladder.** This artifact results when two or more strong reflectors lie in the path of an ultrasound beam and sound ricochets back and forth between the two reflectors before returning to the transducer.

Reference: Savage RM, Aronson S, Thomas JD, Shanewise JS, Shernan SK. *Comprehensive Textbook of Intraoperative Transesophageal Echocardiography.* Philadelphia: Lippincott Williams & Wilkins 2004:40.

101. **Answer = C, A eustachian valve is an embryologic remnant of the sinus venosus.** In the fetus the eustachian valve serves to divert well-oxygenated blood from the inferior vena cava across a patent foramen ovale into the left atrium, where it preferentially flows to the brain and the heart.

Reference: Savage RM, Aronson S, Thomas JD, Shanewise JS, Shernan SK. *Comprehensive Textbook of Intraoperative Transesophageal Echocardiography.* Philadelphia: Lippincott Williams & Wilkins 2004:44.

102. **Answer = C, A chiari network is associated with an aneurysmal interatrial septum and a patent foramen ovale.** This thin mobile web-like structure can be seen in the bicaval view in about 2% of patients.

Reference: Savage RM, Aronson S, Thomas JD, Shanewise JS, Shernan SK. *Comprehensive Textbook of Intraoperative Transesophageal Echocardiography.* Philadelphia: Lippincott Williams & Wilkins 2004:44.

103. **Answer = C, A chiari network is associated with an aneurysmal interatrial septum and a patent foramen ovale.** This thin mobile web-like structure can be seen in the bicaval view in about 2% of patients.

Reference: Savage RM, Aronson S, Thomas JD, Shanewise JS, Shernan SK. *Comprehensive Textbook of Intraoperative Transesophageal Echocardiography.* Philadelphia: Lippincott Williams & Wilkins 2004:44.

104. **Answer = C, The crista terminalis is a muscular ridge that extends anteriorly from the superior vena cava to the inferior vena cava and divides the trabeculated portion of the right atrium from the posterior smooth-walled sinus venarum segment.**

Reference: Savage RM, Aronson S, Thomas JD, Shanewise JS, Shernan SK. *Comprehensive Textbook of Intraoperative Transesophageal Echocardiography.* Philadelphia: Lippincott Williams & Wilkins 2004:44.

105. **Answer = B, The Nyquist limit is the maximum Doppler shift that can be accurately measured. It determines the max velocity that can be measured, is responsible for aliasing artifact, and is infinite with continuous wave Doppler.**

Reference: Edelman SK. *Understanding Ultrasound Physics.* Woodlands, TX: ESP, Inc. 1994:131–137.

106. **Answer = C, Decreasing the depth of the sample volume will decrease aliasing artifact.** Decreasing the depth will decrease the time required to listen for returning echoes and thereby increase the pulse repetition frequency and the Nyquist limit (NL = 1/2 PRF). Other things associated with a decrease in aliasing include decreasing the transmitted frequency, increasing the Nyquist limit, and increasing the pulse repetition frequency.

Reference: Edelman SK. *Understanding Ultrasound Physics.* Woodlands, TX: ESP, Inc. 1994:131–137.

107. **Answer = A, The upper esophageal aortic arch short axis view can be used to estimate the right ventricular stroke volume.**

Reference: Konstadt SN, Shernon S, Oka Y (eds). *Clinical Transesophageal Echocardiography: A Problem-Oriented Approach, Second Edition.* Philadelphia: Lippincott Williams & Wilkins 2003:428.

108. **Answer = A, The midesophageal ascending aortic short axis view allows visualization of the pulmonary artery bifurcation.**

Reference: Konstadt SN, Shernon S, Oka Y (eds). *Clinical Transesophageal Echocardiography: A Problem-Oriented Approach, Second Edition.* Philadelphia: Lippincott Williams & Wilkins 2003:428.

109. **Answer = B, The midesophageal ascending aortic short axis view occasionally allows one to visualize the superior vena cava in cross section (short axis).**

Reference: Perrino AC, Reeves S. *A Practical Approach to TEE.* Philadelphia: Lippincott Williams & Wilkins 2003:332.

110. **Answer = E, SV_{TV} = 72 cm^3.** The calculation is as follows.

$$SV_{TV} = A_{TV} * TVI_{TV}$$

$$SV_{TV} = 6\ cm^2 * 12\ cm$$

$$SV_{TV} = 72\ cm^3$$

Where:

> SV_{TV} = stroke volume of diastolic transtricuspid inflow

> A_{TV} = area of the tricuspid valve

> TVI_{TV} = time velocity integral of transtricuspid inflow

Reference: Perrino AC, Reeves S. *A Practical Approach to TEE.* Philadelphia: Lippincott Williams & Wilkins 2003:150.

111. **Answer = C, 58.8 ml is the best estimate of the stroke volume of blood flow through the pulmonic valve.** The calculation is as follows.

$$SV_{PA} = A_{PA} * TVI_{PA}$$

$$SV_{PA} = \pi r^2 * TVI_{PA}$$

$$SV_{PA} = \pi\ (1.2)^2 * (13\ cm)$$

$$SV_{PA} = 58.8\ ml$$

Where:

> SV_{PA} = stroke volume of blood flow through the main pulmonary artery

> A_{PA} = area of the pulmonic artery

> TVI_{PA} = time velocity integral of blood flow though the pulmonary artery

Reference: Sidebotham D, Merry A, Legget M (eds.). *Practical Perioperative Transoesophageal Echocardiography.* Burlington, MA: Butterworth Heinemann 2003:231.

112. **Answer = D, 13.2 ml is the tricuspid valve regurgitant volume.** The calculation is as follows:

$$TV\ RVol = (SV_{TV} - SV_{PA}) = (72\ cm^3 - 58.8\ ml) = 13.2\ ml$$

$$SV_{PA} = A_{PA} * TVI_{PA}$$

$$SV_{PA} = \pi r^2 * TVI_{PA}$$

$$SV_{PA} = \pi\ (1.2)^2 * (13\ cm)$$

$$SV_{PA} = 58.8\ ml$$

$$SV_{TV} = A_{TV} * TVI_{TV}$$

$$SV_{TV} = 6\ cm^2 * 12\ cm$$

$$SV_{TV} = 72\ cm^3$$

Where:

SV_{PA} = stroke volume of blood flow through the main pulmonary artery

A_{PA} = area of the main pulmonary artery

TV RVol = tricuspid regurgitant volume

TVI_{PA} = time velocity integral of blood flow though the pulmonary artery

SV_{TV} = stroke volume of diastolic transtricuspid inflow

A_{TV} = area of the tricuspid valve

TVI_{TV} = time velocity integral of transtricuspid inflow

Reference: Sidebotham D, Merry A, Legget M (eds.). *Practical Perioperative Transoesophageal Echocardiography.* Burlington, MA: Butterworth Heinemann 2003:235.

113. **Answer = E, 18.3% is the tricuspid valve regurgitant fraction.** The calculation is as follows:

TV regurgitant fraction = TV RVol / SV_{TV}

TV regurgitant fraction = 13.2 ml / 72 ml

TV regurgitant fraction = 18.3%

Where:

TV RVol = tricuspid regurgitant volume

SV_{TV} = stroke volume of diastolic transtricuspid inflow

Reference: Sidebotham D, Merry A, Legget M (eds.). *Practical Perioperative Transoesophageal Echocardiography.* Burlington, MA: Butterworth Heinemann 2003:235.

114. **Answer = C, 0.073 cm² = the tricuspid valve regurgitant orifice area (ROA).** The calculation is as follows.

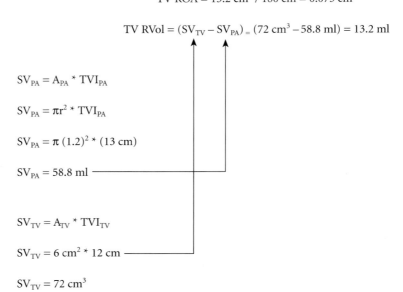

$$TV\ ROA = RVol/TVI_{TRjet}$$

$$TV\ ROA = 13.2\ cm^3\ /\ 180\ cm = 0.073\ cm^2$$

$$TV\ RVol = (SV_{TV} - SV_{PA}) = (72\ cm^3 - 58.8\ ml) = 13.2\ ml$$

$$SV_{PA} = A_{PA} * TVI_{PA}$$

$$SV_{PA} = \pi r^2 * TVI_{PA}$$

$$SV_{PA} = \pi\ (1.2)^2 * (13\ cm)$$

$$SV_{PA} = 58.8\ ml$$

$$SV_{TV} = A_{TV} * TVI_{TV}$$

$$SV_{TV} = 6\ cm^2 * 12\ cm$$

$$SV_{TV} = 72\ cm^3$$

Where:

SV_{PA} = stroke volume of blood flow through the main pulmonary artery

A_{PA} = area of the main pulmonary artery

TVI = time velocity integral of the tricuspid regurgitant jet

TVI_{PA} = time velocity integral of blood flow though the pulmonary artery

SV_{TV} = stroke volume of diastolic transtricuspid inflow

A_{TV} = area of the tricuspid valve

TVI_{TV} = time velocity integral of transtricuspid inflow

TV RVol = tricuspid regurgitant volume

TV ROA = tricuspid valve regurgitant orifice area

Reference: Sidebotham D, Merry A, Legget M (eds.). *Practical Perioperative Transoesophageal Echocardiography.* Burlington, MA: Butterworth Heinemann 2003:235.

115. **Answer = E, An increase in the dynamic range will create more shades of dark black and bright white, with fewer shades of gray on the image.** The dynamic range is the spectrum or range of signals that can be processed by the different components of an ultrasound system. The returning echoes have a large dynamic range, much larger than the components of an ultrasound machine can manage. Thus, the

signals cannot be properly processed until they are compressed into a manageable size. The machine maintains the relative strengths of the signals (i.e., the strongest echo is still the strongest and the smallest echo is still the smallest) but reduces the difference in voltage between the signals (compression). This reduces the range of signals to a manageable size, enabling the machine to process information that is within the confines of the system. Increasing the dynamic range will increase the voltage difference between the strongest and weakest signals, effectively creating more shades of dark black and bright white (with fewer shades of gray on the image).

Reference: Edelman SK. *Understanding Ultrasound Physics.* Woodlands, TX: ESP, Inc. 1994:169.

116. **Answer = B, Stunned myocardium is newly reperfused myocardium with impaired wall motion that reverses following resolution of reperfusion injury and damage due to ischemia.** Regional wall motion abnormalities after cardiopulmonary bypass for CABG can be due to dead myocardium (old scar), ischemic myocardium (not revascularized adequately), or stunned myocardium.

Reference: Savage RM, Aronson S, Thomas JD, Shanewise JS, Shernan SK. *Comprehensive Textbook of Intraoperative Transesophageal Echocardiography.* Philadelphia: Lippincott Williams & Wilkins 2004:360.

117. **Answer = C, Hibernating myocardium is viable myocardium that appears dysfunctional.** This salvageable myocardium has a limited coronary flow reserve and benefits from revascularization. Hibernating myocardium typically displays a biphasic pattern with dobutamine stress echocardiography. Function improves with low-dose dobutamine and then deteriorates again with higher doses.

Reference: Savage RM, Aronson S, Thomas JD, Shanewise JS, Shernan SK. *Comprehensive Textbook of Intraoperative Transesophageal Echocardiography.* Philadelphia: Lippincott Williams & Wilkins 2004:360.

118. **Answer = E, All of the post-revascularization findings listed can be predicted by dobutamine stress echocardiography.**

Reference: Savage RM, Aronson S, Thomas JD, Shanewise JS, Shernan SK. *Comprehensive Textbook of Intraoperative Transesophageal Echocardiography.* Philadelphia: Lippincott Williams & Wilkins 2004:360.

119. **Answer = D, Myocardial contrast echocardiography can be used to distinguish acutely ischemic myocardium from stunned myocardium in the operating room after separation from bypass in CABG patients.** Myocardial contrast echocardiography involves the injection of an echo contrast agent into the aortic root to assess myocardial perfusion. This diagnostic technique visualizes flow in the myocardial microvasculature, which is a marker for viability. This can be used to delineate myocardial perfusion patterns in patients

undergoing CABG surgery. Before cardiopulmonary bypass, it can help distinguish between hibernating myocardium (RWMA with perfusion) from infarcted myocardium (RWMA without perfusion). After separation from cardiopulmonary bypass, it can assist in determining if the cause of a new RWMA is graft incompetence (decreased perfusion and contractility) or stunning (normal perfusion but decreased contractility). This can assist in determining if flow is adequate (stunned myocardium) or if further revascularization may be of benefit (ischemic myocardium). Confirmation of flow into myocardium after revascularization predicts later improvement in global and regional left ventricular function.

- CABG = coronary artery bypass graft
- RWMA = regional wall motion abnormalities

Reference: Savage RM, Aronson S, Thomas JD, Shanewise JS, Shernan SK. *Comprehensive Textbook of Intraoperative Transesophageal Echocardiography.* Philadelphia: Lippincott Williams & Wilkins 2004:360.

120. **Answer = B, Positron emission tomography (PET) imaging is regarded as the gold standard and the final arbiter in decisions regarding myocardial viability.** This imaging technique tracks markers of perfusion and metabolism to compare blood flow and metabolic activity. NH_3 is a marker of perfusion and 18F-fluorodeoxyglucose is a marker of metabolism. Normally blood flow and metabolism match. Table 1.2Q summarizes PET imaging.

Reference: Savage RM, Aronson S, Thomas JD, Shanewise JS, Shernan SK. *Comprehensive Textbook of Intraoperative Transesophageal Echocardiography.* Philadelphia: Lippincott Williams & Wilkins 2004: 360.

Table 1.2Q.   PET IMAGING

Perfusion	Metabolism	Myocardium
Normal	Normal	Normal
Decreased	Decreased	Scar (irreversible damage, nonviable)
Decreased	Normal or increased	Hibernating (viable, needs reperfusion)

121. **Answer = D, 16 mm is consistent with moderate left ventricular hypertrophy** (see Table 1.2R).

Table 1.2R.

Degree LVH	LV Free-wall Thickness
Normal	6–11 mm
Mild LVH	12–14 mm
Moderate LVH	15–19 mm
Severe LVH	≥ 20 mm

LV = left ventricle, LVH = left ventricle hypertrophy.

122. **Answer = A, The X descent corresponds to the hepatic venous systolic wave (S wave).** As the right ventricle contracts, the tricuspid valve descends and the right atrial pressure decreases (X descent), allowing forward systolic flow from the hepatic veins to the right atrium (S wave).

Reference: Otto C. *Textbook of Clinical Echocardiography, Third Edition.* Philadelphia: Elsevier 2004:244.

123. **Answer = E, All of the above are consistent with restrictive cardiomyopathy.** Normal systolic function, thick right and left ventricular walls, and a dilated inferior vena cava would be expected in a patient with restrictive cardiomyopathy.

Reference: Otto C. *Textbook of Clinical Echocardiography, Third Edition.* Philadelphia: Elsevier 2004:241.

124. **Answer = E, All of the above would be expected in a patient with chronic hypertension.** Concentric left ventricular hypertrophy, mitral annular calcification, aortic valve sclerosis, aortic root dilation, left atrial enlargement, and impaired relaxation are findings seen with chronic hypertension. Atrial fibrillation may also occur if left atrial pressure is severely elevated.

Reference: Otto C. *Textbook of Clinical Echocardiography, Third Edition.* Philadelphia: Elsevier 2004:245.

125. **Answer = C, Pulsed-wave Doppler transmitral E/A < 1 is consistent with impaired relaxation, which would be expected in a patient with chronic hypertension.** A wall thickness of greater than 11 mm would be expected, as would an aortic root diameter of greater than 32 mm. A lateral mitral annular tissue Doppler E_M of 8.2 cm/sec and a transmitral color M-mode propagation velocity of 63 cm/sec are normal and would not be expected in a patient with chronic hypertension.

Reference: Otto C. *Textbook of Clinical Echocardiography, Third Edition.* Philadelphia: Elsevier 2004:245.

126. **Answer = C, Phased-array transducers are capable of creating multiple focal zones per scan line.** The other transducers listed do not have this capability. Increasing the number of focal zones per scan line will improve the lateral resolution.

Reference: Edelman SK. *Understanding Ultrasound Physics.* Woodlands, TX: ESP, Inc. 1994:122.

127. **Answer = C, As line density increases frame rate decreases.** Line density equals the number of scan lines per image. As line density increases the number of pulses per image increases, temporal resolution decreases, and frame rate is decreased. Line density does not determine propagation velocity (V). Velocity is determined solely by the stiffness and density of the medium through which the ultrasound beam travels.

Reference: Edelman SK. *Understanding Ultrasound Physics.* Woodlands, TX: ESP, Inc. 1994:122.

128. **Answer = E, All of the above are indications for a dobutamine stress echo.**

Reference: Oh JK, Seward JB, Tajik AJ (eds). *The Echo Manual, Second Edition.* Philadelphia: Lippincott Williams & Wilkins 1999:91.

129. **Answer = C, If the left ventricle becomes hyperdynamic except for the inferior wall during a dobutamine stress echo (DSE), this indicates right coronary artery ischemia.**

Reference: Oh JK, Seward JB, Tajik AJ (eds). *The Echo Manual, Second Edition.* Philadelphia: Lippincott Williams & Wilkins 1999:94.

130. **Answer = E, New regional wall motion abnormalities are the most sensitive sign of myocardial ischemia during a dobutamine stress echo (DSE).**

Reference: Oh JK, Seward JB, Tajik AJ (eds). *The Echo Manual, Second Edition.* Philadelphia: Lippincott Williams & Wilkins 1999:94.

131. **Answer = A, The pulmonic valve is least likely to be affected by the endocarditis.**

Reference: Oh JK, Seward JB, Tajik AJ (eds). *The Echo Manual, Second Edition.* Philadelphia: Lippincott Williams & Wilkins 1999:347.

132. **Answer = C, Of the choices listed, carcinoid heart disease is the most likely cause of both tricuspid and pulmonic valve pathology.** Carcinoid heart disease results from the release of active metabolites from carcinoid tumor cells. These metabolites (serotonin, bradykinin, histamine, and prostaglandins) damage the right-sided valves. The left-sided valves are protected from these substances because they are degraded by monoamine oxidases in the lung. Carcinoid syndrome results in thickened fibrotic leaflets with restricted mobility.

Reference: Perrino AC, Reeves S. *A Practical Approach to TEE.* Philadelphia: Lippincott Williams & Wilkins 2003:226.

133. **Answer = D, Ventricular rupture, although a rare complication, is the most common complication of mitral valve repair listed.** Rupture usually occurs between the papillary muscle insertions and the atrioventricular groove and is obviously a serious (albeit rare) problem. Predisposing factors include severe annular calcification, advanced age, and female sex. Complications of mitral valve repair include damage to the circumflex coronary artery, damage to the left or non-coronary cusps of the aortic valve, decreased cardiac conduction, systolic anterior motion of the anterior mitral valve leaflet, and ventricular rupture.

Reference: Perrino AC, Reeves S. *A Practical Approach to TEE.* Philadelphia: Lippincott Williams & Wilkins 2003:172.

134. **Answer = B, The proximal isovelocity surface area (PISA) method of determining mitral valve area is not influenced by aortic insufficiency or mitral regurgitation.** The continuity equation and the pressure half time method are affected by these valvular abnormalities, but the PISA method is only dependent on flow immediately prior to the valve (at the first aliasing velocity) and at the stenotic mitral orifice.

Reference: Perrino AC, Reeves S. *A Practical Approach to TEE.* Philadelphia: Lippincott Williams & Wilkins 2003:155.

135. **Answer = B, Rheumatic heart disease is the most common cause of mitral stenosis.**

Reference: Otto C. *Textbook of Clinical Echocardiography, Third Edition.* Philadelphia: Elsevier 2004:295.

136. **Answer = A, Mitral regurgitation due to P_2 prolapse is the pathology most amenable to surgical repair listed.**

Reference: Sidebotham D, Merry A, Legget M (eds.). *Practical Perioperative Transoesophageal Echocardiography.* Burlington, MA: Butterworth Heinemann 2003:147.

TEST II PART 1

Video Test Booklet

This product is designed to prepare people for the PTEeXAM. This booklet is to be used with the CD-ROM to practice for the video portion of the PTEeXAM.

Preface

As stated previously, this part of this product is designed to prepare people for the video component of the PTEeXAM. Please do not open this test booklet until you have read the instructions. During the PTEeXAM, instructions similar to these will be written on the back of the test booklet. You will be asked to read these instructions by a proctor at the exam. After you have read these instructions you will be asked to break the seal on the test booklet and to remove an answer sheet.

After you have filled out your name, test number, and other identifying information on the answer sheet you will be instructed to open the test booklet and begin. This test will involve video images shown on a computer monitor. You will share this monitor with 3 other examinees. This portion of the PTEeXAM has about 50 questions. It consists of about 17 cases, with 2 to 5 questions for each case. It is timed. Good luck!

Instructions

This test will consist of several cases, accompanied by 3 to 5 questions per case. Each case will show one or more images. For each case, you are to utilize the information written in this booklet and the information shown in the images to answer questions concerning each case. An audible chime or tone will assist in timing the exam. This tone alerts you when the test advances to the next step.

The order of the exam is as follows.

Tone/chime

    1. Read the questions for case 1.

Tone/chime

    2. View the images for case 1.

Tone/chime

    3. Answer the questions for case 1.

Tone/chime

    4. View the images for case 1 again.

Tone/chime

    5. Check your answers to the questions for case 1.

Tone/chime

    6. Read the questions for case 2.

Tone/chime

The process continues in this manner. In summary: tone, read, tone, view, tone, answer, tone, view, tone, check answers, tone.

Cases

Case 1

A 27-year-old male with an aortic tear at the level of the ligamentum arteriosum following a motor vehicle accident is undergoing femoral-artery/femoral-vein partial cardiopulmonary bypass. The aorta is clamped just proximal to the tear.

    1. Which of the following best describes this patient's systolic function?

        A. Normal

        B. Mildly decreased

        C. Moderately decreased

        D. Severely decreased

        E. Hyperdynamic

2. The patient's right radial arterial line indicates a blood pressure of 65/30. What is the best treatment to pursue at this time?

   A. Tell the perfusionist to decrease the venous cannula drainage.

   B. Administer 500 cc of hydroxyethlystarch.

   C. Administer 100 mcg of phenylephrine.

   D. Administer 500 mg of calcium chloride.

   E. Administer 10 mcg of epinephrine.

Case 2

A 51-year-old male is undergoing an off pump coronary artery bypass grafting procedure. A shunt has been placed in the left anterior descending artery, and the patient is hemodynamically stable.

3. What wall is indicated by the arrow?

   A. Lateral

   B. Septal

   C. Anterior

   D. Inferior

   E. Posterior

4. What is the most likely cause of the regional wall motion abnormality seen in this image?

   A. Right coronary artery ischemia

   B. Circumflex coronary artery ischemia

   C. Left anterior descending artery ischemia

   D. A Left ventricular stabilizing device (octopus) is attached to the epicardium

Case 3

A 63-year-old male with end-stage renal disease and aortic stenosis is scheduled for aortic valve replacement.

5. Which of the following best describes this patient's systolic function?

    A. Normal, LVEF = 55%

    B. Mildly decreased, LVEF = 40–50

    C. Moderately decreased, LVEF = 30–44

    D. Severely decreased, LVEF < 25%

6. If the arterial blood pressure was 70/35, which of the following would be the most appropriate treatment?

    A. 500 cc bolus of 5% albumin

    B. 300 mg bolus of calcium chloride

    C. Ephedrine 10 mg bolus

    D. Epinephrine infusion at 0.03 mcg/kg/min

Case 4

7. What mitral valve scallop is indicated by the arrow shown in image 1 and image 2 for case 4?

    A. P1

    B. P2

    C. P3

    D. A1

    E. A2

8. What mitral valve commissure is indicated by the arrow in image 3 for case 4?

    A. Posterolateral

    B. Posteromedial

    C. Anterolateral

    D. Anteromedial

    E. Lateral

9. What mitral valve leaflet is indicated by the arrow in image 4?

    A. Anterior

    B. Posterior

    C. Lateral

    D. Septal

    E. Inferior

Case 5

The left ventricular outflow tract (LVOT) diameter is 1.9 cm. Given the LVOT diameter and the information shown in the images, answer the following questions. Note: VTI = TVI = velocity time integral, SV = stroke volume, and LVOT = left ventricular outflow tract.

10. Which of the following is the best estimate of the mitral valve stroke volume (the volume of blood traveling through the mitral valve during diastole)?

    A. 39 cm^3

    B. 56 cm^3

    C. 68 cm^3

    D. 87 cm^3

    E. 96 cm^3

11. What is the left ventricular outflow tract (LVOT) stroke volume?

    A. 20 cm^3

    B. 31 cm^3

    C. 42 cm^3

    D. 53 cm^3

    E. 64 cm^3

12. What is the mitral valve regurgitant volume?

   A. 26 cm^3

   B. 33 cm^3

   C. 44 cm^3

   D. 56 cm^3

   E. 65 cm^3

13. What is the regurgitant fraction?

   A. 27%

   B. 34%

   C. 45%

   D. 58%

   E. 64%

14. What is the mitral valve regurgitant orifice area?

   A. 0.20 cm^2

   B. 0.30 cm^2

   C. 0.40 cm^2

   D. 0.50 cm^2

   E. 0.60 cm^2

Case 6

15. What is the mechanism for the mitral regurgitation seen in case 6?

   A. Ruptured chord and flail posterior leaflet

   B. Ruptured chord and flail anterior leaflet

   C. Tethered leaflets from rheumatic mitral disease

   D. Ischemic mitral regurgitation with annular dilation and incomplete leaflet coaptation

   E. Myxomatous mitral valve disease with posterior leaflet prolapse

16. Using the Carpentier classification of leaflet motion, describe the leaflet motion seen in this patient.

   A. Type I leaflet motion

   B. Type II leaflet motion

   C. Type III leaflet motion

   D. Type IV leaflet motion

   E. Type V leaflet motion

Case 7

17. Images 1 through 9 for case 7 were obtained from a patient undergoing abdominal surgery. Which of the following best describes the aortic valve function?

   A. Critical aortic stenosis

   B. Moderate aortic stenosis

   C. Mild aortic stenosis

   D. Aortic valve sclerosis but not stenosis

   E. Normal aortic valve function

18. Which of the following is the best explanation for the aortic transvalular gradient shown?

   A. Severe aortic regurgitation decreases the pressure gradient.

   B. Severe mitral regurgitation decreases the pressure gradient.

   C. Left ventriculare diastolic dysfunction increases the pressure gradient.

   D. Severe mitral regurgitation increases the pressure gradient.

   E. Severe aortic regurgitation increases the pressure gradient.

19. Which of the following measures of aortic valve stenosis is not affected by poor systolic function?

    A. Peak transvalvular velocity

    B. TVI_{LVOT} / TVI_{AV}

    C. Peak transvalvular pressure gradient

    D. Pressure half time method

    E. Proximal isovelocity surface area method

    (LVOT = left ventricular outflow tract, AV = atrioventricular, TVI = time velocity integral)

20. Which of the following measures of aortic valve stenosis is not affected by severe mitral regurgitation?

    A. Peak transvalvular velocity

    B. Peak transvalvular pressure gradient

    C. Continuity equation method

    D. Pressure half time method

    E. Proximal isovelocity surface area method

21. Which of the following will prevent an accurate assessment of the aortic valve area by the continuity equation (LVOT = left ventricular outflow tract, AV = atrioventricular)?

    A. Restrictive diastolic dysfunction

    B. Severe aortic insufficiency

    C. Severe mitral insufficiency

    D. Complete AV canal defect

    E. Inability to measure the LVOT diameter accurately

Case 8

22. What view is shown in image 1 for case 8?

    A. Transgastric two-chamber view

    B. Transgastric right ventricular inflow outflow view

    C. Transgastric right ventricular inflow view

    D. Midesophageal right ventricular inflow outflow

    E. Transgastric right ventricular long axis view

23. The arrow in image 2 for case 8 indicates which of the following?

    A. Pulmonic valve

    B. Tricuspid valve

    C. Mitral valve

    D. Chiari network

    E. Eustachian valve

24. Which of the following is indicated by the arrow in image 3 for case 8?

    A. Intraaortic balloon pump

    B. Retrograde cardiopledgia catheter

    C. Central venous line

    D. Pulmonary artery catheter

    E. Antegrade cardiopledgia catheter

25. What view is shown in image 3 for case 8?

    A. Upper esophageal aortic arch short axis view

    B. Midesophageal ascending aortic short axis view

    C. Midesophageal aortic short axis view

    D. Midesophageal ascending aortic long axis

    E. Upper esophageal aortic arch long axis view

Case 9

26. The arrow in image 1 for case 9 indicates which of the following?

    A. Pulmonic valve

    B. Tricuspid valve

    C. Aortic valve

    D. Chiari network

    E. Eustachian valve

27. Which of the following is indicated by the arrow in image 2 for case 9?

    A. Right ventricle

    B. Pulmonary artery

    C. Pericardial effusion

    D. Right atrium

    E. Coronary sinus

Case 10

28. Which of the following best describes this patient's RV systolic function?

    A. Normal.

    B. Mildly decreased.

    C. Moderately decreased.

    D. Severely decreased.

    E. It cannot be determined from the data given.

29. Arrow 1 in image 4 for case 10 indicates which of the following?

    A. Anterolateral papillary muscle

    B. Posteromedial papillary muscle

    C. Moderator band

    D. Tricuspid valve

    E. Chiari network

30. Which of the following treatments would most likely be of benefit?

   A. Milrinone infusion

   B. Phenylephrine infusion

   C. 500-milliliter hetastarch bolus

   D. Vasopressin infusion

   E. Norepinephrine infusion

31. Which of the following is a normal tricuspid annular plane systolic excursion?

   A. 5–10 mm

   B. 10–15 mm

   C. 15–20 mm

   D. 20–25 mm

   E. 25–30 mm

Case 11

32. Which of the following defects would be expected to result in the image seen?

   A. Atrial septal defect

   B. Ventricular septal defect

   C. Patent ductus arteriosus

   D. Aortic coarctation

   E. Kartagener's syndrome

33. Given the information in image 3 for case 11, what additional information is needed to calculate the pulmonary artery systolic pressure?

   A. RA pressure

   B. Systolic blood pressure

   C. Diastolic blood pressure

   D. Pulmonary flow velocity

   E. Pulmonic valve area

34. Which of the following will affect the accuracy of the calculation of the pulmonary artery systolic pressure from the regurgitant jet shown in image 3 for case 11?

    A. Tricuspid stenosis

    B. Mitral regurgitation

    C. Pulmonic regurgitation

    D. Patent ductus arteriosus

    E. Pulmonic stenosis

Case 12

35. Which of the following is indicated by the arrow shown in image 1 for case 12?

    A. Interatrial septum

    B. Coumadin ridge

    C. Supraventricular membrane

    D. Cor triatriatum

    E. Chiari network

36. Which of the following is indicated by the arrow in image 3 for case 12?

    A. Ostium primum atrial septal defect

    B. Ostium secundum atrial septal defect

    C. Sinus venosus atrial septal defect

    D. Coronary sinus atrial septal defect

    E. Perimembranous atrial septal defect

37. On the color flow map shown, which of the following colors indicates laminar flow going away from the transducer?

    A. Blue

    B. Red

    C. Yellow

    D. Green

    E. Orange

Case 13

38. What is the diagnosis?

    A. Ostium primum atrial septal defect

    B. Ostium secundum atrial septal defect

    C. Sinus venosus atrial septal defect

    D. Coronary sinus atrial septal defect

    E. Perimembranous atrial septal defect

39. Which of the following is associated with this defect?

    A. Bicuspid aortic valve

    B. Cleft mitral valve

    C. Aortic coarctation

    D. Anomalous pulmonary venous return

    E. Persistent left superior vena cava

40. Turbulent blood flow toward the transducer with a 90-degree incident angle (angle between the ultrasound beam and blood flow) will be represented by which of the following colors according to the color map shown in case 13?

    A. Red

    B. Blue

    C. Black

    D. Green

    E. Yellow

Case 14

41. Which of the following best describes the degree of aortic insufficiency?

   A. Trace

   B. Mild

   C. Moderate

   D. Severe

   E. It cannot be determined from the information given

42. Which of the following pressure half time measurements for the aortic insufficiency jet would be expected?

   A. 190 milliseconds

   B. 301 milliseconds

   C. 403 milliseconds

   D. 500 milliseconds

   E. 621 milliseconds

43. Which of the following slopes of the aortic insufficiency jet decay would be consistent with the images seen?

   A. 96 cm/sec

   B. 130 cm/sec

   C. 190 cm/sec

   D. 212 cm/sec

   E. 313 cm/sec

44. Arrow 1 in image 4 for case 14 indicates which of the following?

   A. Right coronary cusp

   B. Left coronary cusp

   C. Noncoronary cusp

   D. Inferior coronary cusp

   E. Lateral coronary cusp

Case 15

45. Which of the following is the best estimate of this patient's LV ejection fraction?

    A. < 15 %

    B. 20–30%

    C. 30–40%

    D. 40–50%

    E. > 55%

46. Which of the following findings would be consistent with the images shown?

    A. Elevated troponin levels

    B. Systolic anterior motion of the anterior mitral valve leaflet

    C. Severe aortic stenosis

    D. Severe mitral stenosis

    E. Decreased brain natriuretic peptide

47. If this patient was hypotensive in the operating room, which of the following would most likely be effective in increasing the systolic blood pressure?

    A. 500 cc of hetastarch bolus

    B. Phenylephrine infusion

    C. Vasopressin infusion

    D. Milrinone infusion

    E. Epinephrine infusion

48. Which of the following best describes the wall motion of the anterior apical left ventricular wall?

    A. Normal

    B. Mildly hypokinetic

    C. Severely hypokinetic

    D. Akinetic

    E. Dyskinetic

Case 16

49. What is the most likely diagnosis?

    A. Endocarditis of the mitral and aortic valves

    B. Rheumatic heart disease

    C. Multiple rhabdomyosarcoma tumors

    D. Thrombus formation on the aortic and mitral valves

    E. Myxomatous valvular degeneration

50. What view is shown in image 2 and image 3?

    A. Midesophageal two-chamber view

    B. Midesophageal mitral valve inflow view

    C. Midesophageal long axis view

    D. Midesophageal mitral valve commissural view

    E. Midesophageal four-chamber view

51. Which of the following is most likely indicated by arrow 1?

    A. Thrombus

    B. Rhabdomyosarcoma tumor

    C. Vegetation

    D. Flail posterior mitral valve leaflet

    E. Myxoma

52. The structure indicated by arrow 1 is attached to which of the following mitral valve scallops?

    A. A_1

    B. A_2

    C. P_1

    D. P_2

    E. P_3

Case 17

53. According to the American Society of Echocardiography 16-segment model, what numerical segment of the left ventricle is described by arrow 1?

   A. 9

   B. 10

   C. 11

   D. 12

   E. 13

54. According to the American Society of Echocardiography 16-segment model, what numerical segment of the left ventricle is described by arrow 2?

   A. 6

   B. 7

   C. 8

   D. 9

   E. 10

55. According to the American Society of Echocardiography 16-segment model, what numerical segment of the left ventricle is described by arrow 3?

   A. 6

   B. 7

   C. 8

   D. 9

   E. 10

56. According to the American Society of Echocardiography 16-segment model, what numerical segment of the left ventricle is described by arrow 4?

   A. 6

   B. 7

   C. 8

   D. 9

   E. 10

Case 18

57. The arrows in image 2 and image 3 for case 18 indicate which of the following?

    A. Posteromedial papillary muscle

    B. Thrombus

    C. Fibroma

    D. Rhabdomyoma

    E. Anterolateral papillary muscle

58. Which of the following treatments is indicated?

    A. Chemotherapy

    B. Surgical removal

    C. Anticoagulation

    D. Radiation treatment

    E. None of the above

59. With which wall is the object indicated by the arrow attached?

    A. Posterior wall

    B. Anteroseptal wall

    C. Lateral wall

    D. Inferior

    E. None of the above

Case 19

60. What do the arrows labeled I in case 19 indicate?

    A. Crista terminalis

    B. Chiari network

    C. Moderator band

    D. Eustachian valve

    E. Thrombus

61. Which of the following treatments is indicated?

    A. Chemotherapy

    B. Surgical removal

    C. Anticoagulation

    D. Radiation treatment

    E. None of the above

62. What is indicated by the arrow labeled 2 in image 6 for case 19?

    A. Left ventricular outflow tract

    B. Main pulmonary artery

    C. Coronary sinus

    D. Sinus of valsalva

    E. Proximal aortic root

Case 20

63. Which of the following is indicated by the arrow in image 2 for case 20?

    A. Coronary sinus

    B. Eustachian valve

    C. Right upper pulmonary vein

    D. Right coronary artery

    E. Left main coronary artery

64. Which of the following is true concerning the structure indicated by the arrow?

    A. It provides blood supply to the anterior wall of the left ventricle.

    B. It provides blood supply to the inferior wall of the left ventricle.

    C. It is dilated in patients with tricuspid stenosis.

    D. It is often found attached to the superior vena cava in sinus venosus ASDs.

    E. It can make placement of a retrograde coronary sinus catheter difficult.

Case 21

65. Arrow 1 indicates which of the following?

    A. Superior vena cava

    B. Inferior vena cava

    C. Aorta

    D. Right pulmonary artery

    E. Coronary sinus

66. Arrow 2 indicates which of the following?

    A. Right upper pulmonary vein

    B. Right lower pulmonary vein

    C. Left upper pulmonary vein

    D. Left lower pulmonary vein

    E. Coronary sinus

67. Arrow 3 indicates which of the following?

    A. Right upper pulmonary vein

    B. Right lower pulmonary vein

    C. Left upper pulmonary vein

    D. Left lower pulmonary vein

    E. Coronary sinus

Answers:

1. E	24. D	47. E
2. A	25. B	48. E
3. C	26. A	49. A
4. D	27. A	50. D
5. A	28. D	51. C
6. A	29. C	52. C
7. E	30. A	53. D
8. C	31. D	54. B
9. B	32. A	55. C
10. D	33. A	56. D
11. B	34. E	57. E
12. D	35. D	58. E
13. E	36. B	59. C
14. B	37. A	60. C
15. B	38. A	61. E
16. B	39. B	62. B
17. A	40. C	63. E
18. B	41. D	64. A
19. B	42. A	65. A
20. C	43. E	66. A
21. E	44. A	67. B
22. C	45. B	
23. B	46. A	

Explanations

Case 1

1. **Answer = E, Hyperdynamic.** This patient's left ventricle is empty and his systolic function is hyperdynamic.

2. **Answer = A, Tell the perfusionist to decrease the venous cannula drainage.** There is a clamp just proximal to the left subclavian artery. During this anesthetic, the heart will supply arterial blood flow to the body above the clamp and the bypass machine will supply arterial blood flow to the body distal to the aortic clamp via the cannula in the femoral artery. Blood removed via the venous cannula is taken from the circulation above the clamp and delivered to the arterial circulation distal to the clamp. If too much blood is drained into the pump, the heart will not have enough blood to effectively provide flow to the circulation (carotids, coronary arteries) proximal to the clamp. The fastest and most effective treatment for hypotension proximal to the clamp is to reduce venous cannula drainage into the pump.

Case 2

3. **Answer = C, The anterior wall is indicated by the arrow.**

4. **Answer = D, A left ventricular stabilizing device (octopus) is attached to the epicardium.** It is unlikely that this hemodynamically stable patient with a stented LAD is having anterior wall ischemia.

Case 3

5. **Answer = A, Normal, LVEF ≥ 55%.**

6. **Answer = A, 500-cc bolus of 5% albumin.** This is the best treatment for a hypotensive hypovolemic patient with aortic stenosis and concentric left ventricular hypertrophy. The patient has normal contractility. Therefore, the other choices (which augment contractility) are not ideal in this case. A bolus of a pure vasoconstrictor such as phenylephrine or vasopressin would also have been an acceptable option.

Case 4

7. **Answer = E, The A2 scallop is indicated by the arrow.** The midesophageal long axis view is shown. The A2 scallop lies adjacent to the left ventricular outflow tract in this view.

Reference: Sidebotham D, Merry A, Legget M (eds.). *Practical Perioperative Transoesophageal Echocardiography.* Burlington, MA: Butterworth Heinemann 2003:137.

8. **Answer = C, The arrow indicates the anterolateral commissure.**
   In the transgastric basal short axis view the commissures shown below are visualized.

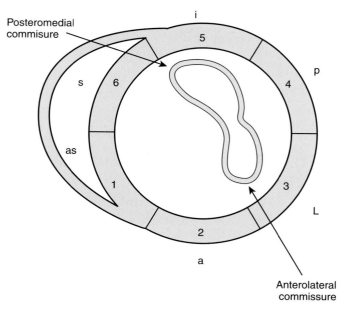

Fig. 2-1

Reference: Sidebotham D, Merry A, Legget M (eds.). *Practical Perioperative Transoesophageal Echocardiography.* Burlington, MA: Butterworth Heinemann 2003:137.

9. **Answer = B, The arrow points to the posterior mitral valve leaflet.**
   Specifically, the P2 scallop is indicated by the arrow.

Reference: Sidebotham D, Merry A, Legget M (eds.). *Practical Perioperative Transoesophageal Echocardiography.* Burlington, MA: Butterworth Heinemann 2003:138.

Case 5

10. **Answer = D, 87 cm³ is the mitral valve stroke volume.** The calculation is as follows:

$$SV_{MV} = TVI_{MV} * MVA \rightarrow SV_{MV} = (94\ cm) * (0.921\ cm^2) = 87\ cm^3$$

Where:

MVA = mitral valve area

SV_{MV} = mitral valve stroke volume

TVI_{MV} = time velocity integral of transmitral flow by continuous wave Doppler

Reference: SCA/ASE Annual Comprehensive Review and Update of Perioperative Hemodynamics Workshop. 17 Feb. 2005, San Diego, CA; discussion led by Stanton Shernon, et al.

11. **Answer = B, 31 cm³ is the stroke volume through the left ventricular outflow tract.** The calculation is as follows:

$$SV_{LVOT} = A_{LVOT} * TVI_{LVOT} = \pi r^2 * TVI_{LVOT} = [(3.14)(1.9/2)^2 * 11cm^2] = 31\ cm^3$$

Where:

VTI = TVI = velocity time integral

SV = stroke volume

LVOT = left ventricular outflow tract

Reference: SCA/ASE Annual Comprehensive Review and Update of Perioperative Hemodynamics Workshop. 17 Feb. 2005, San Diego, CA; discussion led by Stanton Shernon, et al.

12. **Answer = D, 56 cm³ is the mitral valve regurgitant volume (MV$_{RVOL}$).** The calculation is as follows:

$$MV_{RVOL} = SV_{MV} - SV_{LVOT} = 87\ cm^3 - 31\ cm^3 = 56\ cm^3$$

Where:

VTI = TVI = velocity time integral

SV = stroke volume

LVOT = left ventricular outflow tract

Reference: SCA/ASE Annual Comprehensive Review and Update of Perioperative Hemodynamics Workshop. 17 Feb. 2005, San Diego, CA; discussion led by Stanton Shernon, et al.

13. **Answer = E, 64% is the mitral valve regurgitant fraction (MV$_{RF}$).** The calculation is as follows:

$$MV_{RF} = MV_{RVOL} / SV_{MV} = 56\ cm^3 / 87\ cm^3$$

Where:

VTI = TVI = velocity time integral

SV = stroke volume

LVOT = left ventricular outflow tract

Reference: SCA/ASE Annual Comprehensive Review and Update of Perioperative Hemodynamics Workshop. 17 Feb. 2005, San Diego, CA; discussion led by Stanton Shernon, et al.

14. **Answer = B, 0.30 cm² is the mitral valve regurgitant orifice area (MV$_{ROA}$).** The calculation is as follows.

$$MV_{ROA} = MV_{RVOL} / TVI_{MV} = 56\ cm^3 / 184\ cm = 0.30\ cm^2$$

Where:

VTI = TVI = velocity time integral

SV = stroke volume

LVOT = left ventricular outflow tract

Reference: SCA/ASE Annual Comprehensive Review and Update of Perioperative Hemodynamics Workshop. 17 Feb. 2005, San Diego, CA; discussion led by Stanton Shernon, et al.

Case 6

15. **Answer = B, Anterior leaflet prolapse with a ruptured chord is the mechanism of mitral regurgitation in this patient.** Image I for this case clearly shows a ruptured chord attached to an anterior mitral valve leaflet, resulting in a posteriorly directed regurgitant jet.

16. **Answer = B, Type II leaflet motion is present.** Using the Carpentier system of classification, excessive leaflet motion is referred to as type II. The Carpentier classification system of leaflet motion for mitral regurgitation follows.

Reference: Perrino AC, Reeves S. *A Practical Approach to TEE.* Philadelphia: Lippincott Williams & Wilkins 2003:162–163.

Carpentier class:	Leaflet Motion:
Type I	Normal
Type II	Excessive
Type III	Restrictive

Case 7

17. **Answer = A, Critical aortic stenosis is shown.**

Reference: Otto C. *Textbook of Clinical Echocardiography, Third Edition.* Philadelphia: Elsevier 2004:286–293.

18. **Answer = B, Severe mitral regurgitation (MR) decreases the aortic transvalvular pressure gradient.** The aortic transvalvular gradient is dependent on the stroke volume that traverses the valve. Severe MR decreases this aortic transvalvular stroke volume and thereby decreases the peak gradient generated. Decreased systolic function will have a similar effect by the same mechanism. This is why it is important to determine the TVI_{LVOT}/TVI_{AV} ratio or the valve area before assuming that significant aortic valve stenosis is not present in patients with low pressure gradients (TVI = time velocity integral, AV = aortic valve, LVOT = left ventricular outflow tract).

Reference: Otto C. *Textbook of Clinical Echocardiography, Third Edition.* Philadelphia: Elsevier 2004:286–293.

19. **Answer = B, The TVI_{LVOT}/TVI_{AV} ratio is not affected by poor systolic function and is a good method of grading aortic stenosis in patients with decreased aortic transvalvular stroke volume.** The TVI_{LVOT}/TVI_{AV} ratio is equal to the ratio of the aortic valve area to LVOT area. If the area of the aortic valve is equal to the area of the LVOT, the TVI_{LVOT}/TVI_{AV} ratio should equal 1.

$$Q_{AV} = Q_{LVOT}$$

$$A_{AV} * TVI_{AV} = A_{LVOT} * TVI_{LVOT}$$

$$\frac{A_{AV}}{A_{LVOT}} = \frac{TVI_{LVOT}}{TVI_{AV}}$$

A TVI_{LVOT}/TVI_{AV} ratio of < 0.25 indicates severe aortic stenosis. The TVI_{LVOT}/TVI_{AV} ratio has the added advantage of controlling for size differences. It assumes that the patient's aortic valve area should be about the same as the patient's LVOT area without requiring that you actually calculate the LVOT area. Smaller people will have smaller LVOT areas and smaller aortic valve areas, but the ratio of those areas should still be close to 1 (unless aortic stenosis is present). This method involves less error than using the continuity equation to calculate the aortic valve area because LVOT diameter measurements are not required and LVOT diameter measurements are frequently incorrect.

Reference: Otto C. *Textbook of Clinical Echocardiography, Third Edition.* Philadelphia: Elsevier 2004:286–293.

20. **Answer = C, The continuity equation is not affected by severe mitral regurgitation or severe systolic dysfunction.** As long as flow in the left ventricular outflow tract is the same as flow through the aortic valve, the continuity equation will work.

Reference: Otto C. *Textbook of Clinical Echocardiography, Third Edition.* Philadelphia: Elsevier 2004:286–293.

21. **Answer = E, Inability to accurately measure the LVOT diameter will decrease the reliability of the continuity equation.** The other factors listed will not impact the continuity equation. As long as flow in the left ventricular outflow tract is the same as flow through the aortic valve, the continuity equation will work.

Reference: Otto C. *Textbook of Clinical Echocardiography, Third Edition.* Philadelphia: Elsevier 2004:286–293.

Case 8

22. **Answer = C, The transgastric right ventricular inflow view is shown.**

23. **Answer = B, The tricuspid valve is indicated by the arrow in image 2 for case 8.**

24. **Answer = D, A pulmonary artery catheter is shown in the pulmonary artery.**

25. **Answer = B, The midesophageal ascending aortic short axis view is shown.**

Reference: Perrino AC, Reeves S. *A Practical Approach to TEE.* Philadelphia: Lippincott Williams & Wilkins 2003:227.

Case 9

26. Answer = **A, The pulmonic valve is indicated by the arrow.**

27. Answer = **A, The right ventricle is shown.**

Case 10

28. Answer = **D, Severe right ventricular dysfunction is present.**

Reference: Perrino AC, Reeves S. *A Practical Approach to TEE.* Philadelphia: Lippincott Williams & Wilkins 2003:220.

29. Answer = **C, A moderator band is shown.**

Reference: Perrino AC, Reeves S. *A Practical Approach to TEE.* Philadelphia: Lippincott Williams & Wilkins 2003:219.

30. Answer = **A, Milrinone is the best treatment option.** This patient has severe right ventricular dilation and systolic dysfunction. Milrinone is a phosphodiesterase inhibitor that increases contractility while at the same time decreasing pulmonary vascular resistance (inodilator). This drug should help improve right ventricular function and decreased RV chamber size. Right ventricular dysfunction is a frequent occurrence following cardiopulmonary bypass and may result from air traveling down the anteriorly positioned right coronary artery or from inadequate cardioplegia.

Reference: Perrino AC, Reeves S. *A Practical Approach to TEE.* Philadelphia: Lippincott Williams & Wilkins 2003:220.

31. Answer = **D, 20 to 25 mm is the normal tricuspid annular plane systolic excursion.**

Reference: Perrino AC, Reeves S. *A Practical Approach to TEE.* Philadelphia: Lippincott Williams & Wilkins 2003:221.

Case 11

32. Answer = **A, An atrial septal defect is most likely to result in the clinical images seen.** Severe right atrial and right ventricular dilation are present, along with right ventricular hypertrophy from pressure and volume overload. Flow with most ASDs is predominantly diastolic left-to-right flow. This results in right-sided volume overload, causing right atrial and right ventricular dilation. Although a VSD would seem to cause RV dilation, this usually does not occur because the VSD causes left-to-right flow during systole. This left-to-right systolic flow moves blood directly across the VSD into the PA and back to the LA and LV. This creates LA and LV volume overload as the left heart receives excess blood from the pulmonary veins, but RV volume overload does not occur (ASD = atrial septal defect, VSD = ventricular septal defect, RV = right ventricle, LV = left ventricle).

Reference: Otto C. *Textbook of Clinical Echocardiography, Third Edition.* Philadelphia: Elsevier 2004:457.

33. **Answer = A, The right atrial pressure is needed to calculate the pulmonary artery systolic pressure when the max velocity of the tricuspid regurgitant jet is given.** The calculation is as follows.

$$\Delta P = 4V^2$$

$$(RVSP - RAP) = 4V_{TR}^2$$

$$(RVSP - RAP) = 4V^2$$

$$PASP = RVSP = 4V^2 + RAP$$

Where:

RVSP = right ventricular systolic pressure

RAP = right atrial pressure

V_{TR} = peak velocity of the tricuspid valve regurgitant jet

Reference: Otto C. *Textbook of Clinical Echocardiography, Third Edition.* Philadelphia: Elsevier 2004:463.

34. **Answer = E, Pulmonic stenosis will affect the accuracy of estimating the pulmonary artery systolic pressure from a tricuspid valve regurgitant jet because the right ventricular systolic pressure will not equal the pulmonary artery systolic pressure.**

Reference: Otto C. *Textbook of Clinical Echocardiography, Third Edition.* Philadelphia: Elsevier 2004:463.

Case 12

35. **Answer = D, A cor triatriatum is seen.**

36. **Answer = B, An ostium secundum atrial septal defect is shown.**

37. **Answer = A, Blue indicates laminar flow away from the probe on the variance color flow map shown.**

Reference: Edelman SK. *Understanding Ultrasound Physics.* Woodlands, TX: ESP, Inc. 1994:155.

Case 13

38. **Answer = A, An ostium primum atrial septal defect is present.**

39. **Answer = B, A cleft anterior mitral valve leaflet is associated with an ostium primum atrial septal defect.**

Reference: Sidebotham D, Merry A, Legget M (eds.). *Practical Perioperative Transoesophageal Echocardiography.* Burlington, MA: Butterworth Heinemann 2003:223.

40. **Answer = C, Turbulent blood flow toward the transducer with a 90-degree incident angle (angle between the ultrasound beam and blood flow) will be represented by the color black.** This is because no Doppler shift occurs with an incident angle of 90 degrees.

Reference: Edelman SK. *Understanding Ultrasound Physics.* Woodlands, TX: ESP, Inc. 1994:155.

Case 14

41. **Answer = D, Severe aortic insufficiency (AI) is present. Using color flow Doppler in the midesophageal aortic valve long axis view you can determine the ratio of the AI jet height to the height of the left ventricular outflow tract (LVOT).** An AI jet to LVOT ratio of > 2/3 is indicative of severe AI.

Degree of AI:	Trace (0-1+)	Mild (1-2+)	Moderate (2-3+)	Severe (3-4+)
AI jet d/ LVOT d:	1-24%	25-46%	47-64%	> 65%

Where:

AI jet d = aortic insufficiency jet diameter

LVOT d = left ventricular outflow tract diameter

Reference: Perrino AC, Reeves S. *A Practical Approach to TEE.* Philadelphia: Lippincott Williams & Wilkins 2003:180.

42. **Answer = A, A pressure half time of less than 200 milliseconds is indicative of severe aortic insufficiency.** Some books consider < 300 ms (not < 200 ms) to indicate severe AI.

Degree of AI:	Trace (0-1+)	Mild (1-2+)	Moderate (2-3+)	Severe (3-4+)
PHT		> 500 ms	200-500 ms	< 200 (300?)ms

Reference: Perrino AC, Reeves S. *A Practical Approach to TEE.* Philadelphia: Lippincott Williams & Wilkins 2003:180.

43. **Answer = E, A slope of greater than 300 cm/sec (3 m/s) is indicative of severe AI.**

Degree of AI:	Trace (0-1+)	Mild (1-2+)	Moderate (2-3+)	Severe (3-4+)
Slope:			200-300 cm/sec	≥ 300 cm/sec

Reference: Perrino AC, Reeves S. *A Practical Approach to TEE.* Philadelphia: Lippincott Williams & Wilkins 2003:180.

44. **Answer = A, The right coronary cusp is shown.**

Case 15

45. **Answer = B, The left ventricular ejection fraction (LVEF) is 20 to 30%.**

46. **Answer = A, Troponin levels could be elevated given the segmental wall motion abnormalities (SWMA) shown.** TEE has a

high sensitivity for ischemia, which shows up as new segmental wall motion abnormalities. Unfortunately, there are other causes of segmental wall motion abnormalities (conduction problems, and the like) and TEE is most beneficial when comparing new images to recently acquired older images.

47. **Answer = E, Epinephrine is most likely to increase this patient's blood pressure.** With this patient's severely decreased LVEF, a strong inotrope and vasopressor will be needed to increase blood pressure. Unfortunately, epinephrine may also worsen intraoperative ischemia (if the patient is undergoing an intraoperative myocardial infarction) by increasing the myocardial oxygen demand. Treatment with a beta agonist (such as epinephrine) must be undertaken with this in mind. Nonpharmacolic treatment with an intraortic balloon (IABP) would also likely greatly benefit this patient by increasing perfusion pressure while at the same time decreasing afterload. Milrinone alone would not be a good choice in a hypotensive patient because it decreases systemic vascular resistance and would decrease myocardial oxygen supply while increasing myocardial oxygen demand. Milrinone may be helpful in conjunction with a vascular smooth muscle vasoconstrictor (vasopressor).

48. **Answer = E, The apical anterior wall appears dyskinetic.**

Case 16

49. **Answer = A, Mitral and aortic valve endocarditis is the diagnosis.**

50. **Answer = D, The midesophageal mitral valve commissural view is shown.**

51. **Answer = C, A mitral valve vegetation is shown.**

Reference: ASE/SCA Guidelines for Performing a Comprehensive Intraoperative Multiplane Transesophageal Echocardiography Examination. *J Am Soc Echocardiog* 1999;12:884–900.

52. **Answer = C, The P_1 scallop is shown.**

Reference: ASE/SCA Guidelines for Performing a Comprehensive Intraoperative Multiplane Transesophageal Echocardiography Examination. *J Am Soc Echocardiog* 1999;12:884–900.

Case 17

53. **Answer = D, Segment 12 (the mid septal wall segment) is shown.**

Reference: ASE/SCA Guidelines for Performing a Comprehensive Intraoperative Multiplane Transesophageal Echocardiography Examination. *J Am Soc Echocardiog* 1999;12:884–900.

54. **Answer = B, Segment 7 (the mid anteroseptal wall segment) is shown.**

Reference: ASE/SCA Guidelines for Performing a Comprehensive Intraoperative Multiplane Transesophageal Echocardiography Examination. *J Am Soc Echocardiog* 1999;12:884–900.

55. Answer = C, Segment 8 (the mid anterior wall segment) is shown.

Reference: ASE/SCA Guidelines for Performing a Comprehensive Intraoperative Multiplane Transesophageal Echocardiography Examination. *J Am Soc Echocardiog* 1999;12:884–900.

56. Answer = D, Segment 9 (the mid lateral wall segment) is shown.

Reference: ASE/SCA Guidelines for Performing a Comprehensive Intraoperative Multiplane Transesophageal Echocardiography Examination. *J Am Soc Echocardiog* 1999;12:884–900.

Case 18

57. **Answer = E, The anterolateral papillary muscle is shown.** This papillary muscle is less likely to rupture than the posteromedial papillary muscle following an ischemic insult because the anterolateral papillary muscle has a dual blood supply (LAD and circumflex). The posteromedial papillary muscle is supplied by a single coronary artery (the right coronary artery).

58. **Answer = E, No treatment is indicated.**

59. **Answer = C, The lateral wall is shown.**

Case 19

60. **Answer = C, A moderator band is shown.**

61. **Answer = E, None of the above are indicated because this is a normal finding.**

62. **Answer = B, The main pulmonary artery is shown.**

Case 20

63. **Answer = E, The left main coronary artery is shown.**

64. **Answer = A, The left main coronary artery supplies the anterior wall of the left ventricle.**

Case 21

65. **Answer = A, The superior vena cava is shown.**

66. **Answer = A, The right upper pulmonary vein is shown.**

67. **Answer = B, The right lower pulmonary vein is shown.**

TEST II PART 2

Written Test Booklet

1. What is the purpose of the matching layer in an ultrasound transducer?

   A. Limits the ringing of the transducer

   B. Shortens the spatial pulse length

   C. Reduces reflection at the tissue transducer interface

   D. Improves axial resolution

   E. Improves temporal resolution

2. Which of the following is a disadvantage of a focused ultrasound beam?

   A. Decreased temporal resolution in the far field

   B. Decreased azithumal resolution in the near field

   C. Decreased lateral resolution in the far field

   D. Decreased axial resolution in the near field

   E. Decreased radial resolution in the near field

3. Which of the following is an advantage of a focused ultrasound beam?

   A. Improved lateral resolution in the near field

   B. Improved axial resolution in the near field

   C. Improved angular resolution in the far field

   D. Improved spatial resolution in the far field

   E. Improved temporal resolution in the near field

4. Which of the following is determined by the ultrasound beam thickness?

   A. Depth resolution

   B. Longitudinal resolution

   C. Axial resolution

   D. Radial resolution

   E. Elevational resolution

5. Which of the following is the maximum spatial peak temporal average intensity recommended for unfocused ultrasound beams?

   A. 100 mW/cm^2

   B. 1 W/cm^2

   C. 10 W/cm^2

   D. 100 W/cm^2

   E. 1 kW/cm^2

6. Which of the following correctly matches the coronary blood supply to the numerical myocardial segment as described by the 16-segment model found in the ASE/SCA guidelines for perioperative TEE?

   A. Circumflex coronary artery → anterior apical wall

   B. Left anterior descending coronary artery → apical inferior wall

   C. Posterior descending coronary artery → mid interior wall

   D. Right coronary artery → basal lateral wall

   E. Left anterior descending coronary artery → basal posterior wall

7. Which of the following correctly matches the coronary blood supply to the numerical myocardial segment as described by the 16-segment model found in the ASE/SCA guidelines for perioperative TEE?

   A. Left anterior descending coronary artery → basal inferior wall

   B. Left anterior descending coronary artery → basal anterior wall

   C. Circumflex coronary artery → apical anteroseptal wall

   D. Right coronary artery → apical posterior wall

   E. Circumflex coronary artery → apical inferior wall

8. Which of the following correctly matches the coronary blood supply to the numerical myocardial segment as described by the 16-segment model found in the ASE/SCA guidelines for perioperative TEE?

   A. Right coronary artery → mid anteroseptal wall

   B. Left anterior descending coronary artery → mid inferior wall

   C. Circumflex coronary artery → mid posterior wall

   D. Left anterior descending coronary artery → basal posterior wall

   E. Posterior descending coronary artery → mid lateral wall

9. Which of the following correctly matches the coronary blood supply to the numerical myocardial segment as described by the 16-segment model found in the ASE/SCA guidelines for perioperative TEE?

   A. Circumflex coronary artery → apical anterior wall

   B. Right coronary artery → basal inferior wall

   C. Posterior descending coronary artery → basal anterior wall

   D. Diagonal branches → apical inferior wall

   E. Circumflex coronary artery → apical anteroseptal wall

10. Which of the following correctly matches the coronary blood supply to the numerical myocardial segment as described by the 16-segment model found in the ASE/SCA guidelines for perioperative TEE?

    A. Circumflex coronary artery → apical inferior wall

    B. Right coronary artery → apical anteroseptal wall

    C. Left anterior descending coronary artery → apical posterior wall

    D. Posterior descending coronary artery → mid inferior wall

    E. Obtuse marginal branches → basal inferior wall

11. Which of the following mitral valve chordae tendinae attach to the mitral valve leaflet tips?

    A. First-order chordae

    B. Second-order chordae

    C. Third-order chordae

    D. Fourth-order chordae

    E. None of the above

12. Which of the following mitral valve scallops is most likely to be affected by myxomatous degeneration, annular dilation, and regurgitation? Leaflet prolapse occurs more frequently with this scallop.

    A. A_1

    B. P_1

    C. A_2

    D. P_2

    E. A_3

13. Which of the following papillary muscles is most likely to rupture?

    A. Anterolateral

    B. Anteromedial

    C. Posterolateral

    D. Posteromedial

    E. Anteroseptal

14. A patient has a tricuspid regurgitant jet area to right atrial area ratio of 45%. Which of the following best describes the severity of tricuspid regurgitation in this patient?

    A. Trace (grade I).

    B. Mild (grade II).

    C. Moderate (grade III).

    D. Severe (grade IV).

    E. It cannot be determined from the given information.

NOTE: Use Table 2.2A to answer the next six (6) questions.

Table 2.2A.

PHT_{MV} = 62 msec	TVI_{LVOT} = 15 cm	PAP = 40/20 mmHg
$V_{peakMVinflow}$ = 200 cm/sec	TVI_{AV} = 14.8 cm	LAP = 14 mmHg
LA diameter = 43 mm	TVI_{MV} = 20 cm	BP = 120/80 mmHg
RA diameter = 31 mm	TVI_{MRjet} = 100 cm	CVP = 10 mmHg

PHT_{MV} = mitral valve pressure half time, PAP = pulmonary artery pressure,
TVI_{LVOT} = time velocity integral of blood flow in the left ventricular outflow tract,
$V_{peakMVinflow}$ = peak diastolic mitral inflow velocity, LAP = left atrial pressure, RA = right atrial,
TVI_{AV} = time velocity integral of blood flow through the aortic valve, LA = left atrial,
TVI_{MV} = time velocity integral of blood flow through the mitral valve, BP = blood pressure,
TVI_{MRjet} = time velocity integral of the mitral valve regurgitant jet,
CVP = central venous pressure.

15. Which of the following best describes the degree of aortic stenosis?

   A. No stenosis.

   B. Mild.

   C. Moderate.

   D. Severe.

   E. It cannot be determined without additional data.

16. What additional information is needed to determine the aortic valve area?

   A. Aortic valve pressure half time

   B. Left ventricular outflow tract diameter

   C. Mitral valve annulus diameter

   D. Left ventricular end diastolic pressure

   E. None of the above

17. What is the mitral valve stroke volume?

   A. 20 ml

   B. 52 ml

   C. 71 ml

   D. 81 ml

   E. 91 ml

18. If the left ventricular outflow tract diameter is 20 mm, what is the mitral valve regurgitant volume?

    A. 14 ml

    B. 24 ml

    C. 34 ml

    D. 44 ml

    E. 54 ml

19. What is the mitral valve regurgitant orifice area?

    A. 0.14 cm^2

    B. 0.24 cm^2

    C. 0.34 cm^2

    D. 0.44 cm^2

    E. 0.54 cm^2

20. Which of the following best describes the degree of mitral regurgitation?

    A. Trace.

    B. Mild.

    C. Moderate.

    D. Severe.

    E. It cannot be determined from the given information.

21. Which of the following is true concerning TEE compared to TTE (TEE = transesophageal echocardiography, TTE = transthoracic echocardiography)?

    A. TEE allows better assessment of the left ventricular apex.

    B. TEE has superior Doppler beam alignment.

    C. TEE is less invasive.

    D. TTE offers superior assessment of the interatrial septum.

    E. TEE provides superior images in ventilated patients.

22. In which of the following situations is TEE most likely to provide a more accurate estimate of left ventricular end diastolic volume than a pulmonary artery catheter?

   A. Lateral mitral annular tissue Doppler E_M = 10 cm/sec

   B. Transmitral peak velocities: E >> A

   C. Color M-mode propagation velocity (VP) > 50 cm/sec

   D. Isovolumic relaxation time = 100 milliseconds

   E. Peak E-wave deceleration time = 190 milliseconds

23. In which of the following types of ultrasound imaging is the amplitude of returning echoes plotted as brightness along ventricle lines drawn for each transmitted pulse and graphed on the display with distance (depth) on the Y axis versus time on the X axis?

   A. A-mode

   B. B-mode

   C. C-mode

   D. M-mode

   E. Two-dimensional grayscale imaging

24. In which of the following is the amplitude of returning echoes plotted as brightness (stronger echoes appear brighter)?

   A. A-mode only

   B. B-mode only

   C. B-mode and C-mode

   D. B-mode, M-mode, and two-dimensional imaging

   E. A-mode, B-mode, M-mode, and two-dimensional imaging

25. Which of the following ultrasound modes plots amplitude of returning echoes on the Y axis versus depth on the X axis?

    A. A-mode

    B. B-mode

    C. C-mode

    D. M-mode

    E. None of the above

26. Which of the following correctly describes the pulse repetition period?

    A. It increases with decreasing pulse repetition frequency.

    B. It decreases as imaging depth increases.

    C. It increases when pulse duration increases.

    D. It decreases as the ultrasound beam travels through tissue.

27. Which of the following is the correct formula for pressure?

    A. $dB = Log\, p_2 / p_1$

    B. $dB = 10\, Log\, p_2 / p_1$

    C. $dB = 20\, Log\, p_2 / p_1$

    D. $dB = 30\, Log\, p_2 / p_1$

28. Which of the following most closely estimates the thickness of tissue required to reduce the intensity of a 6-MHz TEE transducer ultrasound beam by half?

    A. 1 cm

    B. 3 cm

    C. 6 cm

    D. 12 cm

    E. 18 cm

29. The half value layer thickness is the thickness of tissue required to reduce the *intensity* of a sound beam by half. How many dB of attenuation does this represent?

A. 3 dB

B. 6 dB

C. 9 dB

D. 10 dB

E. 12 dB

30. Which of the following is *most* likely true concerning the frequency of a piezoelectric crystal?

A. As frequency increases attenuation increases.

B. As frequency increases focal length decreases.

C. As frequency increases half power distance increases.

D. As frequency increases piezoelectric crystal thickness increases.

E. As frequency increases scattering decreases.

31. An ultrasound beam travels from one medium into another with an incident angle of 90 degrees. Which of the following properties of the media is *most* important in determining if *reflection* will occur at the interface of the two media?

A. Specific heat

B. Density

C. Conductivity

D. Hydrophilicity

E. Critical temperature

32. Which of the following is true concerning the angle of incidence of an ultrasound beam?

A. Oblique = less than or greater than 90 degrees

B. Normal = less than 90 degrees

C. Orthogonal = greater than 90 degrees

D. Obtuse = less than 90 degrees

33. Which of the following is **most** likely to be true concerning the angle of incidence of an ultrasound beam?

    A. Refraction can occur with an orthogonal incidence.

    B. Both acute and obtuse angles are oblique.

    C. Normal incidence is required for reflection to occur.

    D. None of the above is correct.

34. An ultrasound beam with normal incidence strikes a boundary between two media. There is total reflection of the ultrasound beam at this boundary. The velocity of ultrasound in the two media is identical. Which of the following is *most* likely to be true?

    A. The acoustic impedance of the two media are similar.

    B. The intensity transmission coefficient is > 10%.

    C. The intensity reflection coefficient is < 10%.

    D. The incident intensity is greater than the reflected intensity.

    E. The density of the two media is different.

35. A TEE ultrasound pulse travels from the probe to a reflector in soft tissue and then back to the probe. If this round-trip takes 26 microseconds, which of the following most closely estimates the depth of the reflector?

    A. 5 mm

    B. 10 mm

    C. 20 mm

    D. 40 mm

36. Which of the following is true concerning a piezoelectric crystal in a TEE probe?

    A. If its temperature is increased above the critical temperature it will lose the ability to generate an ultrasound pulse.

    B. It is composed of lead zirconate titanate.

    C. As crystal thickness increases wavelength decreases.

    D. It is arranged in a linear switched-array transducer.

37. Which of the following is the *most* commonly found piezoelectric material in diagnostic imaging transducers?

A. Lead zirconate titanate (PZT)

B. Barium titanate (BT)

C. Lead titanate (PBT)

D. Lead metaniobate titanate (PMT)

38. Which of the following is a disadvantage of the backing material?

A. It decreases the Q factor (quality factor).

B. It shortens the spatial pulse length.

C. It decreases axial resolution.

D. It decreases the transducer's sensitivity to reflected echoes.

NOTE: Use Table 2.2B to answer the following question.

Table 2.2B.

	Crystal A	Crystal B	Crystal C	Crystal D
Crystal thickness	1.0	1.0	0.5	2.0
Density	1.0	2.0	1.0	2.0
Elasticity	0.5	3.0	0.5	3.0

39. Of the piezoelectric crystals shown in Table 2.2B, which will have the *lowest* resonant frequency?

A. Crystal A

B. Crystal B

C. Crystal C

D. Crystal D

40. Which of the following is most likely true concerning bandwidth?

A. The shorter the pulse the wider the bandwidth.

B. The damping material tends to decrease the bandwidth of the ultrasound transducer.

C. As bandwidth increases the Q factor increases.

D. Imaging transducers tend to have narrower bandwidths than transducers used in therapeutic ultrasound.

41. If the resonant frequency of the electrical excitation voltage of a continuous-wave TEE transducer is 8 MHz, what is the frequency of the continuous-wave ultrasound beam?

A. 2 MHz.

B. 4 MHz.

C. 8 MHz.

D. 16 MHz.

E. It cannot be determined from the given information.

42. Which of the following is a synonym of *axial resolution?*

A. Longitudinal resolution

B. Angular resolution

C. Transverse resolution

D. Lateral resolution

43. A piezoelectric crystal is exchanged for a larger-diameter crystal. The frequency and all other properties of the new crystal are the same as the old crystal. Which of the following is *most* likely true?

A. The near-zone length decreases.

B. The beam diameter in the near zone increases.

C. The beam diameter in the far zone increases.

D. The pulse repetition period (PRP) increases.

44. An increase in which of the following is *most* likely to increase temporal resolution?

A. Line density

B. Pulse repetition frequency (PRF)

C. Imaging depth

D. The number of foci per scan line

E. Heart rate

45. For which type of Doppler ultrasound is aliasing artifact impossible?

   A. Continuous-wave Doppler.

   B. Pulsed-wave Doppler.

   C. Color flow Doppler.

   D. 2D Doppler.

   E. Aliasing occurs with all forms of Doppler ultrasound.

46. Which of the following is true of color flow Doppler?

   A. It is a form of pulsed-wave Doppler.

   B. It superimposes a color representation of blood flow onto a 2D image,
      and it is subjected to low frame rates and reduced temporal resolution.

   C. Colors represent the velocity of blood flow.

   D. Colors represent the direction of blood flow.

   E. All of the above are true.

47. Blood flows through the left ventricular outflow tract at a velocity of
    100 cm/s. A Doppler system calculates a velocity of 50 cm/s. What is the
    angle between the direction of blood flow and the TEE transducer beam?

   A. 90 degrees

   B. 70 degrees

   C. 60 degrees

   D. 30 degrees

   E. 0 degrees

NOTE: Use Table 2.2C to answer the next three (3) questions.

Table 2.2C.

	Transducer A	Transducer B	Transducer C	Transducer D	Transducer E
Incident angle:	90 degrees	0 degrees	90 degrees	0 degrees	90 degrees
Frequency:	8 MHz	4 MHz	12 MHz	4 MHz	4 MHz
Sample volume depth:	10 cm	5 cm	8 cm	2 cm	10 cm
Max. imaging depth:	10 cm	9 cm	10 cm	9 cm	12 cm

48. Which of the transducers is best suited for 2D imaging?

    A. A

    B. B

    C. C

    D. D

    E. E

49. Which of the transducers is *most* likely to be subject to aliasing artifact?

    A. A.

    B. B.

    C. C.

    D. D.

    E. The transducers all have the same propensity for aliasing artifact.

50. Which of the following is *most* likely to provide the highest-quality pulsed-wave Doppler determinations?

    A. A

    B. B

    C. C

    D. D

    E. E

51. Which of the following atrial septal defects is associated with a persistent left superior vena cava?

    A. Ostium secundum

    B. Ostium primum

    C. Sinus venosus

    D. Coronary sinus

    E. Perimembranous

52. Which of the following is the least common atrial septal defect?

    A. Ostium secundum

    B. Ostium primum

    C. Sinus venosus

    D. Coronary sinus

    E. Perimembranous

53. Which of the following ventricular septal defects (VSDs) is *most* likely to be associated with herniation of an aortic valve cusp?

    A. Perimembranous

    B. Aortic outflow

    C Subarterial

    D. Trabecular (muscular)

    E. Inlet

54. Which of the following ventricular septal defects is commonly seen in patients with Down's syndrome?

    A. Perimembranous

    B. Aortic outflow

    C. Subarterial

    D. Trabecular (muscular)

    E. Inlet

55. The modified Bernoulli equation ($\Delta P = 4V^2$) is inaccurate when continuous-wave Doppler is utilized in which of the following situations/conditions?

    A. Doppler examination of the MV in a patient with severe rheumatic MS and elevated left atrial pressures secondary to severe MR

    B. Doppler examination of the PV in a patient with congenital PS and anatomic narrowing of the RVOT, creating elevated flow velocities in the RVOT proximal to the PV

    C. Doppler examination of the TV in a patient with TS and a marked increase in the A-wave on hepatic venous pulsed-wave Doppler exam

    D. Doppler exam of the AV in a patient with AS, MR, and MS due to rheumatic heart disease

    E. Doppler determinations of right ventricular systolic pressure in a patient with a left-to-right shunt across a restrictive muscular VSD

    (MR = mitral regurgitation, MS = mitral stenosis, MV = mitral valve, PV = pulmonic valve, PS = pulmonic stenosis, RVOT = right ventricular outflow tract, TV = tricuspid valve, TS = tricuspid stenosis, AV = aortic valve, AS = aortic stenosis, VSD = ventricular septal defect)

56. Which of the following defects would **most** likely result in right ventricular dilation and paradoxical septal motion?

    A. Secundum atrial septal defect

    B. Perimembranous ventricular septal defect

    C. Cortriatriatum

    D. Aortic coarctation

    E. Patent ductus arteriosus

57. Irreversible pulmonary hypertension with equalization of systemic and pulmonary artery pressures due to a intracardiac shunt is know as which of the following?

    A. Zvara's physiology

    B. Noonan's physiology

    C. Eisenmenger's physiology

    D. Bernoulli's physiology

    E. Miller's physiology

58. Which of the following describes a heart located in the right hemithorax with the apex in the right midclavicular line?

   A. Dextroversion

   B. Situs inversus

   C. Dextrocardia

   D. Dextroinversus

   E. Dextrotransposition

NOTE: The information in Table 2.2D was obtained from a 47-year-old with no AI scheduled for CABG surgery. Use this information to answer the following six (6) questions.

Table 2.2D.

$TVI_{MV} = 12$ cm	HR = 100 beats/min	MV annulus diameter = 30 mm
$TVI_{LVOT} = 15$ cm	BP = 130/80 mmHg	LVOT diameter = 20 mm
$TVI_{MRjet} = 180$ cm	CVP = 10 mmHg	Sinus of valsalva diameter = 32 mm

TVI_{MV} = time velocity integral of flow through the mitral valve (diastolic mitral inflow TVI), TVI_{LVOT} = time velocity integral of flow through the left ventricular outflow tract by pulsed-wave Doppler, TVI_{MRjet} = time velocity integral of the mitral insufficiency jet (regurgitant mitral valve flow TVI), HR = heart rate, BP = blood pressure, CVP = central venous pressure, AI = aortic insufficiency, LVOT = left ventricular outflow tract, CABG = coronary artery bypass graft surgery.

59. Given the data in Table 2.2D, what is the best estimate of the stroke volume of diastolic blood flow through the mitral valve?

   A. 64.8 cm^3

   B. 74.8 cm^3

   C. 84.8 cm^3

   D. 94.8 cm^3

   E. 104.8 cm^3

60. Given the data in Table 2.2D, what is the best estimate of the stroke volume through the left ventricular outflow tract?

   A. 37.1 cm^3

   B. 47.1 cm^3

   C. 57.1 cm^3

   D. 67.1 cm^3

   E. 77.1 cm^3

61. What is the regurgitant volume of flow through the mitral valve?

    A. 37.7 cm^3

    B. 47.7 cm^3

    C. 57.7 cm^3

    D. 67.7 cm^3

    E. 77.7 cm^3

62. What is the mitral valve regurgitant fraction?

    A. 14.4%

    B. 24.4%

    C. 34.4%

    D. 44.4%

    E. 54.4%

63. What is the mitral valve regurgitant orifice area?

    A. 0.11 cm^2 (11 mm^2)

    B. 0.15 cm^2 (15 mm^2)

    C. 0.21 cm^2 (21 mm^2)

    D. 0.33 cm^2 (33 mm^2)

    E. 0.51 cm^2 (51 mm^2)

64. Which of the following best describes the severity of this patient's mitral regurgitation?

    A. Trace.

    B. Mild.

    C. Moderate.

    D. Severe.

    E. It cannot be determined from the information given.

NOTE: Use Table 2.2E to answer the next five (5) questions.

Table 2.2E.

$V_{VSDPeak} = 350$ cm/sec	HR = 100 beats/min	LVOT diameter = 2.0 cm
$TVI_{PA} = 22$ cm	BP = 100/60 mmHg	PA diameter = 2.4 cm
$TVI_{LVOT} = 16$ cm	CVP = 10 mmHg	Aortic valve side = 2.2 cm

$V_{VSDPeak}$ = peak velocity of left to right flow across a ventricular septal defect, HR = heart rate,
TVI_{PA} = time velocity integral of flow through the pulmonary artery, PA = pulmonary artery,
TVI_{LVOT} = time velocity integral of flow through the left ventricular outflow tract, BP = blood pressure,
CVP = central venous pressure, LVOT = left ventricular outflow tract.

65. Which of the following is the best estimate of the aortic valve area as calculated from the data in Table 2.2E?

A. 2.1 cm^2

B. 2.5 cm^2

C. 3.1 cm^2

D. 3.5 cm^2

E. 4.1 cm^2

66. Which of the following is the best estimate of the right ventricular stroke volume as calculated from the data in Table 2.2E?

A. 59.5 cm^3

B. 69.5 cm^3

C. 79.5 cm^3

D. 89.5 cm^3

E. 99.5 cm^3

67. Which of the following is the best estimate of the left ventricular stroke volume as calculated from the data in Table 2.2E?

A. 40.2 cm^3

B. 50.2 cm^3

C. 60.2 cm^3

D. 70.2 cm^3

E. 80.2 cm^3

68. Which of the following is the best estimate of the ratio of pulmonary to systemic flow (Q_p/Q_s) as calculated from the data in Table 2.2E?

    A. 1:1

    B. 1.5:1

    C. 2:1

    D. 2.5:1

    E. 3:1

69. Which of the following is the best estimate of the pulmonary artery systolic pressure (PASP)?

    A. 41 mmHg

    B. 51 mmHg

    C. 61 mmHg

    D. 71 mmHg

    E. 81 mmHg

70. An aortic aneurysm extends from 1 cm below the left subcalvian artery to the aortic bifurcation. How would this aneurysm be best described according to the Crawford classification system?

    A. Crawford type I

    B. Crawford type II

    C. Crawford type III

    D. Crawford type IV

    E. Crawford type V

NOTE: Use Figure 2.2A to answer the next question.

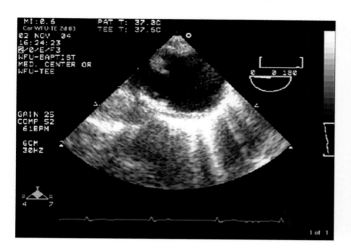

Fig. 2-2A1

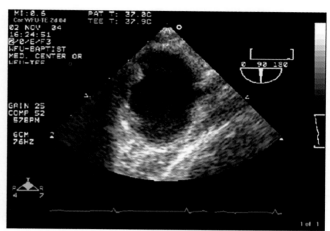

Fig. 2-2A2

71. Given the findings in the TEE images of the aorta in Figure 2.2A, what additional treatment would you recommend for this patient undergoing CABG?

  A. An epiaortic ultrasound scan of the ascending aorta prior to aortic cannulation

  B. An aortic root replacement

  C. Lower extremity Doppler ultrasound

  D. Aortic valve replacement

  E. Aortic angiography looking at distal lower extremity runoff

72. Which of the following aspects of the aorta is the **most** difficult to evaluate using transesophageal echocardiography?

  A. The sinus of valsalva

  B. The distal aortic arch at the level of the left subclavian

  C. The proximal ascending aorta 2 cm distal to the sinotubular ridge

  D. The distal ascending aorta and proximal aortic arch

  E. The descending thoracic aorta at the level of the diaphragm

73. Congestive heart failure is the most common diagnosis among in-patients in the United States. What percentage of these patients has a normal ejection fraction with diastolic dysfunction (diastolic heart failure)?

    A. 20%

    B. 30%

    C. 40%

    D. 50%

    E. 60%

74. Which of the following places the four phases of diastole in the correct order?

    A. Isovolumic left ventricular relaxation, early filling, atrial contraction, diastasis

    B. Isovolumic left ventricular relaxation, early filling, diastasis, atrial contraction

    C. Isovolumic left ventricular relaxation, diastasis, early filling, atrial contraction

    D. Diastasis, isovolumic ventricular relaxation, early filling, atrial contraction

    E. Early filling, atrial contraction, diastasis, isovolumic left ventricular relaxation

75. Which of the following is indicative of high filling pressures (E = early diastolic transmitral filling velocity via pulsed-wave Doppler, E_M = E´ = early diastolic lateral mitral annular tissue Doppler velocity)?

    A. $E/E_M > 5$

    B. $E/E_M > 10$

    C. $E/E_M > 15$

    D. $E/E_M > 20$

    E. $E/E_M > 25$

76. Which of the following best describes the incidence of oropharyngeal, esophageal, and gastric trauma occurring with the insertion of the TEE probe in cardiac surgery patients?

    A. 0.01%

    B. 0.02%

    C. 0.1%

    D. 0.2%

    E. 0.5%

77. What is the incidence of esophageal perforation secondary to TEE in the emergency room and intensive care unit?

    A. 0.002 to 0.003%

    B. 0.02 to 0.03%

    C. 0.2 to 0.3%

    D. 0.5 to 1.0%

    E. None of the above

78. Which of the following is true concerning the isovolumic relaxation time (IVRT)?

    A. IVRT is increased during acute new-onset myocardial ischemia.

    B. IVRT is increased with increased left atrial filling pressures.

    C. IVRT is decreased with impaired relaxation.

    D. IVRT is increased with pseudonormal diastolic dysfunction.

    E. IVRT is increased with restrictive diastolic dysfunction.

79. Which of the following would be expected in a patient with reduced left ventricular compliance due to infiltrative amyloidosis?

    A. Increased isovolumic relaxation time (IVRT)

    B. Transmitral E >>A

    C. E_M = increased

    D. V_P = normal

    E. Prolonged transmitral E-wave deceleration time (DT)

80. How does heart rate affect diastolic transmitral inflow velocities, assuming a constant sweep speed?

   A. As heart rate increases max A velocity decreases.

   B. As heart rate increases E/A ratio decreases.

   C. As heart rate increases max E velocity increases.

   D. As heart rate increases the distance between the E and A waves increases.

   E. None of the above.

81. Which of the following *best* describes how mitral regurgitation affects diastolic transmitral flow velocities?

   A. A is increased.

   B. E/A is decreased.

   C. E/A does not change.

   D. E/A is increased.

   E. None of the above.

NOTE: Use the hepatic venous flow profile shown in Figure 2.2B to answer the next three (3) questions.

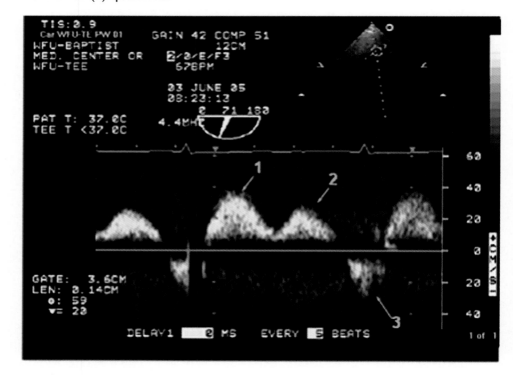

Fig. 2-2B

82. Which of the following **best** describes the hepatic venous flow wave labeled 1?

A. A wave

B. D wave

C. E wave

D. S wave

E. V wave

83. Which of the following *best* describes the hepatic venous flow wave labeled 2?

A. A wave

B. D wave

C. E wave

D. S wave

E. V wave

84. Which of the following *best* describes the hepatic venous flow wave labeled 3?

A. A wave

B. D wave

C. E wave

D. S wave

E. V wave

NOTE: Use Figure 2.2C to answer the next question.

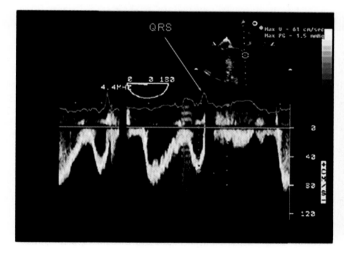 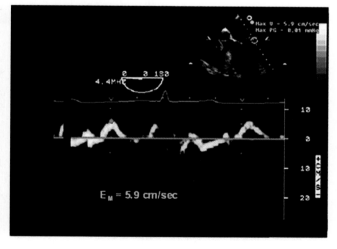

Fig. 2-2C1   Fig. 2-2C2

85. Given the transmitral pulsed-wave Doppler flow velocities and the lateral mitral annular tissue Doppler E_M velocity shown in Figure 2.2C, which of the following *best* describes this patient's diastolic function?

   A. Normal

   B. Pseudonormal

   C. Impaired relaxation

   D. Constrictive

   E. Restrictive

NOTE: Use the pulsed-wave Doppler transmitral flow velocity profile shown in Figure 2.2D to answer the next three (3) questions.

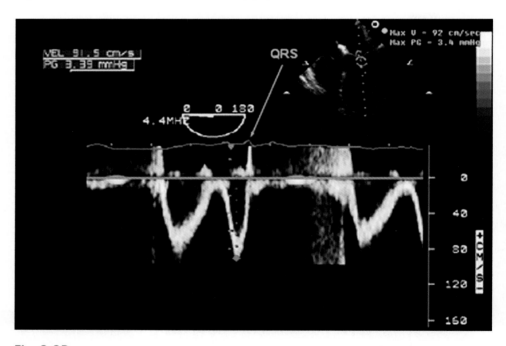

Fig. 2-2D

86. Given the transmitral pulsed-wave Doppler flow velocities shown in Figure 2.2D, which of the following *best* describes this patient's diastolic function?

   A. Normal

   B. Pseudonormal

   C. Impaired relaxation

   D. Constrictive

   E. Restrictive

87. Which of the following patients would most likely have a transmitral Doppler flow velocity profile similar to that shown in Figure 2.2D?

    A. A healthy 42-year-old

    B. A patient with end-stage infiltrative amyloidosis

    C. A patient with constrictive pericarditis

    D. A patient with acute myocardial ischemia

    E. A patient with a 34-mm pericardial effusion with RV diastolic collapse

88. Which of the following *best* describes other findings that would be expected in this patient?

    A. Left atrial pressure catheter pressure > 13 mmHg

    B. Lateral mitral annular tissue Doppler E_M = 9.3 cm/sec

    C. Transmitral color M-mode propagation velocity (V_P) = 64 cm/sec

    D. Pulmonary vein S wave > D wave

    E. Pulmonary vein PV_{AR}-wave duration greater than transmitral E-wave duration

NOTE: Use the transmitral inflow pulsed-wave Doppler and lateral mitral annular tissue E_M velocity profiles shown in Figure 2.2E to answer the following two (2) questions.

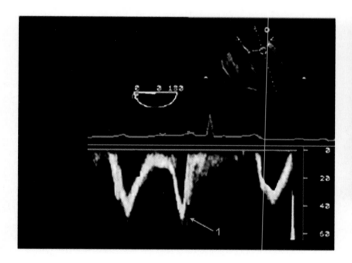

Fig. 2-2E1

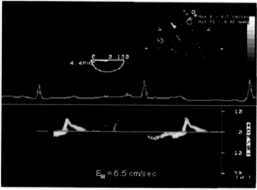

Fig. 2-2E2

89. Which of the following *best* describes this patient's diastolic function?

   A. Normal

   B. Pseudonormal

   C. Impaired relaxation

   D. Constrictive

   E. Restrictive

90. Which of the following *best* describes the wave labeled 1?

   A. PV_{AR} wave

   B. S wave

   C. D wave

   D. E wave

   E. A wave

NOTE: Use the continuous-wave Doppler shown in Figure 2.2F to answer the next three (3) questions.

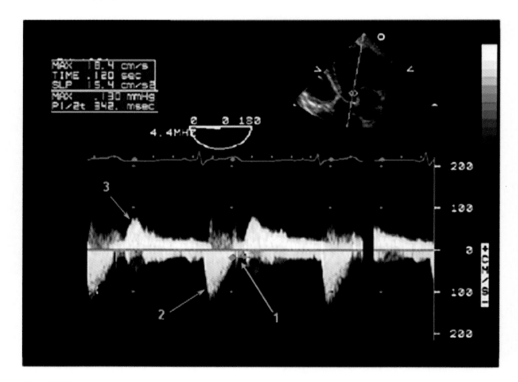

Fig. 2-2F

91. Which of the following time periods is represented by arrow 1?

A. Deceleration time (DT)

B. Isovolumic relaxation time (IVRT)

C. Pressure half time (PHT)

D. Ejection time (ET)

E. Coffee break time (CBT)

92. The wave indicated by arrow 2 results from which of the following?

A. Flow through the left ventricular outflow tract and aorta

B. Flow through the mitral valve into the left ventricle

C. Flow through the tricuspid valve into the right ventricle

D. Flow through the right ventricular outflow tract and the aortic valve

E. Flow through the descending thoracic aorta

93. The wave indicated by arrow 3 results from which of the following?

A. Flow through the left ventricular outflow tract and aorta

B. Flow through the mitral valve into the left ventricle

C. Flow through the tricuspid valve into the right ventricle

D. Flow through the right ventricular outflow tract and the aortic valve

E. Flow through the descending thoracic aorta

NOTE: Use Table 2.2F to answer the next four (4) questions.

Table 2.2F.

LVEDd = 65 mm	TVI_{LVOT} = 11 cm	BP = 110/60 mmHg	HR = 100 beats/min
LVESd = 50 mm	LA diameter = 52 mm	CVP = 10 mmHg	BSA = 2 M^2
LVEDA = 30 mm	LV free wall thickness = 13 mm	V_{AVpeak} = 200 cm/sec	WT = 75 kg
LVESA = 20 mm	LVOT diameter = 20 mm	V_{MRpeak} = 450 cm/sec	V_{TRpeak} = 300 cm/sec

LVEDd = left ventricular end diastolic dimension, LVESd = left ventricular end systolic dimension,
TVI_{LVOT} = time velocity integral of blood flow through the left ventricular outflow tract,
LVOT = left ventricular outflow tract, BP = blood pressure, CVP = central venous pressure,
V_{AVpeak} = peak velocity of blood flow across the aortic valve, HR = heart rate,
V_{MRpeak} = peak velocity of the mitral regurgitant jet, BSA = body surface area,
V_{TRpeak} = peak velocity of the tricuspid regurgitant jet.

94. Which of the following is the *best* estimate of the fractional shortening?

    A. 13%

    B. 23%

    C. 33%

    D. 43%

    E. 53%

95. Which of the following is the *best* estimate of the fractional area change?

    A. 13%

    B. 23%

    C. 33%

    D. 43%

    E. 53%

96. Which of the following is the *best* estimate of the cardiac output?

    A. 3.45 L/min

    B. 4.45 L/min

    C. 5.45 L/min

    D. 6.45 L/min

    E. 7.45 L/min

97. Which of the following is the *best* estimate of the peak instantaneous pressure gradient across the aortic valve?

    A. 16 mmHg

    B. 26 mmHg

    C. 36 mmHg

    D. 46 mmHg

    E. 56 mmHg

98. How long should a TEE probe be soaked in a glutaraldehyde-based solution during the cleaning process?

   A. 10 min

   B. 12 min

   C. 17 min

   D. 20 min

   E. 30 min

99. Which of the following can be used to differentiate between pseudonormal and normal diastolic function in patients with moderate mitral regurgitation?

   A. Transmitral E and A waves

   B. Pulmonary vein S and D waves

   C. Lateral mitral annular tissue Doppler E_M

   D. Pulmonary vein E and A waves

   E. Hepatic venous S and D waves

100. In which of the following would an increase in left ventricular free wall thickness *not* be expected?

   A. Dilated cardiomyopathy

   B. Hypertrophic cardiomyopathy

   C. Restrictive cardiomyopathy

   D. Hypertensive heart disease

   E. Aortic stenosis

101. Which of the following is *not* an etiology of pericarditis?

   A. Bacterial infection.

   B. Trauma.

   C. Uremia.

   D. Transmural myocardial infarction.

   E. All of the above are potential causes of pericarditis.

102. What is Dressler's syndrome?

    A. Pericardial effusion due to myocardial infarction

    B. Pericardial effusion due to tuberculosis infection

    C. Pericardial effusion due to malignancy

    D. Pericardial effusion due to viral pericarditis

    E. Pericardial effusion due to uremia

103. Which of the following would be consistent with large pericardial effusion?

    A. > 0.5 cm

    B. > 1.0 cm

    C. > 1.5 cm

    D. > 2 cm

    E. > 2.5 cm

104. Which of the following would be expected to increase with spontaneous inspiration in constrictive pericarditis?

    A. Pulmonary venous D-wave peak velocity

    B. Pulmonary venous S-wave peak velocity

    C. Transmitral peak E-wave velocity

    D. Transtricuspid peak E-wave velocity

    E. Hepatic venous A wave

105. Which of the following is an absolute contraindication to perioperative TEE?

    A. Esophageal varices

    B. Recent esophageal or gastric surgery

    C. Severe coagulopathy

    D. Cervical spine instability

    E. History of dysphagia or odynophagia

106. An ultrasound probe interrogates a blood vessel with an incident angle of 60 degrees. The probe emits a frequency of 10 MHz and the returning echoes have a frequency of 10.5 MHz. What is the velocity of blood flow in the vessel?

   A. 17 m/s

   B. 37 m/s

   C. 57 m/s

   D. 77 m/s

   E. 97 m/s

107. Which of the following is an advantage of continuous-wave Doppler over pulsed-wave Doppler?

   A. Improved lateral resolution

   B. Improved spatial resolution

   C. Improved temporal resolution

   D. Improved range resolution

   E. Ability to measure high velocities

108. Which of the following is an advantage of pulsed-wave Doppler over continuous-wave Doppler?

   A. Range resolution

   B. Ability to measure high velocities

   C. Higher Nyquist limit

   D. Less aliasing artifact

   E. None of the above

109. Which of the following is true concerning the Nyquist limit?

   A. It determines the max velocity that can be measured.

   B. It is the max Doppler shift.

   C. It is infinite with continuous-wave Doppler.

   D. Above this limit aliasing artifact occurs.

   E. All of the above.

110. A decrease in which of the following will create more shades of gray with less bright white and dark black on the image?

   A. Gain

   B. Focus

   C. Time gain compensation

   D. Power

   E. Dynamic range

111. A rapidly moving cardiac valve produces flashes of color on a color flow Doppler exam. Which of the following *best* describes this artifact?

   A. Ghosting

   B. Aliasing

   C. Reverberation

   D. Doppler flashing

   E. Acoustic interference

112. Pectinate muscles can appear thick and hypertrophied and can be mistaken for thrombus in which of the following?

   A. Transverse sinus

   B. Left atrial appendage

   C. Left ventricular apex

   D. Right ventricular outflow tract

   E. Main pulmonary artery

113. What percentage of the general population has a persistent left superior vena cava?

   A. < 0.5%

   B. 0.5%

   C. 1%

   D. 2%

   E. 4%

114. A persistent left superior vena cava is associated with which of the following?

   A. Dilated left atrial appendage

   B. Dilated right atrium

   C. Dilated coronary sinus

   D. Dilated sinus of valsalva

   E. Dilated left upper pulmonary vein

115. Which of the following is formed by fibrous bands at the opening of the coronary sinus (which can make coronary sinus cannulation difficult)?

   A. Eustachian valve

   B. Thebesian valve

   C. Christa terminalis

   D. Chiari network

   E. Pectinate muscles

NOTE: Use the dobutamine stress echocardiography results outlined in Table 2.2G to answer the next four (4) questions.

Table 2.2G.

Dobutamine Dose	Inferior Wall	Anterior Wall	Posterior Wall
0 mcg/kg/min	Akinesis	Akinesis	Normal
5 mcg/kg/min	Mild hypokinesis	Akinesis	Normal
15 mcg/kg/min	Moderate hypokinesis	Akinesis	Hypokinesis
35 mcg/kg/min	Akinesis	Akinesis	Hypokinesis

116. Given the dobutamine stress echocardiography results in Table 2.2G, which of the following best describes the inferior wall?

   A. Scar

   B. Hibernating myocardium

   C. Infarcted myocardium

   D. Stunned myocardium

   E. Somnolent myocardium

117. Given the dobutamine stress echocardiography results in Table 2.2G, which of the following *best* describes the *anterior* wall?

A. Scar

B. Hibernating myocardium

C. Normal myocardium

D. Stunned myocardium

E. Somnolent myocardium

118. Which of the following walls is likely to benefit from revascularization?

A. Anterior only

B. Anterior and inferior

C. Anterior, inferior, and posterior

D. Inferior and posterior

E. Inferior only

119. Which of the following coronary arteries are likely significantly occluded?

A. Circumflex coronary artery

B. Left anterior descending coronary artery (LAD)

C. Right coronary artery

D. Circumflex and right coronary arteries

E. Circumflex, left anterior descending, and right coronary arteries

120. M-mode analysis of the aortic valve showing midsystolic closure of aortic valve followed by coarse fluttering of the aortic valve leaflets is indicative of which of the following?

A. Severe aortic insufficiency

B. Severe mitral insufficiency

C. Hypertrophic cardiomyopathy

D. Amyloidosis

E. Bicuspid aortic valve

121. Which of the following is a potential cause of dilated cardiomyopathy?

   A. Chagas disease

   B. Thiamine deficiency

   C. Viral infections

   D. Duchenne's muscular dystrophy

   E. All of the above

122. Which of the following left ventricular wall thickness measurements is consistent with mild left ventricular hypertrophy in an adult?

   A. 5 mm

   B. 11 mm

   C. 13 mm

   D. 16 mm

   E. 19 mm

123. Which of the following *cannot* be measured or estimated reliably by echocardiography in patients with dilated cardiomyopathy?

   A. Cardiac index (CI)

   B. Pulmonary artery mean pressure (PAMP)

   C. Pulmonary artery diastolic pressure (PADP)

   D. Mixed venous oxygen saturation (SVO_2)

   E. Pulmonary artery systolic pressure (PASP)

124. Using the Carpentier classification of leaflet motion, describe the leaflet motion seen with mitral regurgitation due to systolic anterior motion in a patient with hypertrophic cardiomyopathy.

   A. Type I leaflet motion

   B. Type II leaflet motion

   C. Type III leaflet motion

   D. Type IV leaflet motion

   E. Type V leaflet motion

125. Which of the following left ventricular wall segments is always spared (not hypertrophic) in patients with hypertrophic cardiomyopathy?

    A. Mid posterior wall

    B. Basal posterior wall

    C. Apical posterior wall

    D. Mid lateral wall

    E. Basal lateral wall

126. Which of the following transmitral flow velocity patterns is *most* common in patients with hypertrophic cardiomyopathy?

    A. Normal

    B. Pseudonormal

    C. Impaired relaxation

    D. Restrictive

    E. Constrictive

127. Which of the following would be expected in a patient with restrictive cardiomyopathy due to amyloidosis?

    A. Nondilated thick left ventricle

    B. Fractional area change (FAC) = 18%

    C. Lateral mitral annulular tissue Doppler E_M = 8.6 cm/sec

    D. Fractional shortening (FS) = 14%

    E. Transmitral pulsed-wave Doppler E/A < 1

128. Which of the following is *most* likely to result in an increase in the frame rate?

    A. An increase in the imaging depth

    B. An increase in the line density

    C. Changing from grayscale imaging to color flow Doppler imaging

    D. Narrowing the sector depth

129. In patients with left main coronary artery disease, which of the following is a difference between exercise stress echocardiography (ESE) and dobutamine stress echocardiography (DSE)?

   A. Patients are more likely to have an increase in LVEF with DSE.

   B. Patients are less likely to have left ventricular dilation with exercise.

   C. Patients are more likely to exhibit RWMA with exercise.

   D. Patients are less likely to have ST-segment depression with exercise.

   E. DSE and ESE are very similar in patients with left main disease.

   (LVEF = left ventricular ejection fraction, RWMA = regional wall motion abnormality)

130. Which of the following is the *best* estimate of the sensitivity of dobutamine stress echocardiography?

   A. 68%

   B. 78%

   C. 85%

   D. 95%

   E. 99%

131. Which of the following is the *best* estimate of the specificity of dobutamine stress echocardiography?

   A. 65%

   B. 76%

   C. 88%

   D. 95%

132. Holodiastolic flow reversal in the main pulmonary artery may result from which of the following?

   A. Moderate pulmonic regurgitation

   B. A patent ductus arteriosus

   C. Severe pulmonic stenosis

   D. Ebstein's anomaly

   E. Noonan's syndrome

133. The intensity of the tricuspid valve regurgitant signal relative to the intensity of the antegrade diastolic transtricuspid inflow signal reflects which of the following?

    A. The regurgitant volume of blood traversing the valve

    B. Parallel alignment of the ultrasound beam with blood flow

    C. The velocity of the tricuspid blood flow

    D. The depth of the sample volume

    E. The Nyquist limit of the continuous-wave Doppler ultrasound beam

Answers:

1. C	22. B	43. B
2. C	23. D	44. B
3. A	24. D	45. A
4. E	25. A	46. E
5. B	26. A	47. C
6. C	27. C	48. C
7. B	28. D	49. B
8. C	29. A	50. D
9. B	30. A	51. D
10. D	31. B	52. D
11. A	32. A	53. C
12. D	33. B	54. E
13. D	34. E	55. B
14. C	35. C	56. A
15. A	36. B	57. C
16. B	37. A	58. C
17. C	38. D	59. C
18. B	39. D	60. B
19. B	40. A	61. A
20. C	41. C	62. D
21. E	42. A	63. C

Answers:—continued

64. C	88. D	112. B
65. A	89. C	113. B
66. E	90. E	114. C
67. B	91. B	115. B
68. C	92. A	116. B
69. B	93. B	117. A
70. B	94. B	118. D
71. A	95. C	119. E
72. D	96. A	120. C
73. D	97. A	121. E
74. B	98. D	122. C
75. C	99. C	123. D
76. D	100. A	124. C
77. B	101. E	125. B
78. A	102. A	126. C
79. B	103. D	127. A
80. B	104. D	128. D
81. D	105. D	129. A
82. D	106. D	130. C
83. B	107. E	131. C
84. A	108. A	132. B
85. B	109. E	133. A
86. C	110. E	
87. D	111. A	

Explanations

1. **Answer = C, The purpose of the matching layer is to reduce the reflection at the tissue transducer interface.** The matching layer has acoustic impedance between that of the piezoelectric crystal and soft tissue, and thereby reduces the difference in acoustic impedance at the interface of the probe and soft tissue. Because the amount of reflection at an interface is related to the difference in acoustic impedance between the two media this matching layer will decrease the amount of reflection that occurs at the interface.

Reference: Sidebotham D, Merry A, Legget M (eds.). *Practical Perioperative Transoesophageal Echocardiography.* Burlington, MA: Butterworth Heinemann 2003:19.

2. **Answer = C, Decreased lateral resolution in the far field is a disadvantage of a focused ultrasound beam.** With a focused ultrasound beam the beam diverges rapidly in the far field, increasing the beam width and decreasing lateral resolution.

Reference: Sidebotham D, Merry A, Legget M (eds.). *Practical Perioperative Transoesophageal Echocardiography.* Burlington, MA: Butterworth Heinemann 2003:20.

3. **Answer = A, Improved lateral resolution in the near field is an advantage of a focused ultrasound beam.** Focusing an ultrasound beam creates a narrow beam width in the near field and improves lateral resolution in the near field at the expense of lateral resolution in the far field.

Reference: Sidebotham D, Merry A, Legget M (eds.). *Practical Perioperative Transoesophageal Echocardiography.* Burlington, MA: Butterworth Heinemann 2003:19.

4. **Answer = E, Elevational resolution is determined by the ultrasound beam thickness.**

Reference: Sidebotham D, Merry A, Legget M (eds.). *Practical Perioperative Transoesophageal Echocardiography.* Burlington, MA: Butterworth Heinemann 2003:25.

5. **Answer = B, 1 W/cm^2 is the maximum spatial peak temporal average intensity recommended for unfocused ultrasound beams.**

Reference: Sidebotham D, Merry A, Legget M (eds.). *Practical Perioperative Transoesophageal Echocardiography.* Burlington, MA: Butterworth Heinemann 2003:31.

6. **Answer = C, The posterior descending coronary artery supplies the mid inferior wall.**

References: ASE/SCA Guidelines for Performing a Comprehensive Intraoperative Multiplane Transesophageal Echocardiography Examination. *J Am Soc Echocardiog* 1999;12:884-900; Konstadt SN, Shernon S, Oka Y (eds). *Clinical Transesophageal Echocardiography: A Problem-Oriented Approach, Second Edition.* Philadelphia: Lippincott Williams & Wilkins 2003:45.

7. **Answer = B, The left anterior descending coronary artery supplies the basal anterior wall.**

References: ASE/SCA Guidelines for Performing a Comprehensive Intraoperative Multiplane Transesophageal Echocardiography Examination. *J Am Soc Echocardiog* 1999;12:884-900; Konstadt SN, Shernon S, Oka Y (eds). *Clinical Transesophageal Echocardiography: A Problem-Oriented Approach, Second Edition.* Philadelphia: Lippincott Williams & Wilkins 2003:45.

8. **Answer = C, The circumflex coronary artery supplies the mid posterior wall.**

References: ASE/SCA Guidelines for Performing a Comprehensive Intraoperative Multiplane Transesophageal Echocardiography Examination. *J Am Soc Echocardiog* 1999;12:884-900; Konstadt SN, Shernon S, Oka Y (eds). *Clinical Transesophageal Echocardiography: A Problem-Oriented Approach, Second Edition.* Philadelphia: Lippincott Williams & Wilkins 2003:45.

9. **Answer = B, The right coronary artery supplies the basal inferior wall.**

References: *ASE/SCA* Guidelines for Performing a Comprehensive Intraoperative Multiplane Transesophageal Echocardiography Examination. *J Am Soc Echocardiog* 1999;12:884–900; Konstadt SN, Shernon S, Oka Y (eds). *Clinical Transesophageal Echocardiography: A Problem-Oriented Approach, Second Edition.* Philadelphia: Lippincott Williams & Wilkins 2003:45.

10. **Answer = D, The posterior descending coronary artery supplies the mid inferior wall.**

References: ASE/SCA Guidelines for Performing a Comprehensive Intraoperative Multiplane Transesophageal Echocardiography Examination. *J Am Soc Echocardiog* 1999;12:884–900; Konstadt SN, Shernon S, Oka Y (eds). *Clinical Transesophageal Echocardiography: A Problem-Oriented Approach, Second Edition.* Philadelphia: Lippincott Williams & Wilkins 2003:45.

11. **Answer = A, First-order chordae tendinae arise from papillary muscles and attach to the mitral valve leaflet tips.** Second-order chordae tendinae arise from the papillary muscles and attach to the undersurface of the mitral valve leaflets. Third-order chordae tendinae arise from the ventricular wall (not the papillary muscles) and are present only on the posterior mitral valve, where they attach to the base of the mitral leaflets.

Reference: Sidebotham D, Merry A, Legget M (eds.). *Practical Perioperative Transoesophageal Echocardiography.* Burlington, MA: Butterworth Heinemann 2003:133.

12. **Answer = D, P_2 is the mitral valve scallop most likely to be affected by myxomatous degeneration, annular dilation, and regurgitation.** Leaflet prolapse occurs more frequently with this scallop.

Reference: Sidebotham D, Merry A, Legget M (eds.). *Practical Perioperative Transoesophageal Echocardiography.* Burlington, MA: Butterworth Heinemann 2003:138–141.

13. **Answer = D, The posteromedial papillary muscle is most likely to rupture.** It has a single blood supply (usually the right coronary artery), unlike the anterolateral papillary muscle (which is supplied by both the left anterior descending and circumflex coronary arteries).

Reference: Sidebotham D, Merry A, Legget M (eds.). *Practical Perioperative Transoesophageal Echocardiography.* Burlington, MA: Butterworth Heinemann 2003:138–141.

14. **Answer = C, A TR jet area to RA area of 45% is indicative of moderate (grade III) tricuspid regurgitation.**

Reference: Konstadt SN, Shernon S, Oka Y (eds). Clinical Transesophageal Echocardiography: A Problem-Oriented Approach, Second Edition. Philadelphia: Lippincott Williams & Wilkins 2003:429.

Degree of TR	Trace (grade I)	Mild (grade II)	Moderate (grade III)	Severe (grade IV)
TR jet area/ RA area	< 15 %	16-30 %	31-60 %	> 60 %

15. **Answer = A, No stenosis is present.** The ratio of TVI_{AV} to TVI_{LVOT} is greater than 1, indicating a normal aortic valve area. Although we cannot determine the numerical value for the aortic valve area, we can use this ratio to determine the degree of aortic stenosis. This method is useful because it is not influenced by patient size and errors due to left ventricular outflow tract radius measurements influencing the values adversely.

Reference: Otto C. *Textbook of Clinical Echocardiography, Third Edition.* Philadelphia: Elsevier 2004:287.

16. **Answer = B, The left ventricular outflow tract diameter is needed to calculate the aortic valve area via the continuity equation.**

Reference: Otto C. *Textbook of Clinical Echocardiography, Third Edition.* Philadelphia: Elsevier 2004:287.

17. **Answer = C, 71 ml is the mitral valve stroke volume.** The calculation is as follows:

$$SV_{MV} = A_{MV} * TVI_{MV}$$
$$SV_{MV} = 220/PHT_{MV} * TVI_{MV} = 220/_{62} * 20 \text{ cm} = 71 \text{ mL}$$

Where:

SV_{MV} = mitral valve stroke volume

TVI_{MV} = time velocity integral of mitral valve inflow

PHT_{MV} = mitral valve pressure half time

Reference: SCA/ASE Annual Comprehensive Review and Update of Perioperative Hemodynamics Workshop. 17 Feb. 2005, San Diego, CA; discussion led by Stanton Shernon, et al.

18. **Answer = B, 24 ml is the mitral valve regurgitant volume.** The calculation is as follows:

$$MV\ Rvol = SV_{MV} - SV_{LVOT}$$

$$MV\ Rvol = 71\ ml - [A_{LVOT} * TVI_{LVOT}]$$

$$MV\ Rvol = 71\ ml - [(\pi(1.0\ cm)^2 * (15\ cm)] = \underline{\textbf{24 ml}}$$

$$SV_{MV} = 220/PHT_{MV} * TVI_{MV} = 220/62 * 20\ cm = 71ml$$

Where:

SV_{MV} = mitral valve stroke volume

TVI_{MV} = time velocity integral of mitral valve inflow

PHT_{MV} = mitral valve pressure half time

SV_{LVOT} = stroke volume in the left ventricular outflow tract

A_{LVOT} = area of the left ventricular outflow tract

MV Rvol = mitral valve regurgitant volume

TVI_{LVOT} = time velocity integral of flow through the left ventricular outflow tract

Reference: SCA/ASE Annual Comprehensive Review and Update of Perioperative Hemodynamics Workshop. 17 Feb. 2005, San Diego, CA; discussion led by Stanton Shernon, et al.

19. **Answer = B, 24 mm² or 0.24 cm² is the mitral valve regurgitant orifice area (MV ROA).** The calculation is as follows:

$$MV\ ROA = MVRVol\ /\ TVI_{MRjet} = (24\ cm^3\ /\ 100\ cm) = \underline{\textbf{0.24 cm}^2}$$

$$MV\ Rvol = SV_{MV} - SV_{LVOT}$$

$$MV\ Rvol = 71\ ml - [A_{LVOT} * TVI_{LVOT}]$$

$$MV\ Rvol = 71\ ml - [(\pi(1.0\ cm)^2 * (15\ cm)] = 24\ ml$$

$$SV_{MV} = 220/PHT_{MV} * TVI_{MV} = 220/62 * 20\ cm = 71\ ml$$

Where:

SV_{MV} = mitral valve stroke volume

TVI_{MV} = time velocity integral of mitral valve inflow

PHT_{MV} = mitral valve pressure half time

SV_{LVOT} = stroke volume in the left ventricular outflow tract

A_{LVOT} = area of the left ventricular outflow tract

MV Rvol = mitral valve regurgitant volume

TVI_{LVOT} = time velocity integral of flow through the left ventricular outflow tract

TVI_{MRjet} = time velocity integral of the mitral regurgitant jet

Reference: SCA/ASE Annual Comprehensive Review and Update of Perioperative Hemodynamics Workshop. 17 Feb. 2005, San Diego, CA; discussion led by Stanton Shernon, et al.

20. **Answer = C, A mitral regurgitant orifice area of 23 mm² indicates moderate mitral regurgitation** (see Table 2.2H).

Reference: Perrino AC, Reeves S. *A Practical Approach to TEE.* Philadelphia: Lippincott Williams & Wilkins 2003:137.

Table 2.2H.

Degree of MR	Mild	Moderate	Severe
Regurgitant orifice area (PISA)	< 10 mm²	10-25 mm²	> 25 mm²
Regurgitant fraction	20-30%	30-50%	> 55%

21. **Answer = E, TEE provides superior images in ventilated patients.**

Reference: Sidebotham D, Merry A, Legget M (eds.). *Practical Perioperative Transoesophageal Echocardiography.* Burlington, MA: Butterworth Heinemann 2003:6.

22. **Answer = B, When transmitral E >> A, this indicates restrictive diastolic dysfunction and during this state of decreased left ventricular compliance, TEE provides a better estimate of a patient's intravascular volume status than a pulmonary artery catheter.**

Reference: Sidebotham D, Merry A, Legget M (eds.). *Practical Perioperative Transoesophageal Echocardiography.* Burlington, MA: Butterworth Heinemann 2003:4.

23. **Answer = D, M-mode (motion mode) is described as an ultrasound imaging mode in which the amplitude of returning echoes are plotted as brightness along vertical lines drawn for each transmitted pulse and graphed on the display with depth (distance) on the Y axis versus time on the X axis.**

References: Sidebotham D, Merry A, Legget M (eds.). *Practical Perioperative Transoesophageal Echocardiography.* Burlington, MA: Butterworth Heinemann 2003:96–97.

24. **Answer = D, In B-mode, M-mode, and two-dimensional ultrasound imaging the amplitude of returning echoes is plotted as brightness (with stronger echoes appearing brighter).**

References: Sidebotham D, Merry A, Legget M (eds.). *Practical Perioperative Transoesophageal Echocardiography.* Burlington, MA: Butterworth Heinemann 2003:96–97.

25. **Answer = A, A-mode (amplitude mode) is an antiquated form of obsolete ultrasound imaging in which amplitude is plotted on the Y axis versus depth on the X axis.** It is unlikely that A-mode will be tested, but it is included here for completeness. B-mode (brightness mode) is another older form of ultrasound in which returning echoes are plotted according to depth and amplitude (with stronger echoes appearing brighter, and deeper echoes appearing deeper on the image). M-mode is essentially B-mode plotted versus time. M-mode allows visualization of the movement

of cardiac structures. M-mode has outstanding temporal resolution because only one scan line of information is analyzed over time.

References: Sidebotham D, Merry A, Legget M (eds.). *Practical Perioperative Transoesophageal Echocardiography.* Burlington, MA: Butterworth Heinemann 2003:24–25; Edelman SK. *Understanding Ultrasound Physics.* Woodlands, TX: ESP, Inc. 1994:96–97.

26. **Answer = A, PRP increases with decreasing pulse repetition frequency.** The pulse repetition period (PRP) is the time from the start of one pulse to the start of the next pulse. It increases as imaging depth increases. It does not change when pulse length or duration is changed. Attenuation does not alter the PRP and therefore it does not change as the sound beam travels through tissue.

Reference: Edelman SK. *Understanding Ultrasound Physics.* Woodlands, TX: ESP, Inc. 1994:30.

27. **Answer = C, Pressure: dB = 20 Log p_2 / p_1.** The following are the correct formulas:
    - Pressure: dB = 20 Log p_2 / p_1
    - Intensity: dB = 10 Log I_2 / I_1
    - Amplitude: dB = 20 Log A_2 / A_1
    - Power: dB = 10 Log P_2 / P_1

Reference: http://www.phys.unsw.edu.au/~jw/dB.html.

28. **Answer = A, 1 cm = the thickness required to reduce the intensity of a 6-MHz TEE transducer ultrasound beam by half (the half-value layer thickness).** In soft tissue the *half-value layer thickness* = 3dB / AC = 3dB / 3dB / cm = 1 cm. For ultrasound in soft tissue: attenuation coefficient (AC) = 1/2 freq.

Reference: Edelman SK. *Understanding Ultrasound Physics.* Woodlands, TX: ESP, Inc. 1994:56.

29. **Answer = A, 3 dB of attenuation.** The *half-value layer thickness* is the thickness required to reduce the intensity of a sound beam by half. This represents 3 dB of attenuation. Note that for ultrasound in soft tissue intensity dB = 10 log I_2 / I_1. When I_2 = 1/2 I_1, this represents 10 log 1/2 (or −3dB). Note that the negative sign (−3) implies a reduction in intensity. For the previous equation, I_1 = initial or reference intensity and I_2 = final intensity or intensity at a given depth. I_2 is always less than I_1.

Reference: Edelman SK. *Understanding Ultrasound Physics.* Woodlands, TX: ESP, Inc. 1994:56.

30. **Answer = A, As frequency increases attenuation increases, focal length increases, and scattering increases.** As crystal thickness increases frequency decreases. As frequency increases attenuation increases and therefore the half-power distance decreases.

Reference: Edelman SK. *Understanding Ultrasound Physics.* Woodlands, TX: ESP, Inc. 1994:56, 60, 81.

31. **Answer = B, Density is the most important property of the media in determining if reflection will occur at the interface.** When an ultrasound beam has normal incidence, while traveling from one medium into another the amount of reflection that occurs at the interface depends on the difference in acoustic impedance of the two media. The greater the difference in the impedance the more reflection will occur. Impedance = density * velocity.

References: Kremkau FW. *Diagnostic Ultrasound: Principles Instruments and Exercises, Third Edition.* Philadelphia: Saunders 1989:293; Perrino AC, Reeves S. *A Practical Approach to TEE.* Philadelphia: Lippincott Williams & Wilkins 2003:6.

32. **Answer = A, Oblique = less than or greater than 90 degrees.** Oblique means not normal. This can be less than 90 degrees (acute) or more than 90 degrees (obtuse). Refraction only occurs with oblique incidence. All obtuse angles are oblique, but not all oblique angles are obtuse because oblique also includes acute angles. Oblique = *not* 90 degrees. Normal = perpendicular = orthogonal = right = 90 degrees.

Reference: Edelman SK. *Understanding Ultrasound Physics.* Woodlands, TX: ESP, Inc. 1994:61.

33. **Answer = B, Both acute and obtuse angles are oblique.** Refraction cannot occur with perpendicular = orthogonal incidence. Oblique means *not* normal. This can be less than 90 degrees (acute) or more than 90 degrees (obtuse). Refraction only occurs with oblique incidence. Reflection sometimes occurs with oblique incidence.

Reference: Edelman SK. *Understanding Ultrasound Physics.* Woodlands, TX: ESP, Inc. 1994:61.

34. **Answer = E, The density of the two media is different.** With normal incidence, reflection only occurs when two media have different acoustic impedance. Acoustic impedance (Z) = density * velocity. Given that the velocity of ultrasound in the two media is the same, for reflection to occur the media must have different density. The intensity reflection coefficient is 100% with total reflection. Total reflection implies that all of the ultrasound is reflected back to the transducer. This only occurs when there is a very large difference in the acoustic impedance of the media. If the entire ultrasound beam is reflected, no ultrasound is transmitted and the reflected intensity = 100% of the incident intensity. Therefore, the reflected intensity coefficient is 100% and the transmitted intensity coefficient is 0%.

Reference: Edelman SK. *Understanding Ultrasound Physics.* Woodlands, TX: ESP, Inc. 1994:63.

35. **Answer = C, The distance for a round-trip = (26 μsec) (1.54 mm/μsec) = 40 mm. Therefore, the depth is 1/2 (round-trip dist.) = 20 mm 1.54 mm/μsec = 1540 m/sec = speed of sound in soft tissue.**

Reference: Edelman SK. *Understanding Ultrasound Physics.* Woodlands, TX: ESP, Inc. 1994:71.

36. **Answer = B, Most diagnostic imaging transducers have crystals made of lead zirconate titanate (PZT).** The high temperature at which a crystal loses its function is called the curie temperature (*not* the critical temperature). As crystal thickness increases wavelength increases (frequency decreases).The crystals in TEE probes are arranged in a linear phased array.

Reference: Edelman SK. *Understanding Ultrasound Physics.* Woodlands, TX: ESP, Inc. 1994:72, 73, 75, 103.

37. **Answer = A, Lead zirconate titanate is the most common piezoelectric material found in modern ultrasound transducers.**

Reference: Edelman SK. *Understanding Ultrasound Physics.* Woodlands, TX: ESP, Inc. 1994:73.

38. **Answer = D, The backing material decreases the transducer's sensitivity to reflected echoes.** The backing material functions to improve the image quality. It does this by decreasing the spatial pulse length (SPL). Decreasing spatial pulse length improves axial resolution, as axial resolution = 1/2 * SPL, and the smaller the numerical value for axial resolution the better the image quality. Quality factor (Q factor) = resonant frequency / bandwidth. The backing material decreases the Q factor by decreasing the resonant frequency and increasing the bandwidth. Good imaging transducers have high frequencies, small spatial pulse lengths, and low Q factors.

Reference: Edelman SK. *Understanding Ultrasound Physics.* Woodlands, TX: ESP, Inc. 1994:73.

39. **Answer = D, Crystal D will have the lowest resonant frequency.** Resonant frequency (RF) is determined by the thickness (T) of the crystal and the velocity of ultrasound in the crystal (V). The formula is *RF = V/2T.* Velocity is determined by density and stiffness. The stiffer (less elastic) a material the higher the velocity. The lower the density the higher the velocity. We want the lowest-frequency crystal, so we are looking for the most elastic (least stiff), most dense, thickest crystal: crystal D.

Reference: Edelman SK. *Understanding Ultrasound Physics.* Woodlands, TX: ESP, Inc. 1994:76.

40. **Answer = A, The shorter the pulse the wider the bandwidth.** The damping material tends to decrease the pulse length and increase the bandwidth. As bandwidth increases the quality factor decreases. Q factor = RF / bandwidth. Imaging transducers tend to have wider bandwidths than transducers used for therapeutic ultrasound. RF = resonant frequency.

Reference: Edelman SK. *Understanding Ultrasound Physics.* Woodlands, TX: ESP, Inc. 1994:77.

41. **Answer = C, 8 MHz.** The frequency of a continuous-wave Doppler beam is determined by the frequency of the excitation voltage applied to the TEE crystal.

Reference: Edelman SK. *Understanding Ultrasound Physics.* Woodlands, TX: ESP, Inc. 1994:75.

42. **Answer = A,** *Longitudinal resolution* **is a synonym of** *axial resolution.* *Angular resolution, transverse resolution,* and *lateral resolution* are not synonyms of *axial resolution.*

Reference: Edelman SK. *Understanding Ultrasound Physics.* Woodlands, TX: ESP, Inc. 1994:90.

43. **Answer = B, The beam diameter in the near zone increases if the crystal diameter increases.** With a larger diameter crystal the near zone length is increased and the beam diverges less in the far field, and thus the beam diameter in the far field decreases. The pulse repetition period (PRP) is not related to the crystal diameter.

Reference: Edelman SK. *Understanding Ultrasound Physics.* Woodlands, TX: ESP, Inc. 1994:83–85.

44. **Answer = B, An increase in pulse repetition frequency (PRF) will increase temporal resolution.** PRF = pulses/sec. The higher the PRF the more images can be formed per second. Therefore, the higher the frame rate the greater number of images per second. Increasing the frame rate will improve temporal resolution = the ability to accurately locate the position of moving structures at particular instants in time.

Reference: Edelman SK. *Understanding Ultrasound Physics.* Woodlands, TX: ESP, Inc. 1994:122–124.

45. **Answer = A, Continuous-wave Doppler is not subject to aliasing.** This is why it can be used to measure high velocities, such as the velocity of blood flow through a stenotic aortic valve. Pulsed-wave Doppler is subject to aliasing when the Doppler shift exceeds the Nyquist limit (1/2 the pulse repetition frequency). Color flow Doppler is a form of pulsed-wave Doppler and is subject to aliasing. *2D Doppler* is a fake term.

Reference: Edelman SK. *Understanding Ultrasound Physics.* Woodlands, TX: ESP, Inc. 1994:134–137.

46. **Answer = E, These are all true statements.** Color flow Doppler (CFD) is a form of pulsed-wave Doppler and as such is subject to aliasing artifact. CFD superimposes measurements of blood flow velocity on a two-dimensional grayscale image. It is subject to low frame rates and decreased temporal resolution. Colors represent the speed and direction of blood flow (velocity).

Reference: Edelman SK. *Understanding Ultrasound Physics.* Woodlands, TX: ESP, Inc. 1994: 134–137.

47. **Answer = C, 60 degrees.**

The estimated/measured velocity = actual velocity $* \cos\theta \rightarrow$

$\cos\theta$ = measured velocity / actual velocity = 50 / 100 = 0.5 $\rightarrow \theta$ = 60 degrees.

Note that the arrow ($\rightarrow$) means/symbolizes "implies" or "this rearranges to give."

Reference: Sidebotham D, Merry A, Legget M (eds.). *Practical Perioperative Transoesophageal Echocardiography.* Burlington, MA: Butterworth Heinemann 2003:35.

48. **Answer = C, Transducer C will provide the best two-dimensional grayscale images.** An incident angle of 90 degrees is the best angle for two-dimensional imaging. Both transducer A and transducer C have 90-degree incident angles, but transducer C has a higher frequency and thus should produce higher-quality images. Image quality also increases as imaging depth decreases. Both transducer A and transducer C have identical imaging depths (10 cm).

Reference: Edelman SK. *Understanding Ultrasound Physics.* Woodlands, TX: ESP, Inc. 1994: 134–137.

49. **Answer = B, Transducer B is the most likely transducer to be subject to aliasing artifact.** Transducers A, C, and E will not detect a Doppler shift because the angle of incidence is 90 degrees and cos (90) = 0. Both transducer B and transducer D will detect a Doppler shift, as the ultrasound beam is parallel to blood flow (incident angle = 0). The sample volume depth for transducer B is greater than that for transducer D. Therefore, the pulse repetition frequency (PRF) will be lower for transducer D. Because the Nyquist limit = 1/2 PRF, the probe with the lowest PRF will be the most likely to alias.

Reference: Edelman SK. *Understanding Ultrasound Physics.* Woodlands, TX: ESP, Inc. 1994:134–137.

50. **Answer = D, Transducer D will most likely provide the highest-quality pulsed-wave Doppler determinations.** Transducers D and B both have an incident angle parallel to blood flow (0 degrees) and will thus detect a Doppler shift. Transducer D has a lower sample volume depth than transducer B and is therefore less likely to alias (higher Nyquist limit = 1/2 PRF). Therefore, transducer D will be able to accurately measure higher velocities than transducer B and will provide the highest-quality pulsed-wave Doppler determinations.

Reference: Edelman SK. *Understanding Ultrasound Physics.* Woodlands, TX: ESP, Inc. 1994:137.

51. **Answer = D, Coronary sinus atrial septal defects (ASDs) are frequently associated with a persistent left superior vena cava.** The defect is between the coronary sinus and the left atrium. When a dilated coronary sinus exists (diameter ≥ 14 mm), a persistent superior vena cava must be excluded because this can prevent adequate retrograde cardioplegia. Agitated saline (echo contrast) injected into a left arm peripheral IV can be used to detect this defect. The echo contrast will show in the left atrium before the right atrium if a persistent left superior vena cava and a coronary sinus ASD are present. Coronary sinus ASDs are the least common type of ASD (< 5%).

Reference: Perrino AC, Reeves S. *A Practical Approach to TEE.* Philadelphia: Lippincott Williams & Wilkins 2003:287.

52. **Answer = D, Coronary sinus atrial septal defects (ASDs) are very rare (< 5%).** They are frequently associated with a persistent left superior vena cava. The defect is between the coronary sinus and the left atrium. When a dilated coronary sinus exists (diameter ≥ 14 mm), a persistent superior vena cava must be excluded because this can prevent adequate retrograde cardioplegia. Agitated saline (echo contrast) injected into a left arm peripheral IV can be used to detect this defect. The echo contrast will show in the left atrium before the right atrium if a persistent left superior vena cava and a coronary sinus ASD are present.

Reference: Sidebotham D, Merry A, Legget M (eds.). *Practical Perioperative Transoesophageal Echocardiography.* Burlington, MA: Butterworth Heinemann 2003:224.

53. **Answer = C, Subarterial (doubly committed subarterial) ventricular septal defects (VSDs) are most likely to be associated with herniation of an aortic valve cusp.** Perimembranous VSDs can also cause aortic valve cusp herniation, but not as frequently.

Reference: Perrino AC, Reeves S. *A Practical Approach to TEE.* Philadelphia: Lippincott Williams & Wilkins 2003:287.

54. **Answer = E, Inlet ventricular septal defects are more frequent in patients with Down's syndrome.** These defects sometimes occur in conjunction with an ostium primum atrial septal defect creating a complete AV canal defect (AV septal defect).

Reference: Otto C. *Textbook of Clinical Echocardiography, Third Edition.* Philadelphia: Elsevier 2004:466.

55. **Answer = B, The modified Bernoulli equation ($\Delta P = 4V^2$) is inaccurate when continuous-wave Doppler is utilized in the Doppler examination of the PV in a patient with congenital PS and anatomic narrowing of the RVOT (creating elevated flow velocities in the RVOT proximal to the PV).** When flow velocities proximal to the valve are high, they cannot be ignored and the modified Bernoulli equation ($\Delta P = 4V^2$) is inaccurate. In this case, the following equation must be used to determine the pressure gradient across the PV: $\Delta P = 4 [(V_{jet})^2 - (V_{RVOT})^2]$.

Reference: Otto C. *Textbook of Clinical Echocardiography, Third Edition.* Philadelphia: Elsevier 2004:456.

56. **Answer = A, A secundum atrial septal defect (ASD) is the lesion most likely to result in right ventricular dilation and paradoxical septal motion.** Flow with most ASDs is predominantly diastolic left-to-right flow. This results in right-sided volume overload, causing right atrial and right ventricular dilation and paradoxical septal motion. Although a VSD would seem to cause RV dilation, this usually does not occur because the VSD causes left-to-right flow during systole. This left-to-right systolic flow moves blood directly across the VSD into the PA and back to the LA

and LV. This creates LA and LV volume overload because the left heart receives excess blood from the pulmonary veins.

Reference: Otto C. *Textbook of Clinical Echocardiography, Third Edition.* Philadelphia: Elsevier 2004:457.

57. **Answer = C, Eisenmenger's physiology occurs when irreversible pulmonary hypertension causes equalization of systemic and pulmonary artery pressures.** This is due to an intracardiac defect that results in increased pulmonary blood flow and damage to the pulmonary vasculature. After equalization of pressures, flow reversal across the defect occurs (left-to-right flow reverses to become right-to-left flow). This shunt flow decreases oxygenation and results in cyanosis. The development of Eisenmenger's physiology makes many patients with congenital heart disease inoperable. Thus, intervention to prevent excess pulmonary flow must be implemented early.

Reference: Otto C. *Textbook of Clinical Echocardiography, Third Edition.* Philadelphia: Elsevier 2004:457.

58. **Answer = C, Dextrocardia describes a heart located in the right hemithorax with the apex in the right midclavicular line.**

Reference: Otto C. *Textbook of Clinical Echocardiography, Third Edition.* Philadelphia: Elsevier 2004:457.

59. **Answer = C, 84.8 cm^3 is the stroke volume of diastolic flow through the mitral valve (SV$_{MV}$).** The calculation is as follows:

$$SV_{MV} = A_{MV} * TVI_{MV}$$

$$SV_{MV} = \pi r^2 * TVI_{MV}$$

$$SV_{MV} = 3.14 \, (1.5 \text{ cm})^2 * 12 \text{ cm}$$

$$SV_{MV} = 84.8 \text{ cm}^3$$

Reference: Perrino AC, Reeves S. *A Practical Approach to TEE.* Philadelphia: Lippincott Williams & Wilkins 2003:99.

60. **Answer = B, 47.1 cm^3 = the stroke volume through the left ventricular outflow tract (LVOT).** The calculation is as follows:

$$SV_{LVOT} = A_{LVOT} * TVI_{LVOT}$$

$$SV_{LVOT} = \pi r^2 * TVI_{LVOT}$$

$$SV_{LVOT} = \pi \, (1 \text{ cm})^2 * 15 \text{ cm}$$

$$SV_{LVOT} = 47.1 \text{ cm}^3$$

Reference: Perrino AC, Reeves S. *A Practical Approach to TEE.* Philadelphia: Lippincott Williams & Wilkins 2003:99.

61. **Answer = A, 37.7 cm³ = the regurgitant volume (RVol$_{MV}$) of flow through the mitral valve.** The calculation is as follows:

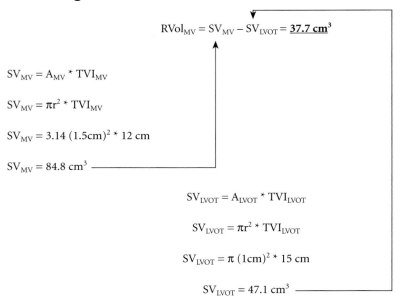

$$RVol_{MV} = SV_{MV} - SV_{LVOT} = \underline{\textbf{37.7 cm}^3}$$

$SV_{MV} = A_{MV} * TVI_{MV}$

$SV_{MV} = \pi r^2 * TVI_{MV}$

$SV_{MV} = 3.14\,(1.5cm)^2 * 12\ cm$

$SV_{MV} = 84.8\ cm^3$

$SV_{LVOT} = A_{LVOT} * TVI_{LVOT}$

$SV_{LVOT} = \pi r^2 * TVI_{LVOT}$

$SV_{LVOT} = \pi\,(1cm)^2 * 15\ cm$

$SV_{LVOT} = 47.1\ cm^3$

Reference: Perrino AC, Reeves S. *A Practical Approach to TEE.* Philadelphia: Lippincott Williams & Wilkins 2003:99.

62. **Answer = D, 44.4% = the mitral valve regurgitant fraction (MV Reg Fx).** The calculation is as follows:

MV Reg Fx = RVol$_{MV}$ / SV$_{MV}$

MV Reg Fx = 37.7 cm³ / 84.8 cm³

MV Reg Fx = 44.4%

Reference: Perrino AC, Reeves S. *A Practical Approach to TEE.* Philadelphia: Lippincott Williams & Wilkins 2003:99.

63. **Answer = C, 0.21 cm² (21 mm²) is the mitral valve regurgitant orifice area (effective regurgitant orifice area) (MV$_{ROA}$).** The calculation is as follows:

MV$_{ROA}$ = RVol$_{MV}$ / TVI$_{MRjet}$

MV$_{ROA}$ = 37.7 cm³ / 180 cm

MV$_{ROA}$ = 0.21 cm² (21 mm²)

Reference: Perrino AC, Reeves S. *A Practical Approach to TEE.* Philadelphia: Lippincott Williams & Wilkins 2003:99.

64. **Answer = C, Moderate mitral regurgitation is present.** A mitral valve regurgitant orifice area of 21 mm² and a regurgitant fraction of 44.4% are consistent with moderate mitral regurgitation (see Table 2.2I).

Reference: Perrino AC, Reeves S. *A Practical Approach to TEE.* Philadelphia: Lippincott Williams & Wilkins 2003:137.

Table 2.21.

Method	Mild	Moderate	Severe
Regurgitant orifice area (MV_{ROA})	$< 10 \text{ mm}^2$	$10\text{-}25 \text{ mm}^2$	$> 25 \text{ mm}^2$
Mitral valve regurgitant fraction	$< 30\%$	$30\text{-}50\%$	$> 50\%$

65. **Answer = A, 2.1 cm² is the aortic valve area (AVA) (A_{AV}).** The calculation is as follows:

$A_{AV} = (\text{aortic valve side})^2 * 0.433$

$A_{AV} = (2.2 \text{ cm})^2 * 0.433$

$A_{AV} = 2.1 \text{ cm}^2$

Reference: Sidebotham D, Merry A, Legget M (eds.). *Practical Perioperative Transoesophageal Echocardiography.* Burlington, MA: Butterworth Heinemann 2003:232.

66. **Answer = E, 99.5 cm³ is the right ventricular stroke volume.** The calculation is as follows:

$SV_{PA} = A_{PA} {}^* TVI_{PA}$

$SV_{PA} = \pi r^2 * TVI_{PA}$

$SV_{PA} = \pi (1.2 \text{ cm})^2 * 22 \text{ cm}$

$SV_{PA} = 99.5 \text{ cm}^3$

Reference: SCA/ASE Annual Comprehensive Review and Update of Perioperative Hemodynamics Workshop. 17 Feb. 2005, San Diego, CA; discussion led by Stanton Shernon, et al.

67. **Answer = B, 50.2 cm³ is the left ventricular stroke volume.** The calculation is as follows:

$SV_{LVOT} = A_{LVOT} {}^* TVI_{LVOT}$

$SV_{LVOT} = \pi r^2 {}^* TVI_{LVOT}$

$SV_{LVOT} = \pi (1.0 \text{ cm})^2 * 16 \text{ cm}$

$SV_{LVOT} = 50.2 \text{ cm}^3$

Reference: SCA/ASE Annual Comprehensive Review and Update of Perioperative Hemodynamics Workshop. 17 Feb. 2005, San Diego, CA; discussion led by Stanton Shernon, et al.

68. **Answer = C, 2:1 = Q_p/Q_s.** The calculation is as follows:

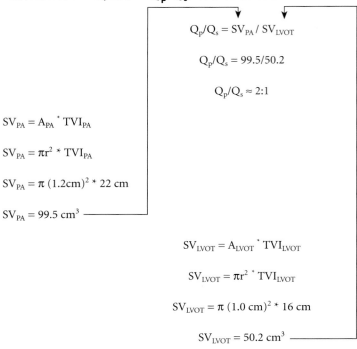

$$Q_p/Q_s = SV_{PA} / SV_{LVOT}$$

$$Q_p/Q_s = 99.5/50.2$$

$$Q_p/Q_s \approx 2:1$$

$$SV_{PA} = A_{PA} {}^* TVI_{PA}$$

$$SV_{PA} = \pi r^2 {}^* TVI_{PA}$$

$$SV_{PA} = \pi (1.2cm)^2 {}^* 22\ cm$$

$$SV_{PA} = 99.5\ cm^3$$

$$SV_{LVOT} = A_{LVOT} {}^* TVI_{LVOT}$$

$$SV_{LVOT} = \pi r^2 {}^* TVI_{LVOT}$$

$$SV_{LVOT} = \pi (1.0\ cm)^2 {}^* 16\ cm$$

$$SV_{LVOT} = 50.2\ cm^3$$

Reference: Sidebotham D, Merry A, Legget M (eds.). *Practical Perioperative Transoesophageal Echocardiography.* Burlington, MA: Butterworth Heinemann 2003:231.

69. **Answer = B, 51 mmHg = the pulmonary artery systolic pressure (PASP).** The calculation is as follows:

$$\Delta P = 4V^2$$

$$(LVSP - RVSP) = 4(V_{VSD})^2$$

$$RVSP = LVSP - 4(V_{VSD})^2$$

$$RVSP = SBP - 4(V_{VSD})^2$$

$$RVSP = 100 - 4(3.5)^2$$

$$RVSP = 51\ mmHg$$

$$PASP = RVSP = 51\ mmHg$$

Where:

LVSP = left ventricular systolic pressure

RVSP = right ventricular systolic pressure

V_{VSD} = peak velocity of the left-to-right flow across the ventricular septal defect

SBP = systemic systolic blood pressure

Reference: Perrino AC, Reeves S. *A Practical Approach to TEE.* Philadelphia: Lippincott Williams & Wilkins 2003:103.

70. **Answer = B, A Crawford type II aortic aneurysm is described.** This thoracoabdominal aneurysm begins near the left subclavian artery and extends distally to a location below the renal arteries (see Table 2.2J).

Reference: Perrino AC, Reeves S. *A Practical Approach to TEE.* Philadelphia: Lippincott Williams & Wilkins 2003:252.

Table 2.2J.	CRAWFORD CLASSIFICATION FOR THORACOABDOMINAL ANEURYSMS	
Type	**Origin**	**Extends Distally:**
I	Near left subclavian artery	Above renal arteries
II	Near left subclavian artery	Below renal arteries
III	More distal than types I or II but above the diaphragm	Below renal arteries
IV	Below the diaphragm (abdominal)	Below renal arteries

71. **Answer = A, An epiaortic ultrasound scan of the ascending aorta prior to aortic cannulation is indicated because this patient has severe atherosclerosis of the descending thoracic aorta** (see Tables 2.2K and 2.2L).

Reference: Katz ES, et al. Grading of atherosclerotic plaques. Journal of American Cardiology 1992;20:70–77.

Table 2.2K.	GRADING OF ATHEROSCLEROTIC PLAQUES (WAKE FOREST GRADING SYSTEM)
Size/Description	**Severity**
< 3 mm	Mild
3-5 mm	Moderate
> 5 mm	Severe
Mobile	Mobile

Table 2.2L.	
Grade	**Size/Description**
I	Normal aorta
II	Extensive intimal thickening
III	Protrudes < 5 mm into aortic lumen
IV	Protrudes > 5 mm into aortic lumen
V	Mobile atheroma

72. **Answer = D, The distal ascending aorta and proximal aortic arch are difficult to image with TEE because the air-filled trachea and left main bronchus lie between the esophagus and the aorta and obstruct the ultrasound beam (making imaging impossible).**

Reference: Otto C. *Textbook of Clinical Echocardiography, Third Edition.* Philadelphia: Elsevier 2004:437.

73. **Answer = D, 50% of in-patients with a diagnosis of congestive heart failure have diastolic heart failure with normal systolic function (LVEF > 55%).**

Reference: Perrino AC, Reeves S. *A Practical Approach to TEE.* Philadelphia: Lippincott Williams & Wilkins 2003:110.

74. **Answer = B, The correct order of the four phases of diastole is: isovolumic left ventricular relaxation, early filling, diastasis, atrial contraction.**

75. **Answer = C, An E/E$_M$ > 15 is indicative of high left atrial filling pressures.**

76. **Answer = D, 0.2% is the incidence of oropharyngeal and gastric trauma occurring with insertion and manipulation of the TEE probe in cardiac surgery patients.** Note that this is not the incidence of esophageal perforation, which is much less (0.02 to 0.03%).

Reference: Kallmeyer IJ, Collard CD, Fox JA, Body SC, Shernan SK. The safety of intraoperative TEE: A case series of 7200 cardiac surgical patients. *Anesthesia and Analgesia* 2001;92:1126–1130.

77. **Answer = B, 0.02 to 0.03% is the incidence of esophageal perforation secondary to TEE in the emergency room and the ICU.** This is likely similar to the incidence of esophageal perforation in the operating room. This serious complication has a high mortality rate, and is associated with difficult probe insertion, increased age, and history of esophageal disease.

Reference: Kallmeyer IJ, Collard CD, Fox JA, Body SC, Shernan SK. The safety of intraoperative TEE: A case series of 7200 cardiac surgical patients. *Anesthesia and Analgesia* 2001;92:1126–1130.

78. **Answer = A, The isovolumic relaxation time (IVRT) is increased during new-onset acute myocardial ischemia.** New-onset ischemia is associated with impaired relaxation, which results in the following: increased IVRT, decreased E, increased A, and a prolonged E-wave deceleration time.

Reference: Sidebotham D, Merry A, Legget M (eds.). *Practical Perioperative Transoesophageal Echocardiography.* Burlington, MA: Butterworth Heinemann 2003:117.

79. **Answer = B, The transmitral E >> A in patients with reduced left ventricular compliance due to infiltrative amyloidosis.** In restrictive diastolic dysfunction, transmitral E >> A, and IVRT, E$_M$, DT, and V$_P$ are decreased.

V$_P$ = transmitral color M-mode Doppler flow propagation velocity

E = pulsed-wave Doppler transmitral early filling velocity

A = pulsed-wave Doppler transmitral peak A-wave velocity

E$_M$ = lateral mitral annular tissue Doppler E wave (E$_M$ = E´ = E prime)

IVRT = isovolumic relaxation time

DT = deceleration time

Reference: Sidebotham D, Merry A, Legget M (eds.). *Practical Perioperative Transoesophageal Echocardiography.* Burlington, MA: Butterworth Heinemann 2003:119.

80. **Answer = B, As heart rate increases the transmitral E/A ratio decreases.** As heart rate increases the distance between the E and A wave (diastasis) decreases. If this distance is obliterated by an elevation of heart rate, the A wave is superimposed or merged with the E wave. With this elevated heart rate there is not enough time for early filling to complete before left atrial contraction occurs. As a result of this incomplete early filling, atrial contraction contributes more to LV filling and the A wave is increased at the expense of the E wave (which is decreased). Thus, tachycardia results in a decreased E wave and an increased A wave (creating a decreased E/A ratio).

Reference: Otto C. *Textbook of Clinical Echocardiography, Third Edition.* Philadelphia: Elsevier 2004:179.

81. **Answer = D, E/A is increased with mitral regurgitation (MR).** With MR left atrial pressure is increased. This increased pressure gradient between the left atrium and the left ventricle increases early left ventricular filling. This increase in early left ventricular filling increases the transmitral E wave and thus increases the E/A ratio.

Reference: Otto C. *Textbook of Clinical Echocardiography, Third Edition.* Philadelphia: Elsevier 2004:179.

82. **Answer = D, The hepatic venous systolic flow wave (S wave) is shown.** This wave results from forward flow into the right atrium during ventricular systole. During systole, the right atrial pressure decreases with atrial relaxation and descent of the tricuspid valve apparatus.

Reference: Perrino AC, Reeves S. *A Practical Approach to TEE.* Philadelphia: Lippincott Williams & Wilkins 2003:124.

83. **Answer = B, The hepatic venous diastolic flow wave (D wave) is shown.** This wave results from forward flow after the tricuspid valve opens and right atrial pressure decreases.

Reference: Perrino AC, Reeves S. *A Practical Approach to TEE.* Philadelphia: Lippincott Williams & Wilkins 2003:124.

84. **Answer = A, The hepatic venous atrial flow reversal wave (A wave) is shown.** This wave is created by retrograde flow into the inferior vena cava from atrial contraction.

Reference: Perrino AC, Reeves S. *A Practical Approach to TEE.* Philadelphia: Lippincott Williams & Wilkins 2003:124.

85. **Answer = B, Pseudonormal diastolic dysfunction is present.** The transmitral pulsed-wave Doppler diastolic velocity profile appears normal. This normal-appearing E- and A-wave profile could result from normal or pseudonormal diastolic function. A decreased lateral mitral annular tissue

Doppler E_M peak velocity is also present (E_M < 8 cm/sec) and this confirms the diagnosis of normal diastolic function. If normal diastolic function was present, the lateral mitral annular tissue Doppler E_M peak velocity would be ≥ 8 cm/sec.

Reference: Groban L, Dolinski SY. Transesophageal echocardiographic evaluation of diastolic function. *Chest* 2005;128:3652–3663.

86. **Answer = C, Impaired relaxation is shown.** The transmitral pulsed-wave Doppler profile shows the following: E = A, prolonged E-wave DT, increased IVRT, and decreased E-wave peak velocity.
   Where:

   DT = transmitral early filling wave (E wave) deceleration time

   E = pulsed-wave Doppler transmitral early filling velocity

   A = pulsed-wave Doppler transmitral late filling velocity (associated with atrial contraction)

   IVRT = isovolumic relaxation time

Reference: Groban L, Dolinski SY. Transesophageal echocardiographic evaluation of diastolic function. *Chest* 2005;128:3652–3663.

87. **Answer = D, A patient with new-onset acute myocardial ischemia is most likely to present with an impaired relaxation pattern of diastolic dysfunction.** A healthy young adult should have normal transmitral pulsed-wave Doppler inflow velocities. The other choices listed will likely present with a restrictive diastolic transmitral inflow velocity profile.

Reference: Groban L, Dolinski SY. Transesophageal echocardiographic evaluation of diastolic function. *Chest* 2005;128:3652–3663.

88. **Answer = D, The pulmonary vein S-wave peak velocity > D-wave peak velocity.** This would be expected in a patient with impaired relaxation. An elevated left atrial pressure is unlikely, as this would produce a pseudonormal or restrictive transmitral inflow pattern. With impaired relaxation, the lateral mitral annular tissue Doppler E_M would be expected to be low (< 8 cm/sec), as would the transmitral color M-mode propagation velocity (V_P) (normal ≥ 50 cm/sec). An elevated PV_{AR} duration is seen in pseudonormal diastolic dysfunction when left ventricular compliance is decreased and retrograde flow dominates following left atrial contraction.

Reference: Groban L, Dolinski SY. Transesophageal echocardiographic evaluation of diastolic function. *Chest* 2005;128:3652–3663.

89. **Answer = C, Impaired relaxation is shown.** The transmitral pulsed-wave Doppler inflow E/A ratio ≤ 1 and the lateral mitral annular tissue Doppler E_M is less than 8 cm/sec.

Reference: Groban L, Dolinski SY. Transesophageal echocardiographic evaluation of diastolic function. *Chest* 2005;128:3652–3663.

90. **Answer = E, The arrow indicates the transmitral pulsed-wave Doppler A wave.**

Reference: Groban L, Dolinski SY. Transesophageal echocardiographic evaluation of diastolic function. *Chest* 2005;128:3652–3663.

91. **Answer = B, Arrow 1 indicates the isovolumic relaxation time (IVRT).** The continuous-wave Doppler beam is positioned such that both transmitral LV inflow and aortic LV outflow are observed. The time between aortic outflow and mitral inflow is the IVRT. During this time period, the aortic and mitral valves are closed and the left ventricle is actively relaxing. The Doppler velocity profile indicated by arrow 2 is due to aortic left ventricular outflow. Arrow 3 indicates transmitral inflow.

Reference: Groban L, Dolinski SY. Transesophageal echocardiographic evaluation of diastolic function. *Chest* 2005;128:3652–3663.

92. **Answer = A, The Doppler velocity profile indicated by arrow 2 is due to left ventricular outflow. Arrow 3 indicates transmitral inflow.**

Reference: Groban L, Dolinski SY. Transesophageal echocardiographic evaluation of diastolic function. *Chest* 2005;128:3652–3663.

93. **Answer = B, The Doppler velocity profile indicated by arrow 3 is due to transmitral inflow. The velocity profile indicated by arrow 2 is due to left ventricular outflow.**

Reference: Groban L, Dolinski SY. Transesophageal echocardiographic evaluation of diastolic function. *Chest* 2005;128:3652–3663.

94. **Answer = B, Fractional shortening (FS) = 23%.** The calculation is as follows.

FS = (LVEDd – LVESd) / LVEDd

FS = (65 – 50) / 65

FS = 23%

Where:

   LVEDd = left ventricular end diastolic diameter

   LVESd = left ventricular end systolic diameter

Reference: Perrino AC, Reeves S. *A Practical Approach to TEE.* Philadelphia: Lippincott Williams & Wilkins 2003:38.

95. **Answer = C, 33% = the fractional area change (FAC).** The calculation is as follows:

FAC = (LVEDA − LVESA) / LVEDA

FAC = (30 − 20) / 30 = 33%

Where:

LVEDA = left ventricular end diastolic area

LVESA = left ventricular end systolic area

Reference: Perrino AC, Reeves S. *A Practical Approach to TEE.* Philadelphia: Lippincott Williams & Wilkins 2003: 41.

96. **Answer = A, 3.45 L/min is the cardiac output.** The calculation is as follows:

$SV_{LVOT} = TVI_{LVOT} * A_{LVOT}$

$SV_{LVOT} = (11 \text{ cm}) * (\pi r^2)$

$SV_{LVOT} = (11 \text{ cm}) * (3.14 \text{ cm}^2)$

$SV_{LVOT} = 34.5 \text{ cc}$

CO = SV * HR = (34.5 cc/beat) * (100 beats/min) = 3.45 L/min

Where:

CO = cardiac output

SV = stroke volume

TVI_{LVOT} = time velocity integral of blood flow through the left ventricular outflow tract

A_{LVOT} = area of the left ventricular outflow tract

Reference: Perrino AC, Reeves S. *A Practical Approach to TEE.* Philadelphia: Lippincott Williams & Wilkins 2003:42.

97. **Answer = A, The peak instantaneous gradient across the aortic valve is 16 mmHg.** The calculation is as follows:

$\Delta P = 4V^2$

$\Delta P = 4(V_{AVpeak})^2$

$\Delta P = 4(2)^2$

$\Delta P = 16 \text{ mmHg}$

Where:

VAV peak = peak instantaneous velocity across the aortic valve

Reference: Perrino AC, Reeves S. *A Practical Approach to TEE.* Philadelphia: Lippincott Williams & Wilkins 2003:43.

98. **Answer = D, A TEE probe should be soaked in a glutaraldehyde solution for at least 20 minutes to eliminate bacterial and viral contaminants during the cleaning process.**

Reference: Savage RM, Aronson S, Thomas JD, Shanewise JS, Shernan SK. *Comprehensive Textbook of Intraoperative Transesophageal Echocardiography.* Philadelphia: Lippincott Williams & Wilkins 2004:109.

99. **Answer = C, Lateral mitral annular tissue Doppler E_M can be used to distinguish between normal and pseudonormal diastolic function in a patient with moderate mitral regurgitation.** Moderate mitral regurgitation will cause systolic suppression of the pulmonary vein S wave. Pseudonormal diastolic dysfunction will also cause the S wave to be decreased. Therefore, pulmonary vein S > D would be expected and may or may not be due pseudonormal diastolic function.

Reference: Groban L, Dolinski SY. Transesophageal echocardiographic evaluation of diastolic function. *Chest* 2005;128:3652–3663.

100. **Answer = A, Increased left ventricular free wall thickness would not be expected in dilated cardiomyopathy.**

Reference: Otto C. *Textbook of Clinical Echocardiography, Third Edition.* Philadelphia: Elsevier 2004:257.

101. **Answer = E, All of the above are potential causes of pericarditis.**

Reference: Otto C. *Textbook of Clinical Echocardiography, Third Edition.* Philadelphia: Elsevier 2004:257.

102. **Answer = A, A post myocardial infarction pericardial effusion is known as Dressler's syndrome.**

Reference: Otto C. *Textbook of Clinical Echocardiography, Third Edition.* Philadelphia: Elsevier 2004:260.

103. **Answer = D, A large pericardial effusion is > 2 cm** (see Table 2.2M).

Reference: Otto C. *Textbook of Clinical Echocardiography, Third Edition.* Philadelphia: Elsevier 2004:262.

Table 2.2M.   PERICARDIAL EFFUSION SEVERITY ACCORDING TO SIZE

Mild	Moderate	Severe
< 0.5 cm	0.5-2.0 cm	> 2.0 cm

104. **Answer = D, During spontaneous inspiration the transtricuspid E-wave peak velocity would be expected to increase in a patient with constrictive pericarditis.** With spontaneous inspiration the negative intrathoracic pressure dilates the thin-walled right ventricle and favors RV filling at the expense of LV filling and LV stroke volume (a reciprocal respiratory filling pattern).

Reference: Otto C. *Textbook of Clinical Echocardiography, Third Edition.* Philadelphia: Elsevier 2004:270–272.

105. **Answer = D, Cervical spine instability is an absolute contraindication to TEE.** Absolute contraindications to TEE include esophageal strictures, webs or rings, patient refusal, esophageal perforation, obstruction esophageal neoplasms, and cervical spin instability.

Reference: Savage RM, Aronson S, Thomas JD, Shanewise JS, Shernan SK. *Comprehensive Textbook of Intraoperative Transesophageal Echocardiography.* Philadelphia: Lippincott Williams & Wilkins 2004:108.

106. **Answer = D, 77 m/s is the velocity of blood flow in the vessel.** The calculation is as follows:

$$V = \Delta F / \cos\theta * C / 2F_T$$

$$V = (0.5\ \text{MHz}) / 0.5 * 1540\ \text{m/s} / (20\ \text{MHz})$$

$$V = 77\ \text{m/s}$$

Note that the TEE machine assumes a parallel angle of incidence (0 degrees) between blood flow and the ultrasound probe. If $\theta > 0°$, the velocity reported by the TEE machine will be underestimated.

(V = velocity of blood flow, ΔF = Doppler shift ($F_T - F_R$), F_T = transmitted frequency, F_R = reflected frequency.)

Reference: Edelman SK. *Understanding Ultrasound Physics.* Woodlands, TX: ESP, Inc. 1994:131.

107. **Answer = E, Continuous-wave Doppler has the ability to measure very high blood flow velocities and this is an advantage of continuous-wave Doppler over pulsed-wave Doppler.** Continuous-wave Doppler (CWD) can measure very high velocities because it is not subject to aliasing. Aliasing occurs with pulsed-wave Doppler when the Doppler shift exceeds the Nyquist limit. The Nyquist limit is the highest Doppler shift (ΔF) that can be measured before aliasing occurs. The Nyquist limit is equal to 1/2 PRF. The pulse repetition frequency (PRF) is the number of pulses per second. Continuous-wave Doppler is by definition continuously producing pulses and therefore has an infinite PRF and an infinite Nyquist limit. Continuous-wave Doppler cannot produce images (only pulsed ultrasound can produce images). There are two definitions for range resolution: (1) Range resolution = depth or axial resolution, and (2) Range resolution = the ability to determine the location/origin of a returning echo. In neither case is range resolution a property of continuous-wave ultrasound. Spatial, lateral, and temporal resolution refers to image quality, and continuous-wave ultrasound cannot make images. In addition, continuous-wave ultrasound cannot determine the origin of echoes (range ambiguity).

Reference: Edelman SK. *Understanding Ultrasound Physics.* Woodlands, TX: ESP, Inc. 1994:131–137.

108. **Answer = A, Range resolution is an advantage of pulsed-wave Doppler.** There are two definitions for range resolution: (1) Range

resolution = depth or axial resolution, and (2) Range resolution = the ability to determine the location/origin of a returning echo. In this question, range resolution refers to the second definition: the ability to determine the location/origin of a returning echo. With pulsed-wave Doppler the ultrasound machine waits for all echoes from an initial pulse to return before sending out another pulse, thereby allowing depth determination of reflectors. Continuous-wave Doppler does not wait for echoes on one pulse to return before it sends out a new pulse. Continuous-wave Doppler is continuously emitting pulses and therefore cannot determine the location of reflectors (range ambiguity).

Reference: Edelman SK. *Understanding Ultrasound Physics.* Woodlands, TX: ESP, Inc. 1994: 131–137.

109. **Answer = E, All of the above are true concerning the Nyquist limit.** The Nyquist limit (Nyquist frequency) is the maximum Doppler shift that can be measured. It determines the max velocity that can be measured, is responsible for aliasing artifact, and is infinite with continuous-wave Doppler.

Reference: Edelman SK. *Understanding Ultrasound Physics.* Woodlands, TX: ESP, Inc. 1994:131–137.

110. **Answer = E, A decrease in the dynamic range will create more shades of gray, and less shades of bright white and dark black on the image.** The dynamic range is the spectrum or range of signals that can be processed by the different components of an ultrasound system. The returning echoes have a large dynamic range, much larger than the components of an ultrasound machine can manage. Thus, the signals cannot be properly processed until they are compressed into a manageable size. The machine maintains the relative strengths of the signals (i.e., the strongest echo is still the strongest and the smallest echo is still the smallest) but reduces the difference in voltage between the signals (compression). This reduces the range of signals to a manageable size, enabling the machine to process information that is within the confines of the system. Decreasing the dynamic range will decrease the voltage difference between the strongest and weakest signals, effectively creating more shades of gray with less bright white and dark on the image.

Reference: Edelman SK. *Understanding Ultrasound Physics.* Woodlands, TX: ESP, Inc. 1994:169.

111. **Answer = A, Ghosting.** Color flow Doppler is intended to measure the velocities of blood flow. The blood flow velocities are color coded and displayed on a two-dimensional grayscale background. Normally, two-dimensional structures do not create colors. However, sometimes rapidly moving structures such as cardiac valves can produce flashes of color (this phenomenon is known as "ghosting").

Reference: Konstadt SN, Shernon S, Oka Y (eds). *Clinical Transesophageal Echocardiography: A Problem-Oriented Approach, Second Edition.* Philadelphia: Lippincott Williams & Wilkins 2003:54.

112. **Answer = B, Pectinate muscles can appear thick and hypertrophied and can be mistaken for thrombus in the left atrial appendage.**

Reference: Konstadt SN, Shernon S, Oka Y (eds). *Clinical Transesophageal Echocardiography: A Problem-Oriented Approach, Second Edition.* Philadelphia: Lippincott Williams & Wilkins 2003:54.

113. **Answer = B, 0.5% of the general population has a persistent left superior vena cava.** The incidence is higher in patients with congenital heart disease (3 to 10%).

Reference: Konstadt SN, Shernon S, Oka Y (eds). *Clinical Transesophageal Echocardiography: A Problem-Oriented Approach, Second Edition.* Philadelphia: Lippincott Williams & Wilkins 2003:55.

114. **Answer = C, A persistent left superior vena cava is associated with a dilated coronary sinus.**

Reference: Konstadt SN, Shernon S, Oka Y (eds). *Clinical Transesophageal Echocardiography: A Problem-Oriented Approach, Second Edition.* Philadelphia: Lippincott Williams & Wilkins 2003:55.

115. **Answer = B, The thebesian valve is a fibrous band at the opening of the coronary sinus, which can make coronary sinus cannulation difficult.**

Reference: Sidebotham D, Merry A, Legget M (eds.). *Practical Perioperative Transoesophageal Echocardiography.* Burlington, MA: Butterworth Heinemann 2003:70.

116. **Answer = B, The inferior wall can be classified as hibernating myocardium, given its biphasic response to dobutamine.** With low doses this viable myocardium's function improves, but with high doses it deteriorates (becoming akinetic again).

Reference: Savage RM, Aronson S, Thomas JD, Shanewise JS, Shernan SK. *Comprehensive Textbook of Intraoperative Transesophageal Echocardiography.* Philadelphia: Lippincott Williams & Wilkins 2004:360.

117. **Answer = A, The anterior wall is infracted, containing scar tissue.** It does not improve with dobutamine, and is not likely to benefit from revascularization because it does not contain viable tissue.

Reference: Savage RM, Aronson S, Thomas JD, Shanewise JS, Shernan SK. *Comprehensive Textbook of Intraoperative Transesophageal Echocardiography.* Philadelphia: Lippincott Williams & Wilkins 2004:360.

118. **Answer = D, Both the posterior and inferior wall have viable myocardium that becomes ischemic with high-dose dobutamine.** Both of these myocardial segments have limited coronary flow reserves and will likely benefit from revascularization.

Reference: Savage RM, Aronson S, Thomas JD, Shanewise JS, Shernan SK. *Comprehensive Textbook of Intraoperative Transesophageal Echocardiography.* Philadelphia: Lippincott Williams & Wilkins 2004:360.

119. **Answer = E, The circumflex right and left anterior descending coronary arteries likely have significant occlusive coronary artery disease, given the dobutamine stress echo findings shown.**

Reference: Savage RM, Aronson S, Thomas JD, Shanewise JS, Shernan SK. *Comprehensive Textbook of Intraoperative Transesophageal Echocardiography.* Philadelphia: Lippincott Williams & Wilkins 2004:360.

120. **Answer = C, M-mode analysis of the aortic valve showing midsystolic closure of the aortic valve followed by coarse fluttering of the aortic valve leaflets is indicative of hypertrophic cardiomyopathy with systolic anterior motion of the anterior mitral valve leaflet and left ventricular outflow tract (LVOT) obstruction.** The LVOT obstruction impedes forward flow through the aortic valve, resulting in early aortic valve closure with leaflet fluttering.

Reference: Otto C. *Textbook of Clinical Echocardiography, Third Edition.* Philadelphia: Elsevier 2004: 237.

121. **Answer = E, All of the choices listed are potential causes of dilated cardiomyopathy.** Chagas disease is endemic in South and Central America.

Reference: Otto C. *Textbook of Clinical Echocardiography, Third Edition.* Philadelphia: Elsevier 2004:228.

122. **Answer = C, 13 mm is consistent with mild left ventricular hypertrophy** (see Table 2.2N).

Table 2.2N.	
Degree of LVH	**LV Free Wall Thickness**
Normal	6-11 mm
Mild LVH	12-14 mm
Moderate LVH	15-19 mm
Severe LVH	≥ 20 mm

LV = left ventricle, LVH = left ventricle hypertrophy.

123. **Answer = D, The mixed venous oxygen saturation (SVO_2) cannot be determined by echocardiography but must be measured with a pulmonary artery catheter.**

Reference: Otto C. *Textbook of Clinical Echocardiography, Third Edition.* Philadelphia: Elsevier 2004:231.

124. **Answer = C, Type III leaflet motion is present.** Using the Carpentier system of classification, restrictive leaflet motion is referred to as type III. The Carpentier classification system of leaflet motion for mitral regurgitation is outlined in Table 2.2O.

Table 2.20.

Carpentier Class	Leaflet Motion
Type I	Normal
Type II	Excessive
Type III	Restrictive

Reference: Perrino AC, Reeves S. *A Practical Approach to TEE.* Philadelphia: Lippincott Williams & Wilkins 2003:162–163.

125. **Answer = B, The basal posterior wall between the papillary muscles and the mid mitral annulus is always spared (never hypertrophied) in patients with hypertrophic cardiomyopathy.** There are four types of hypertrophic cardiomyopathy based on the location of the hypertrophy, but in every type the basal posterior wall is not hypertrophied.

Reference: Otto C. *Textbook of Clinical Echocardiography, Third Edition.* Philadelphia: Elsevier 2004:233.

126. **Answer = C, Impaired relaxation is the most common transmitral flow velocity pattern seen in patients with hypertrophic cardiomyopathy.**

Reference: Otto C. *Textbook of Clinical Echocardiography, Third Edition.* Philadelphia: Elsevier 2004:236.

127. **Answer = A, A nondilated thick left ventricle will be present in a restrictive cardiomyopathy due to amyloidosis.** A lateral mitral annular tissue Doppler E_M = 8.6 cm/sec and an transmitral E/A < 1 would not be expected in a patient with restrictive diastolic dysfunction. Systolic function is typically normal, and the low fractional area change and fractional shortening listed would not be expected.

Reference: Otto C. *Textbook of Clinical Echocardiography, Third Edition.* Philadelphia: Elsevier 2004:241.

128. **Answer = D, Narrowing the sector width is likely to result in an increase in the frame rate.** Increasing the imaging depth and/or the line density will decrease the frame rate. Changing from grayscale imaging to color flow Doppler imaging will also decrease the frame rate.

Reference: Edelman SK. *Understanding Ultrasound Physics.* Woodlands, TX: ESP, Inc. 1994:123.

129. **Answer = A, Patients with left main coronary artery disease are more likely to have an increased ejection fraction during dobutamine stress echocardiography (DSE).** Even in patients with severe coronary artery disease (including left main disease), the left ventricle may not dilate and systolic function may improve despite the appearance of new regional wall motion abnormalities. When compared with DSE, patients with left main disease undergoing exercise echocardiography are more likely to show left ventricular dilation, decreased systolic function, and ST-segment depression. Both DSE and exercise echocardiography will show wall motion abnormalities in patients with severe disease.

Reference: Oh JK, Seward JB, Tajik AJ (eds). *The Echo Manual, Second Edition.* Philadelphia: Lippincott Williams & Wilkins 1999:94.

130. **Answer = C, 85% = the sensitivity of dobutamine stress echocardiography (DSE).**

Reference: Oh JK, Seward JB, Tajik AJ (eds). *The Echo Manual, Second Edition.* Philadelphia: Lippincott Williams & Wilkins 1999:94.

131. **Answer = C, 88% = the specificity of dobutamine stress echocardiography (DSE).**

Reference: Oh JK, Seward JB, Tajik AJ (eds). *The Echo Manual, Second Edition.* Philadelphia: Lippincott Williams & Wilkins 1999:94.

132. **Answer = B, A patent ductus arteriosus may result in holodiastolic reversal of flow in the main pulmonary artery.** Severe pulmonary regurgitation will also result in holodiastolic flow reversal.

Reference: Sidebotham D, Merry A, Legget M (eds.). *Practical Perioperative Transoesophageal Echocardiography.* Burlington, MA: Butterworth Heinemann 2003:213.

133. **Answer = A, The intensity of the tricuspid valve regurgitant signal relative to the intensity of the antegrade diastolic transtricuspid inflow signal reflects the regurgitant volume of blood traversing the valve.**

Reference: Otto C. *Textbook of Clinical Echocardiography, Third Edition.* Philadelphia: Elsevier 2004:348.

TEST III PART 1

Video Test Booklet

This product is designed to prepare people for the PTEeXAM. This booklet is to be used with the CD-ROM to practice for the video portion of the PTEeXAM.

Preface

As stated previously, this part of this product is designed to prepare people for the video component of the PTEeXAM. Please do not open this test booklet until you have read the instructions. During the PTEeXAM, instructions similar to these will be written on the back of the test booklet. You will be asked to read these instructions by a proctor at the exam. After you have read these instructions you will be asked to break the seal on the test booklet and to remove an answer sheet, similar to the one included with this practice test.

After you have filled out your name, test number, and other identifying information on the answer sheet you will be instructed to open the test booklet and begin. This test will involve video images shown on a computer monitor. You will share this monitor with three other examinees. This portion of the PTEeXAM has about 50 questions. It consists of about 17 cases, with 2 to 5 questions for each case. It is timed. Good luck!

Instructions

This test will consist of several cases, accompanied by 3 to 5 questions per case. Each case will show one or more images. For each case, you are to utilize the information written in this booklet and the information shown in the images to answer questions concerning each case. An audible chime or tone will assist in timing the exam. This tone alerts you when the test advances to the next step.

The order of the exam is as follows.

Tone/chime

    1. Read the questions for case 1.

Tone/chime

    2. View the images for case 1.

Tone/chime

    3. Answer the questions for case 1.

Tone/chime

    4. View the images for case 1 again.

Tone/chime

    5. Check your answers to the questions for case 1.

Tone/chime

    6. Read the questions for case 2.

Tone/chime

    The process continues in this manner. In summary: tone, read, tone, view, tone, answer, tone, view, tone, check answers, tone.

Cases

Case 1

1. What would you expect to see on this patient's electrocardiogram (EKG)?

    A. Q waves in leads V4 and V5

    B. Q waves in leads II, III, and AVF

    C. ST segment elevation in leads V1 and V2

    D. ST segment elevation in leads II, III, and AVF

    E. None of the above

2. Which of the following is true concerning the images shown for case 1?

    A. A large basal mid-anterior wall left ventricular aneurysm is shown.

    B. A large basal mid-anterior wall left ventricular pseudoaneurysm is shown.

    C. A large basal mid-inferior wall left ventricular aneurysm is shown.

    D. A large basal mid-inferior wall left ventricular pseudoaneurysm is shown.

3. Which of the following is the best method of determining this patient's systolic function?

A. Simpson's method of discs

B. FAC

C. FS

D. Qualitative estimate of EF

Case 2

A continuous-wave Doppler flow velocity profile of a mitral valve regurgitant jet is shown (CWD of MR jet). Use this flow velocity profile to answer the following question.

4. Which of the following best describes this patient's systolic function?

A. Normal

B. Severely decreased

C. Mildly decreased

D. Increased

Case 3

A continuous-wave Doppler flow velocity profile of a mitral valve regurgitant jet is shown (CWD of MR jet). Use this flow velocity profile to answer the following question.

5. Which of the following best estimates this patient's change in pressure with respect to time during isovolumetric left ventricular contraction: dp/dt.

A. dp/dt = 757

B. dp/dt = 1311

C. dp/dt = 1066

D. dp/dt < 500

E. None of the above

6. Which of the following estimates of systolic function is the most load independent?

   A. The change in pressure with respect to time during isovolumetric LV contraction (dp/dt)

   B. Fractional shortening (FS)

   C. Fractional area change (FAC)

   D. Corrected velocity of circumferential shortening (Vcfc)

   E. Index of myocardial performance (IMP)

7. Which of the following estimates of systolic function is heart rate independent?

   A. Ejection fraction (EF)

   B. Fractional shortening (FS)

   C. Fractional area change (FAC)

   D. Corrected velocity of circumferential shortening (Vcfc)

Case 4

8. What phenomenon is illustrated in image 1 for case 4?

   A. The Groban effect

   B. The Serpentine effect

   C. The Carpentier effect

   D. The Coanda effect

   E. The Pisa effect

9. Which of the following best describes the degree of mitral regurgitation seen in this patient?

   A. Trace.

   B. Mild.

   C. Moderate.

   D. Severe.

   E. It cannot be determined from the given information.

10. What mitral valve commissure is indicated by the arrow in image 2 for case 4?

   A. Posterolateral

   B. Posteromedial

   C. Anterolateral

   D. Anteromedial

   E. Inferior

11. Which of the following best describes the degree of mitral regurgitation shown in image 3 for case 4?

   A. Trace.

   B. Mild.

   C. Moderate.

   D. Severe.

   E. The mitral valve is not shown in this image.

12. What view is shown in image 3 for case 4?

   A. Transgastric left ventricular outflow view

   B. Deep transgastric long axis view

   C. Transgastric long axis view

   D. Midesophageal long axis view

   E. None of the above

13. Using the Carpentier classification system for mitral valve leaflet motion in mitral regurgitation, describe the leaflet motion seen in image 3 for case 4.

   A. Type I leaflet motion

   B. Type II leaflet motion

   C. Type III leaflet motion

   D. Type IV leaflet motion

   E. Type V leaflet motion

Case 5

14. Which of the following best describes the mitral valve disease seen in case 5?

    A. Calcific mitral valve disease

    B. Degenerative mitral valve disease

    C. Rheumatic mitral valve disease

    D. Carcinoid syndrome

    E. Ebstein anomaly

15. Using the Carpentier classification system for mitral valve leaflet motion in mitral regurgitation, describe the leaflet motion seen in case 5.

    A. Type I leaflet motion

    B. Type II leaflet motion

    C. Type III leaflet motion

    D. Type IV leaflet motion

    E. Type V leaflet motion

16. What mitral valve scallop is indicated by the arrow labeled A in image 10 for case 5?

    A. A1

    B. A2

    C. A3

    D. P1

    E. P2

17. What mitral valve scallop is indicated by the arrow labeled B in image 10 for case 5?

    A. A1

    B. A2

    C. A3

    D. P1

    E. P2

    F. P3

18. Using the pressure half time method, what is the mitral valve area for the patient shown in case 5?

A. 0.62 cm²

B. 0.72 cm²

C. 0.82 cm²

D. 0.92 cm²

E. 1.2 cm²

Case 6

19. Which of the following is indicated by arrow 1 shown in image 2 for case 6?

A. Right pulmonary artery

B. Coronary sinus

C. Left main coronary artery

D. Right coronary artery

E. Circumflex coronary artery

20. Given the information shown in images 3 and 4, what is the diagnosis?

A. Carcinoid syndrome

B. Secundum atrial septal defect

C. Interatrial septal aneurysm

D. Chiari network

E. Ostium primum atrial septal defect

21. This patient may be at increased risk for which of the following?

A. Pulmonary embolus

B. Cerebrovascular accident

C. Atrial fibrillation

D. Post operative renal failure

E. Mitral stenosis

Case 7

22. Which of the following is indicated by the arrow shown in image 1 for case 7?

   A. Venous cannula

   B. Aortic cannula

   C. Coronary sinus catheter

   D. Central venous line

   E. Pulmonary artery catheter

23. The arrow in image 2 for case 7 indicates which of the following?

   A. Inferior vena cava

   B. Superior vena cava

   C. Right atrial appendage

   D. Left atrial appendage

   E. Dilated coronary sinus

24. What view is shown in images 1 through 3 for case 7?

   A. Midesophageal right ventricular inflow outflow view

   B. Midesophageal right ventricular inflow view

   C. Midesophageal bicaval view

   D. Mid esophageal long axis view

   E. Mid esophageal two-chamber view

Case 8

25. What is indicated by the arrow in images 1 and 2 for case 8?

   A. Christa terminalis

   B. Right atrial tumor

   C. Thrombus

   D. Eustachian valve

   E. Chiari network

26. What treatment is necessary for this patient?

   A. Anticoagulation

   B. Surgery for tumor resection

   C. CT scan to determine the extent of the disease process

   D. Echo guided percuataneous biopsy for tumor identification

   E. No treatment needed

27. Arrow 1 in image 4 for case 8 indicates which of the following?

   A. Right pulmonary artery

   B. Right atrium

   C. Left atrium

   D. Left pulmonary artery

   E. Left atrial appendage

28. Arrow 2 in image 4 for case 8 indicates which of the following?

   A. Pulmonic valve

   B. Eustachian valve

   C. Chiari network

   D. Aortic valve

   E. Christa terminalis

29. Arrow 3 in image 4 for case 8 indicates which of the following?

   A. Left coronary cusp

   B. Right coronary cusp

   C. Non coronary cusp

   D. Anterior coronary cusp

   E. Posterior coronary cusp

Case 9

30. What is the diagnosis?

    A. Ostium primum atrial septal defect

    B. Ostium secundum atrial septal defect

    C. Sinus venosus atrial septal defect

    D. Coronary sinus atrial septal defect

    E. Perimembranous atrial septal defect

31. Mitral regurgitation in this patient is most likely due to which of the following?

    A. Cleft anterior mitral valve leaflet

    B. Cleft posterior mitral valve leaflet

    C. Mitral valve prolapse

    D. Restricted mitral valve leaflet motion

    E. Mitral regurgitation is not associated with this defect

32. Which of the following is true concerning the color flow seen in image 3?

    A. The blue color indicates a left-to-right shunt.

    B. The red color indicates a left-to-right shunt.

    C. The blue color indicates a right-to-left shunt.

    D. The red color indicates a right-to-left shunt.

    E. The black color indicates flow parallel to the transducer.

33. Which of the following is true concerning the defect shown?

    A. It is the most common type of atrial septal defect.

    B. It is associated with anomalous pulmonary venous return.

    C. It is associated with a dilated coronary sinus.

    D. It is commonly seen in Down's syndrome.

    E. It is associated with a persistent left superior vena cava.

Case 10

34. What is the diagnosis?

    A. Complete atrioventricular canal defect

    B. Truncus arteriosus

    C. Aortic coarctation

    D. Tetralogy of fallot

    E. Dextrocardia

35. Which of the following is the best agent to utilize during this anesthetic?

    A. Sevoflurane

    B. Isoflurane

    C. Desflurane

    D. Halothane

    E. Enflurane

Case 11

36. What is the diagnosis?

    A. Ostium primum atrial septal defect

    B. Patent foramen ovale

    C. Sinus venosus atrial septal defect

    D. Coronary sinus atrial septal defect

    E. Perimembranous atrial septal defect

37. Which of the following is true concerning the color flow Doppler shown?

    A. The blue color indicates a left-to-right shunt.

    B. The red color indicates a left-to-right shunt.

    C. The blue color indicates a right-to-left shunt.

    D. The red color indicates a right-to-left shunt.

    E. The black color indicates flow parallel to the transducer.

Case 12

38. What is the diagnosis?

    A. Perimembranous ventricular septal defect

    B. Supracristal ventricular septal defect

    C. Subarterial ventricular septal defect

    D. Trabecular (muscular) ventricular septal defect

    E. Inlet ventricular septal defect

39. Which of the following is true concerning the defect shown?

    A. It is the most common type of ventricular septal defect.

    B. It is also known as a conal ventricular septal defect.

    C. It is associated with anomalous pulmonary venous return.

    D. It is the most common type of VSD seen in Down's syndrome.

    E. It is associated with an ostium primum atrial septal defect.

40. Which of the following is associated with this defect?

    A. Cleft anterior mitral valve leaflet

    B. Ventricular septal aneurysms

    C. Dilated coronary sinus

    D. Atrioventricular canal defect

    E. Persistent left superior vena cava

Case 13

41. What is the diagnosis?

    A. Coronary artery aneurysm

    B. Dilated coronary sinus

    C. Persistent left superior vena cava

    D. Sinus venosus ventricular septal defect

    E. Kartagener's syndrome

42. Arrow 1 in image 6 for case 13 indicates which of the following walls?

    A. Anterior

    B. Posterior

    C. Inferior

    D. Lateral

    E. Septal

Case 14

43. Which of the following best describes this patient's volume status?

    A. Normal (euvolemic)

    B. Mildly hypovolemic

    C. Severely hypovolemic

    D. Mildly volume overloaded

    E. Severely volume overloaded

44. Which of the following best describes this patient's systolic function?

    A. Normal.

    B. Mildly decreased.

    C. Moderately decreased.

    D. Severely decreased.

    E. It cannot be determined from the images shown.

45. What view is shown in image 1 for case 14?

    A. Midesophageal five-chamber view

    B. Midesophageal two-chamber view

    C. Midesophageal left ventricular inflow/outflow view

    D. Midesophageal aortic valve long axis view

    E. Midesophageal long axis view

46. Arrow 1 indicates which of the following?

   A. Anterior wall

   B. Inferior wall

   C. Septal wall

   D. Lateral wall

   E. Posterior wall

47. Which of the following best describes the left ventricular wall thickness seen?

   A. Normal.

   B. Mild left ventricular hypertrophy.

   C. Moderate left ventricular hypertrophy.

   D. Severe left ventricular hypertrophy.

   E. It cannot be determined from the images shown.

Case 15

48. What valve is being interrogated in case 15?

   A. Tricuspid valve

   B. Pulmonic valve

   C. Aortic valve

   D. Mitral valve

   E. Eustachian valve

49. Which of the following best describes the degree of regurgitation seen in case 15?

   A. Trace.

   B. Mild.

   C. Moderate.

   D. Severe.

   E. It cannot be determined from the images shown.

Case 16

50. According to the American Society of Echocardiography 16-segment model, what numerical segment of the left ventricle is described by arrow 1?

    A. 5

    B. 6

    C. 7

    D. 8

    E. 9

51. According to the American Society of Echocardiography 16-segment model, what numerical segment of the left ventricle is described by arrow 2?

    A. 9

    B. 10

    C. 11

    D. 12

    E. 13

52. According to the American Society of Echocardiography 16-segment model, what numerical segment of the left ventricle is described by arrow 3?

    A. 12

    B. 13

    C. 14

    D. 15

    E. 16

53. According to the American Society of Echocardiography 16-segment model, what numerical segment of the left ventricle is described by arrow 4?

    A. 12

    B. 13

    C. 14

    D. 15

    E. 16

54. According to the American Society of Echocardiography 16-segment model, what numerical segment of the left ventricle is described by arrow 5?

   A. 9

   B. 10

   C. 11

   D. 12

   E. 13

Case 17

55. A 70-year-old female presents with acute diplopia lasting 30 minutes. What is the most likely diagnosis in this patient?

   A. Myxoma

   B. Rhabdomyoma

   C. Intracardiac thrombus

   D. Liposarcoma

   E. Papillary fibroelastoma

56. Which of the following best describes the interatrial septum?

   A. Aneurysmal interatrial septum with a coronary sinus atrial septal defect

   B. Aneurysmal interatrial septum with a patent foramen ovale

   C. Aneurysmal interatrial septum with a perimembranous atrial septal defect

   D. Aneurysmal interatrial septum with a sinus venosus atrial septal defect

   E. Aneurysmal interatrial septum with an ostium primum atrial septal defect

57. What treatment is indicated?

   A. Thrombolytic therapy

   B. Surgical excision

   C. Heparin drip followed by long-term Coumadin therapy

   D. Cardiac catheterization and removal via a snare device

   E. Chemotherapy

58. A wire entering the heart from which of the following sites is most likely to dislodge the mass?

  A. Right internal jugular vein

  B. Left subclavian vein

  C. Right femoral vein

  D. Right femoral artery

  E. Right subclavian vein

59. What view is shown in image 4?

  A. Midesophageal bicaval view

  B. Midesophageal right atrial inflow view

  C. Midesophageal right ventricular inflow/outflow view

  D. Transgastric right ventricular inflow view

  E. Transgastric right atrial inflow view

Case 18

60. What wall is being measured?

  A. Anterior

  B. Lateral

  C. Septal

  D. Anteroseptal

  E. Posterior

61. How would you describe the degree of hypertrophy of this wall?

  A. None, normal wall thickness.

  B. Mild hypertrophy.

  C. Moderate hypertrophy.

  D. Severe hypertrophy.

  E. It cannot be determined from the image shown.

62. What left ventricular wall segment is always spared (not hypertrophied) in patients with hypertrophic cardiomyopathy?

    A. Basal inferior wall

    B. Basal posterior wall

    C. Mid inferior wall

    D. Mid posterior wall

    E. Mid lateral wall

63. According to the American Society of Echocardiography 16-segment model, what numerical segment of the left ventricle is always spared (not hypertrophied) in patients with hypertrophic obstructive cardiomyopathy?

    A. Segment 4

    B. Segment 5

    C. Segment 7

    D. Segment 9

    E. Segment 10

64. According to the American Society of Echocardiography 16-segment model, what numerical segment of the left ventricle is described by arrow 1?

    A. Segment 7

    B. Segment 8

    C. Segment 9

    D. Segment 10

    E. Segment 11

Case 19

65. Given the epiaortic scan of the ascending thoracic aorta, how would you describe the degree of aortic atherosclerosis seen?

    A. Mild.

    B. Moderate.

    C. Severe.

    D. Epiaortic scanning cannot be used for this determination.

66. Given the epiaortic images of the ascending thoracic aorta shown, what is indicated by arrow 1?

A. Superior vena cava

B. Inferior vena cava

C. Azygos vein

D. Coronary sinus

E. Thebesian vein

Answers:

1. B	23. B	45. A
2. C	24. C	46. C
3. D	25. E	47. D
4. B	26. E	48. C
5. B	27. C	49. D
6. B	28. A	50. B
7. C	29. B	51. D
8. D	30. B	52. E
9. D	31. C	53. C
10. B	32. A	54. A
11. A	33. A	55. C
12. B	34. D	56. B
13. A	35. D	57. B
14. C	36. B	58. C
15. C	37. A	59. A
16. B	38. A	60. D
17. E	39. A	61. D
18. D	40. B	62. B
19. B	41. A	63. A
20. C	42. D	64. A
21. B	43. C	65. A
22. A	44. A	66. C

Explanations

Case 1

1. **Answer = B, Q waves in leads II, III, and AVF.** This patient has a large inferior left ventricular aneurysm. Therefore, inferior Q waves would be expected.

2. **Answer = C, A basal/mid-inferior wall left ventricular aneurysm is shown.** An aneurysm is a dilated portion of the LV wall with a wide neck and an inner wall composed of thinned myocardium. A left ventricular pseudoaneurysm is a chronic contained ventricular rupture. A pseudoaneurysm has a wall composed of pericardium (no myocardial fibers). A pseudoaneurysm is more likely to have flow in and out of it. A pseudoaneurysm has a narrow neck, with the ratio of neck diameter to maximum diameter < 0.5. In addition, a pseudoaneurysm has an acute angle between the normal myocardium and the aneurysm.

Reference: Otto C. *Textbook of Clinical Echocardiography, Third Edition.* Philadelphia: Elsevier 2004:216–218.

3. **Answer = D, Qualitative estimate of EF.** The quantitative methods will not be accurate in this patient.

Reference: Perrino AC, Reeves S. *A Practical Approach to TEE.* Philadelphia: Lippincott Williams & Wilkins 2003:37–53.

Case 2

4. **Answer = B, Severely decreased.** dp/dt is the change in pressure with respect to time during isovolumetric LV contraction. Normal systolic function is associated with a dp/dt $\geq$ 1200 mmHg/s and severely depressed systolic function is associated with a dp/dt < 400 mmHg/s.

Reference: Sidebotham D, Merry A, Legget M (eds.). *Practical Perioperative Transoesophageal Echocardiography.* Burlington, MA: Butterworth Heinemann 2003:107.

Case 3

5. **Answer = C, dp/dt = 1066.** dp/dt is the change in pressure with respect to time. It is calculated using a continuous-wave Doppler flow velocity profile of an MR jet from a velocity of 100cm/s–300cm/s. Given that dt = 0.03 sec → dp/dt = 32 / 0.03 = 1066 mmHg/sec.

Reference: Perrino AC, Reeves S. *A Practical Approach to TEE.* Philadelphia: Lippincott Williams & Wilkins 2003:42–47.

6. **Answer = A, dp/dt is the most load independent measure of systolic function listed.**

Reference: Perrino AC, Reeves S. *A Practical Approach to TEE.* Philadelphia: Lippincott Williams & Wilkins 2003:37–53.

7. **Answer = D, Velocity of circumferential shortening (Vcf, mean rate of circumferential shortening) is usually heart rate corrected and identified as Vcfc.**

Vcf = LVEDd − LVESd / LVEDd ET

LVEDd = left ventricular end diastolic dimension, LVESd = left ventricular end systolic dimension, ET = ejection time

Reference: Feigenbaum H, Armstrong WF, Ryan T. *Feigenbaum's Echocardiography, Sixth Edition.* Philadelphia: Lippincott Williams & Wilkins 2004:140.

Case 4

8. **Answer = D, The coanda effect is seen in image 1 for case 4.** This results from a high-velocity jet, which "hugs" the left atrial wall. It is indicative of a structural defect in the mitral valve, which will require surgical correction. Wall-hugging jets are considered severe.

Reference: Perrino AC, Reeves S. *A Practical Approach to TEE.* Philadelphia: Lippincott Williams & Wilkins 2003:137.

9. **Answer = D, Severe mitral regurgitation is present.** A high-velocity jet, which "hugs" the left atrial wall, results from a structural defect in the mitral valve and requires surgical correction. This phenomenon is called the coanda effect, which is indicative of severe mitral regurgitation.

Reference: Perrino AC, Reeves S. *A Practical Approach to TEE.* Philadelphia: Lippincott Williams & Wilkins 2003:137.

10. **Answer = B, The posteromedial commissure is indicated by the arrow.** In the transgastric basal short axis view, the commissures are visualized as shown in Figure 3.1A.

Reference: Sidebotham D, Merry A, Legget M (eds.). *Practical Perioperative Transoesophageal Echocardiography.* Burlington, MA: Butterworth Heinemann 2003:138.

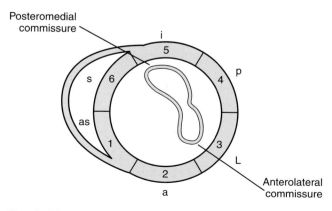

Fig. 3-1A

11. **Answer = A, Trace mitral valve regurgitation is present.**

Reference: Sidebotham D, Merry A, Legget M (eds.). *Practical Perioperative Transoesophageal Echocardiography.* Burlington, MA: Butterworth Heinemann 2003:138.

12. **Answer = B, A deep transgastric long axis view is shown.**

13. **Answer = A, Type I leaflet motion is present.** Using the Carpentier system of classification, normal leaflet motion is referred to as type I. The Carpentier classification system of leaflet motion for mitral regurgitation follows.

Carpentier class, leaflet motion:

- Type I: Normal
- Type II: Excessive
- Type III: Restrictive

Reference: Perrino AC, Reeves S. *A Practical Approach to TEE.* Philadelphia: Lippincott Williams & Wilkins 2003:162–163.

Case 5

14. **Answer = C, Rheumatic mitral valve disease is present.** The classic diastolic doming ("hockey stick") appearance of the anterior mitral valve leaflet in the midesophageal long axis view in addition to leaflet calcification, commissural fusion, and restricted leaflet motion are characteristic of rheumatic disease. This is the most common etiology for mitral stenosis. Epstein's anomaly and carcinoid syndrome predominantly affect the right-sided valves. Calcific mitral stenosis is rare, and is characterized by severe mitral annular calcification, thin mobile leaflet tips, and the absence of commissural fusion.

Reference: Otto C. *Textbook of Clinical Echocardiography, Third Edition.* Philadelphia: Elsevier 2004:295.

15. **Answer = C, Type III leaflet motion is present.** Using the Carpentier system of classification, restricted leaflet motion is referred to as type III. The Carpentier classification system of leaflet motion for mitral regurgitation follows.

Carpentier class, leaflet motion:

- Type I: Normal
- Type II: Excessive
- Type III: Restrictive

Reference: Perrino AC, Reeves S. *A Practical Approach to TEE.* Philadelphia: Lippincott Williams & Wilkins 2003:162–163.

16. **Answer = B, The A2 scallop of the anterior mitral valve leaflet is shown.** The midesophageal long axis view is shown.

Reference: Savage RM, Aronson S, Thomas JD, Shanewise JS, Shernan SK. *Comprehensive Textbook of Intraoperative Transesophageal Echocardiography.* Philadelphia: Lippincott Williams & Wilkins 2004:461.

17. **Answer = E, The P2 scallop of the anterior mitral valve leaflet is shown.** The midesophageal long axis view is shown.

Reference: Savage RM, Aronson S, Thomas JD, Shanewise JS, Shernan SK. *Comprehensive Textbook of Intraoperative Transesophageal Echocardiography.* Philadelphia: Lippincott Williams & Wilkins 2004:461.

18. **Answer = D, 0.92cm^2 = the mitral valve area (MVA) as calculated by the pressure half time (PHT) method.** MVA = 220/PHT = 220/239 = 0.92cm^2.

Reference: Perrino AC, Reeves S. *A Practical Approach to TEE.* Philadelphia: Lippincott Williams & Wilkins 2003:15.

Case 6

19. **Answer = B, The coronary sinus is shown.**

20. **Answer = C, An interatrial septum aneurysm is shown.** Interatrial septum motion of greater than 10 mm is considered excessive, and is associated with defects in the interatrial septum and with cerebrovascular accidents.

Reference: Mas JL, Arquizan C, Lamy C, Zuber M, Cabanes L, Derumeaux G, et al; Patent Foramen Ovale and Atrial Septal Aneurysm Study Group. Recurrent cerebrovascular events associated with patent foramen ovale, atrial septal aneurysm, or both. *N Engl J Med* 2001;345(24):1740–1746.

21. **Answer = B, Cerebrovascular accidents are more common in patients with interatrial aneurysms, which are associated with septal defects such as a patent foramen ovale.**

Reference: Mas JL, Arquizan C, Lamy C, Zuber M, Cabanes L, Derumeaux G, et al; Patent Foramen Ovale and Atrial Septal Aneurysm Study Group.Recurrent cerebrovascular events associated with patent foramen ovale, atrial septal aneurysm, or both. *N Engl J Med* 2001;345(24):1740–1746.

Case 7

22. **Answer = A, A venous cardiopulmonary bypass cannula is shown in the right atrium.**

23. **Answer = B, The arrow indicates the superior vena cava (SVC).**

24. **Answer = C, The midesophageal bicaval view is shown.**

Case 8

25. **Answer = E, A chiari network is shown.**

26. **Answer = E, A chiari network is a normal variant. No treatment is needed.**

27. **Answer = C, Arrow 1 in image 4 for case 8 indicates the left atrium.**

28. **Answer = A, Arrow 2 in image 4 for case 8 indicates the pulmonic valve.**

29. **Answer = B, Arrow 3 indicates the right coronary cusp.**

Case 9

30. **Answer = B, An ostium secundum atrial septal defect is shown.**

31. **Answer = C, Ostium secundum atrial septal defects are associated with mitral regurgitation due to mitral valve prolapse without a cleft anterior mitral valve leaflet.** Ostium primum atrial septal defects are associated with a cleft anterior mitral valve leaflet.

Reference: Sidebotham D, Merry A, Legget M (eds.). *Practical Perioperative Transoesophageal Echocardiography.* Burlington, MA: Butterworth Heinemann 2003:223.

32. **Answer = A, The blue color indicates a left-to-right shunt.**

Reference: Edelman SK. *Understanding Ultrasound Physics.* Woodlands, TX: ESP, Inc. 1994:155.

33. **Answer = A, Ostium secundum atrial septal defects are the most common type of atrial septal defect.**

Case 10

34. **Answer = D, Tetralogy of fallot is shown.** The four classic characteristics are as follows:

   • Ventricular septal defect
   • Right ventricular hypertrophy
   • Overriding aorta
   • Right ventricular outflow obstruction

35. **Answer = D, Tetralogy of fallot can be thought of as IHSS of the right heart.** There is dynamic obstruction of the right ventricular outflow. **Halothane** is the best choice for inhalational anesthesia for a patient with tetralogy of fallot because it best maintains the hemodynamic goals listed in Table 3.1A. Halothane decreases contractility, and it does not decrease SVR or increase heart rate as much as the other inhalational agents.

Table 3.1A.

Hemodynamic parameter:	Goal
Heart rate:	Slow
SVR:	High
Preload:	High
Contractility:	Low

IHSS = idiopathic hypertrophic subaortic stenosis, SVR = systemic vascular resistance.

Reference: Perrino AC, Reeves S. *A Practical Approach to TEE.* Philadelphia: Lippincott Williams & Wilkins 2003:294.

Case 11

36. **Answer = B, A patent foramen ovale (PFO) is shown.** The defect is located in the fossa ovalis. Defects in this region can be due to a PFO or an ostium secundum atrial septal defect.

37. **Answer = A, The blue color indicates a left-to-right shunt.**

Reference: Edelman SK. *Understanding Ultrasound Physics.* Woodlands, TX: ESP, Inc. 1994:155.

Case 12

38. **Answer = A, A perimembranous = infracristal = membranous ventricular septal defect (VSD) is shown.**

39. **Answer = A, Perimembranous or membranous ventricular septal defects (VSDs) are the most common type, composing about 70% of all VSDs.** Conal VSD is not a synonym for this type of defect (conal = subarterial = supracristal VSD). Sinus venosus atrial septal defects are associated with anomalous pulmonary venous return. Down's syndrome patients frequently have an inlet VSD, which (when combined with an ostium primum ASD) can be part of a complete AV canal defect.

VSD = ventricular septal defect, ASD = atrial septal defect, AV = atrioventricular.

Reference: Otto C. *Textbook of Clinical Echocardiography,* Third Edition. Philadelphia: Elsevier 2004:473.

40. **Answer = B, Perimembranous ventricular septal defects are sometimes associated with an aneurysm involving the membranous intraventricular septum composed of tricuspid valve tissue.** This pouch of tissue protrudes into the ventricle.

Reference: Perrino AC, Reeves S. *A Practical Approach to TEE.* Philadelphia: Lippincott Williams & Wilkins 2003:290.

Case 13

41. **Answer = A, A coronary artery aneurysm is shown.**

42. **Answer = D, The lateral wall is shown.**

Case 14

43. **Answer = C, Severe hypovolemia is present.**

44. **Answer = A, Normal systolic function is seen.**

45. **Answer = A, The midesophageal five-chamber view is shown.** When the left ventricular outflow tract (LVOT) is seen from a four-chamber view it is sometimes referred to as a five-chamber view (the LVOT constituting the fifth chamber).

46. **Answer = C, The septal wall is shown.**

47. **Answer = D, Severe left ventricular hypertrophy (LVH) is present.**
    A left ventricular free wall thickness or greater than 20 millimeters is considered severe LVH.

Case 15

48. **Answer = C, The aortic valve is shown from the deep transgastric long axis view.**

49. **Answer = D, Severe aortic insufficiency is present.**

Case 16

50. **Answer = B, Segment 6, the basal septal wall segment, is indicated by arrow 1.**

Reference: Shanewise JS, Cheung AT, Aronson S, Stewart WJ, Weiss RL, Mark JB, et al. ASE/SCA guidelines for performing a comprehensive intraoperative multiplane transesophageal echocardiography examination. *J Am Soc Echocardiog* 1999;12:884–900.

51. **Answer = D, Segment 12, the mid septal wall segment, is indicated by arrow 2.**

Reference: Shanewise JS, Cheung AT, Aronson S, Stewart WJ, Weiss RL, Mark JB, et al. ASE/SCA guidelines for performing a comprehensive intraoperative multiplane transesophageal echocardiography examination. *J Am Soc Echocardiog* 1999;12:884–900.

52. **Answer = E, Segment 16, the apical septal wall segment, is indicated by arrow 3.**

Reference: Shanewise JS, Cheung AT, Aronson S, Stewart WJ, Weiss RL, Mark JB, et al. ASE/SCA guidelines for performing a comprehensive intraoperative multiplane transesophageal echocardiography examination. *J Am Soc Echocardiog* 1999;12:884–900.

53. **Answer = C, Segment 14, the apical lateral wall segment, is indicated by arrow 4.**

Reference: Shanewise JS, Cheung AT, Aronson S, Stewart WJ, Weiss RL, Mark JB, et al. ASE/SCA guidelines for performing a comprehensive intraoperative multiplane transesophageal echocardiography examination. *J Am Soc Echocardiog* 1999;12:884–900.

54. **Answer = A, Segment 9, the mid lateral wall segment, is indicated by arrow 5.**

Reference: Shanewise JS, Cheung AT, Aronson S, Stewart WJ, Weiss RL, Mark JB, et al. ASE/SCA guidelines for performing a comprehensive intraoperative multiplane transesophageal echocardiography examination. *J Am Soc Echocardiog* 1999;12:884–900.

Case 17

55. **Answer = C, An intracardiac thrombus is present.**

56. **Answer = B, An interatrial septum aneurysm and a patent foramen ovale are present. A large thrombus is traversing the interatrial septum.**

57. **Answer = B, Urgent surgical excision is the treatment of choice to avoid embolic injury.**

58. **Answer = C, A wire inserted into the right atrium from the inferior vena cava may be directed toward the foramen ovale by the eustachian valve and therefore would be more likely to dislodge the thrombus.**

59. **Answer = A, The midesophageal bicaval view is shown in image 4.**

Case 18

60. **Answer = D, The anteroseptal wall is being measured.**

61. **Answer = D, Severe left ventricular hypertrophy is present** (see Table 3.1B).

Table 3.1B.

Degree of LVH	LV Free Wall Thickness
Normal	6–11 mm
Mild LVH	12–14 mm
Moderate LVH	15–19 mm
Severe LVH	≥ 20 mm

Abbreviations: LV = left ventricle, LVH = left ventricle hypertrophy.

62. **Answer = B, The basal posterior wall is never hypertrophied in hypertrophic cardiomyopathy.** There are four types of hypertrophic cardiomyopathy defined by the location of left ventricular hypertrophy. These four types have the following common findings: the interventricular septum is always hypertrophied and the basal posterior wall is always spared (not hypertrophied).

Reference: Otto C. *Textbook of Clinical Echocardiography, Third Edition.* Philadelphia: Elsevier 2004:233.

63. **Answer = A, Segment 4, the basal posterior wall, is always spared in hypertrophic cardiomyopathy.**

References: Otto C. *Textbook of Clinical Echocardiography, Third Edition.* Philadelphia: Elsevier 2004:233; Shanewise JS, Cheung AT, Aronson S, Stewart WJ, Weiss RL, Mark JB, et al. ASE/SCA guidelines for performing a comprehensive intraoperative multiplane transesophageal echocardiography examination. *J Am Soc Echocardiog* 1999;12:884–900.

64. **Answer = A, Segment 7, the mid anteroseptal wall, is shown by arrow 1**

Reference: Shanewise JS, Cheung AT, Aronson S, Stewart WJ, Weiss RL, Mark JB, et al. ASE/SCA guidelines for performing a comprehensive intraoperative multiplane transesophageal echocardiography examination. *J Am Soc Echocardiog* 1999;12:884–900.

Case 19

65. **Answer = A, Mild atherosclerosis is seen (< 3 mm).**

66. **Answer = C, The azygos vein is shown.**

TEST III PART 2

Written Test Booklet

1. Which of the following is the maximum spatial peak temporal average intensity recommended for focused ultrasound beams?

   A. 100 mW/cm^2

   B. 1 W/cm^2

   C. 10 W/cm^2

   D. 100 W/cm^2

   E. 1 kW/cm^2

2. A 5-MHz transducer emits a pulse containing two cycles. What is the numerical value of the axial resolution?

   A. 0.21 mm

   B. 0.31 mm

   C. 0.41 mm

   D. 0.51 mm

   E. 0.61 mm

3. Which of the following types of imaging has the best temporal resolution?

   A. A-mode

   B. B-mode

   C. M-mode

   D. Two-dimensional imaging

   E. Continuous-wave Doppler

NOTE: Use Table 3.2A to answer the next four (4) questions.

Table 3.2A.

Echo Parameter	Contractility	EDA	ESA	FAC	CO	E/E′
Scenario A	Normal	Decreased	Decreased	Normal	Decreased	< 15
Scenario B	Normal	Decreased	Decreased	Normal	Decreased	> 15
Scenario C	Normal	Normal	Decreased	Increased	Increased	< 15
Scenario D	Decreased	Increased	Increased	Decreased	Decreased	> 15
Scenario E	Normal	Increased	Increased	Increased	Increased	< 15

Abbreviations: EDA = end diastolic area, ESA = end systolic area, FAC = fractional area change, CO = cardiac output, E/E′ = ratio of transmitral peak E-wave velocity to the early peak lateral mitral annular tissue velocity (E′ = E_M = E "prime").

4. Which of the following scenarios (Table 3.2A) would be expected with decreased systolic function?

   A. Scenario A

   B. Scenario B

   C. Scenario C

   D. Scenario D

   E. Scenario E

5. Which of the following scenarios (Table 3.2A) would be expected with low systemic vascular resistance?

   A. Scenario A

   B. Scenario B

   C. Scenario C

   D. Scenario D

   E. Scenario E

6. Which of the following scenarios (Table 3.2A) would be expected with reduced left ventricular compliance?

   A. Scenario A

   B. Scenario B

   C. Scenario C

   D. Scenario D

   E. Scenario E

7. Which of the following scenarios (Table 3.2A) would be expected with hypovolemia (decreased intravascular volume status)?

   A. Scenario A

   B. Scenario B

   C. Scenario C

   D. Scenario D

   E. Scenario E

8. What percentage of endocardial thickening is consistent with normal segmental wall motion?

   A. > 15%

   B. > 20%

   C. > 25%

   D. > 30%

   E. > 35%

9. What percentage of endocardial thickening is consistent with mild hypokinesis?

   A. 5–15%

   B. 10–20%

   C. 15–25%

   D. 10–30%

   E. 15–35%

10. What percentage of endocardial thickening is consistent with severe hypokinesis?

   A. < 20%

   B. < 15%

   C. < 10%

   D. < 5%

   E. None of the above

11. According to the ASE (American Society of Echocardiography), what numerical grade is given to normal wall motion?

    A. Grade 1

    B. Grade 2

    C. Grade 3

    D. Grade 4

    E. Grade 5

12. According to the ASE (American Society of Echocardiography), what numerical grade is given to mild hypokinesis?

    A. Grade 1

    B. Grade 2

    C. Grade 3

    D. Grade 4

    E. Grade 5

13. Which of the following mitral valve chordae tendinae arise from the papillary muscles and attach to the undersurface of the mitral valve leaflets?

    A. First-order chordae

    B. Second-order chordae

    C. Third-order chordae

    D. Fourth-order chordae

    E. None of the above

14. Which of the following mitral valve scallops is most likely to be supported solely by the anterolateral papillary muscle?

    A. A_3

    B. P_2

    C. P_3

    D. P_1

    E. None of the above

15. Which of the following best describes the most common perfusion of the posteromedial papillary muscle?

   A. Left anterior descending coronary artery

   B. Right coronary artery

   C. Circumflex coronary artery

   D. Circumflex and left anterior descending coronary arteries

   E. Circumflex and right coronary arteries

16. A patient has a tricuspid regurgitant jet area to right atrial area ratio of 63%. Which of the following best describes the severity of tricuspid regurgitation in this patient?

   A. Trace (grade I).

   B. Mild (grade II).

   C. Moderate (grade III).

   D. Severe (grade IV).

   E. It cannot be determined from the given information.

NOTE: Use the information obtained from a patient with no valvular regurgitation (Table 3.2B) to answer the next six (6) questions.

Table 3.2B.

DT_{MV} = 1063 msec	CVP = 10 mmHg	LA diameter = 48 mm
$TVI_{MVinflow}$ = 59 cm	BP = 120/80	RA diameter = 31 mm
TVI_{AV} = 52 cm	LAP = 12 mmHg	Sinus of valsalva diameter = 32 mm
TVI_{TV} = 13 cm	BSA = 2 M^2	ST ridge diameter = 24 mm

Abbreviations: DT_{MV} = mitral valve inflow deceleration time,
$TVI_{MVinflow}$ = mitral valve inflow time velocity integral,
TVI_{AV} = time velocity integral of blood flow through the aortic valve,
TVI_{TV} = time velocity integral of blood flow through the tricuspid valve, CVP = central venous pressure,
BP = systemic blood pressure, LAP = left atrial pressure, BSA = body surface area, LA = left atrial,
RA = right atrial, ST = sinotubular.

17. What is the left ventricular outflow tract stroke volume?

   A. 22 ml

   B. 32 ml

   C. 42 ml

   D. 52 ml

   E. 62 ml

18. What is the aortic valve area?

   A. 0.81 cm^2.

   B. 0.91 cm^2.

   C. 1.1 cm^2.

   D. 2.1 cm^2.

   E. It cannot be determined from the given data.

19. What is the tricuspid valve area?

   A. 0.8 cm^2

   B. 1 cm^2

   C. 2.2 cm^2

   D. 3 cm^2

   E. 3.2 cm^2

20. Which of the following best describes the degree of mitral stenosis?

   A. No stenosis.

   B. Mild.

   C. Moderate.

   D. Severe.

   E. It cannot be determined from the given information.

21. Which of the following best describes the degree of aortic stenosis?

   A. No stenosis.

   B. Mild.

   C. Moderate.

   D. Severe.

   E. It cannot be determined from the given data.

22. Which of the following best describes the degree of tricuspid stenosis?

  A. No stenosis.

  B. Mild.

  C. Moderate.

  D. Severe.

  E. It cannot be determined from the given information.

23. The percentage or fraction of time the ultrasound beam is producing a pulse or transmitting sound is known as the _____.

  A. Bandwidth

  B. Pulse repetition period

  C. Duty factor

  D. Power

  E. Resonant frequency

24. Which of the following is the correct formula for amplitude?

  A. $dB = Log\, A_2/A_1$

  B. $dB = 10\, Log\, A_2/A_1$

  C. $dB = 20\, Log\, A_2/A_1$

  D. $dB = 30\, Log\, A_2/A_1$

25. An *increase* of which of the following will *increase* the amount of *ultrasound attenuation*?

  A. Number of cycles in a pulse

  B. Pulse duration

  C. Image depth

  D. Stiffness of the medium

  E. Density of the medium

26. Which of the following is true concerning attenuation?

   A. As piezoelectric crystal thickness increases, attenuation decreases.

   B. As pulse repetition period increases, attenuation increases.

   C. As frequency increases, attenuation decreases.

   D. As spatial pulse length increases, attenuation increases.

   E. As bandwidth increases, attenuation decreases.

27. Which of the following is the primary form of attenuation in soft tissue?

   A. Scattering

   B. Reflection

   C. Absorption

   D. Refraction

28. The half-value layer thickness is the thickness of tissue required to reduce the *intensity* of a sound beam by half. How many dB of attenuation does this represent?

   A. 3 dB

   B. 6 dB

   C. 9 dB

   D. 10 dB

   E. 12 db

29. Which of the following is true concerning the intensity reflection coefficient?

   A. It is determined by the acoustic impedance of the two media.

   B. It is equal to the reflected intensity / incident intensity $\times$ 100%.

   C. It equals: (incident intensity − transmission intensity) / incident intensity $\times$ 100%.

   D. All of the above.

   E. None of the above.

NOTE: Use the chart in Table 3.2C to answer the next two (2) questions.

Table 3.2C.

Medium 1	Medium 2	Medium 3	Medium 4
Density = 0.5	Density = 0.5	Density = 1	Density = 2
Elasticity = 0.5	Elasticity = 2	Elasticity = 1	Elasticity = 1

30. An ultrasound beam passes from medium 1 to medium 2. The angle of incidence is 72 degrees. Which of the following is **most** likely correct regarding the reflection angle?

   A. Reflection cannot occur.

   B. The reflection angle is less than 72 degrees.

   C. The reflection angle equals 72 degrees.

   D. The reflection angle is greater than 72 degrees.

31. An ultrasound beam travels from medium 1 to medium 2. Which of the following is true concerning refraction?

   A. It is greater when the velocity difference between the two media is small.

   B. It requires oblique incidence.

   C. The transmission angle is greater than the incident angle when the velocity of medium 2 is less than velocity of medium 1.

   D. All of the above.

   E. None of the above.

32. Which of the following is true concerning the damping material?

   A. It decreases bandwidth.

   B. It is also known as the backing material.

   C. It increases the Q factor (quality factor).

   D. It improves the transducers sensitivity to reflected echoes.

33. Which of the following correctly places the given materials in decreasing order of acoustic impedance (from largest to smallest)?

    A. PZT > matching layer > gel > skin

    B. Skin > gel > matching layer > PZT

    C. Skin > matching layer > gel > PZT

    D. PZT > gel > matching layer > skin

    PZT = piezoelectric crystal, gel = ultrasound gel

34. Which of the following is determined by the *thickness* of a piezoelectric crystal?

    A. The frequency of a continuous-wave Doppler beam

    B. The wavelength of a pulsed-wave Doppler beam

    C. The pulse repetition period

    D. The velocity of a pulsed-wave Doppler beam

    E. The velocity of a continuous-wave Doppler beam

35. What determines the frequency of a continuous-wave ultrasound beam?

    A. The thickness of the piezoelectric crystal.

    B. The propagation speed of sound in the ultrasound crystal.

    C. The electrical frequency of the excitation voltage applied to the crystal.

    D. The acoustic impedance of the damping material.

    E. Both A and B are correct.

36. What determines the frequency of a pulsed-wave ultrasound beam?

    A. The thickness of the piezoelectric crystal.

    B. The propagation speed of sound in the ultrasound crystal.

    C. The electrical frequency of the excitation voltage applied to the crystal.

    D. Both A and B are correct.

37. Which of the following is most likely true concerning the resonant frequency of a TEE piezoelectric crystal producing pulsed ultrasound?

    A. It is directly proportional to the crystal thickness.

    B. It increases as crystal density increases.

    C. It is determined by the electrical frequency of the excitation voltage applied to the crystal.

    D. It is directly proportional to the velocity of the sound in the crystal.

38. If the resonant frequency of the electrical excitation voltage of a pulsed-wave TEE transducer is 8 MHz, what is the frequency of the pulsed-wave ultrasound beam?

    A. 2 MHz.

    B. 4 MHz.

    C. 8 MHz.

    D. 16 MHz.

    E. It cannot be determined from the given information.

39. Which of the following is most likely true concerning the Quality factor (Q factor)?

    A. It is inversely related to the resonant frequency.

    B. It is directly related to the bandwidth.

    C. Short pulses contain sound with a broad range of frequencies and a low Q factor.

    D. Therapeutic ultrasound transducers tend to have lower Q factors than imaging transducers.

40. A TEE transducer with a resonant frequency of 10 MHz emits a pulse. The lowest frequency in the pulse is 6 MHz and the highest frequency in the pulse is 14 MHz. What is the bandwidth of the TEE transducer?

    A. 14

    B. 10

    C. 6

    D. 8

    E. 4

41. A TEE transducer with a resonant frequency of 10 MHz emits a pulse. The lowest frequency in the pulse is 6 MHz and the highest frequency in the pulse is 14 MHz. What is the Q factor of the transducer?

    A. 14/6

    B. 6/14

    C. 10/8

    D. 8/10

42. Which of the following is most likely to be true concerning the focal length?

    A. It increases as frequency decreases.

    B. It is proportional to the radius of the transducer face squared.

    C. It is decreased as crystal diameter increases.

    D. It is also known as the Fraunhofer zone length.

43. Which of the following is a synonym for lateral resolution?

    A. Longitudinal resolution

    B. Axial resolution

    C. Radial resolution

    D. Range resolution

    E. Depth resolution

    F. None of the above

44. Which of the following images will most likely have the greatest temporal resolution?

    A. M-mode (motion mode) image

    B. Two-dimensional linear phased-array image

    C. Continuous-wave two-dimensional image of the left ventricular outflow tract

    D. B-mode (brightness mode) image

45. Which of the following is true concerning linear phased-array transducers?

   A. Beam steering is electronic.

   B. Beam focusing is electronic.

   C. The location of the focus can be changed.

   D. All of the above are correct.

46. Which of the following is most likely to *improve* the temporal resolution of a mid esophageal four-chamber-view two-beat loop?

   A. An increase in heart rate from 48 to 110 beats/min

   B. An increase in line density

   C. A decrease in imaging depth

   D. A decrease in the frame rate

   E. An increase in the number of foci per line

47. The imaging depth is increased from 10 to 12 cm. Which of the following is most likely?

   A. Listening time for returning echoes is increased.

   B. Pulse repetition period is decreased.

   C. Pulse repetition frequency is increased.

   D. Decreased time is required to image each scan line.

   E. Temporal resolution is increased.

NOTE: Use the variance map shown in Figure 3.2A to answer the next three (3) color flow Doppler questions.

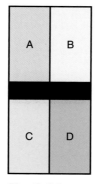

Fig. 3-2A

48. Which letter corresponds to the color that would be expected in color flow Doppler imaging of turbulent flow moving toward the transducer at an angle of 30 degrees?

    A. A

    B. B

    C. C

    D. D

    E. E

49. Which letter corresponds to the color that would be expected in color flow Doppler imaging of laminar flow moving away from the transducer at an angle of 60 degrees?

    A. A

    B. B

    C. C

    D. D

    E. E

50. Which letter corresponds to the color that would be expected in color flow Doppler imaging of turbulent flow moving away from the transducer at an angle of 90 degrees?

    A. A

    B. B

    C. C

    D. D

    E. E

51. Which of the following ventricular septal defects (VSDs) is associated with ventricular septal aneurysms?

    A. Perimembranous

    B. Aortic outflow

    C. Subarterial

    D. Trabecular (muscular)

    E. Inlet

52. Which of the following is the most common type of ventricular septal defect?

   A. Perimembranous

   B. Aortic outflow

   C. Subarterial

   D. Trabecular (muscular)

   E. Inlet

53. Which ventricular septal defect when combined with ostium primum atrial septal defect creates a complete atrioventricular (AV) canal defect (AV septal defect)?

   A. Perimembranous

   B. Aortic outflow

   C. Subarterial

   D. Trabecular (muscular)

   E. Inlet

54. Which type of ventricular septal defect occurs in the muscular portion of the intraventricular septum?

   A. Perimembranous

   B. Aortic outflow

   C. Subarterial

   D. Trabecular

   E. Inlet

NOTE: Use Table 3.2D to answer the following three (3) questions.

Table 3.2D.

$V_{TRjet} = 500$ cm/s	HR = 80 beats/min	LVOT diameter = 22 mm
$V_{PSjet} = 400$ cm/s	SBP = 160 mmHg	PA diameter = 20 mm
$V_{Allate} = 400$ cm/s	DBP = 90 mmHg	Pulmonic valve area = 3.3 cm^3
$V_{MRjet} = 1100$ cm/s	CVP = 10 mmHg	Sinus of valsalva diameter = 32 mm

Abbreviations: RVSP = right ventricular systolic pressure, RAP = right atrial pressure, CVP = central venous pressure, PASP = pulmonary artery systolic pressure, V_{PSjet} = pulmonic stenosis peak flow velocity by Doppler = velocity of systolic flow across the pulmonic valve, V_{TRjet} = peak velocity of the tricuspid valve regurgitant jet, LVEDP = left ventricular end diastolic pressure, SBP = systolic blood pressure, DBP = diastolic blood pressure.

55. Which of the following is the best estimate of the right ventricular systolic pressure?

A. 110 mmHg

B. 100 mmHg

C. 90 mmHg

D. 80 mmHg

E. 60 mmHg

56. Which of the following is the best estimate of the pulmonary artery systolic pressure?

A. 26 mmHg

B. 36 mmHg

C. 46 mmHg

D. 56 mmHg

E. 110 mmHg

57. Which of the following is the best estimate of the left ventricular end diastolic pressure?

A. 8 mmHg

B. 12 mmHg

C. 18 mmHg

D. 26 mmHg

E. 32 mmHg

NOTE: Use Table 3.2E to answer the next five (5) questions.

Table 3.2E.

$TVI_{LVOT} = 30$ cm	BP = 140/75 mmHg	LVOT diameter = 20 mm
$TVI_{MV} = 15$ cm	HR = 100 beats/min	AV side length = 1.3 cm
$V_{AIearly} = 600$ cm/sec	CVP = 10 mmHg	Sinus of valsalva diameter = 33 mm
$V_{AIlate} = 400$ cm/sec	$PHT_{MVinflow} = 60$ msec	Sinotubular ridge diameter = 22 mm
$V_{MVpeak} = 85$ cm/sec	$PHT_{AIjet decay} = 400$ msec	Left atrial diameter = 39 mm

Abbreviations: TVI_{LVOT} = time velocity integral of flow through the mitral valve, $V_{AIearly}$ = early max (peak) velocity of the aortic insufficiency jet, V_{AIlate} = late max (peak) velocity of the aortic insufficiency jet (AI end diastolic V), TVI_{MV} = time velocity integral of diastolic inflow through the mitral valve, $PHT_{AIjet decay}$ = pressure half time of the aortic insufficiency jet decay, $PHT_{MVinflow}$ = pressure half time of diastolic mitral inflow, BP = blood pressure, HR = heart rate, CVP = central venous pressure, LVOT = left ventricular outflow tract, AV = aortic valve.

58. What is the stroke volume of blood flow through the mitral valve?

   A. 45 cm^3

   B. 55 cm^3

   C. 65 cm^3

   D. 75 cm^3

   E. 85 cm^3

59. What is the stroke volume of blood flow through the left ventricular outflow tract?

   A. 54.2 cm^3

   B. 64.2 cm^3

   C. 74.2 cm^3

   D. 84.2 cm^3

   E. 94.2 cm^3

60. What is the aortic valve regurgitant volume?

   A. 39 cm^3

   B. 49 cm^3

   C. 59 cm^3

   D. 69 cm^3

   E. 79 cm^3

61. What is the left ventricular end diastolic pressure?

   A. 11

   B. 14

   C. 17

   D. 19

   E. 22

62. What is the aortic valve regurgitant fraction?

    A. 21%

    B. 31%

    C. 41%

    D. 51%

    E. 61%

63. An aortic aneurysm starts just above the diaphragm several centimeters distal to the left subclavian artery and extends to the aortic bifurcation. How would this aneurysm be best described according to the Crawford classification system?

    A. Crawford type I

    B. Crawford type II

    C. Crawford type III

    D. Crawford type IV

    E. Crawford type V

64. Which of the following has an effect on transmitral pulsed-wave Doppler flow velocity profiles?

    A. Heart rate

    B. Atrial contractility

    C. Left ventricular compliance

    D. Mitral valve disease

    E. All of the above

65. Which of the following is true concerning the isovolumic relaxation time (IVRT)?

    A. It is decreased in restrictive diastolic dysfunction.

    B. It is increased in patients with increased left atrial pressure.

    C. It is decreased in patients with impaired left ventricular relaxation.

    D. In normal diastolic function it is between 110 and 160 milliseconds.

    E. It is decreased in patients with pseudonormal diastolic dysfunction.

66. Which of the following is characteristic of impaired left ventricular relaxation?

   A. Shortened isovolemic relaxation time (IVRT)

   B. Increased E/A ratio

   C. Lateral mitral annular tissue Doppler E´ > 8 cm/sec

   D. Prolonged E-wave deceleration time

   E. Increased transmitral pulsed-wave Doppler E-wave peak velocity

NOTE: Use Figure 3.2B to answer the next two (2) questions.

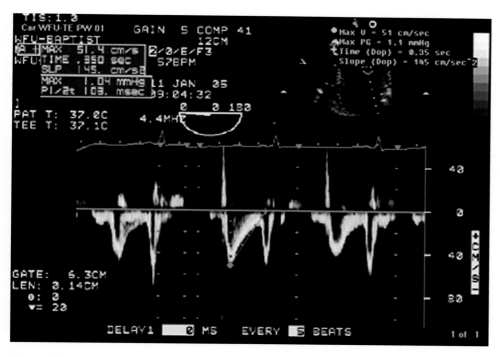

Fig. 3-2B

67. Given the transmitral flow velocities, which of the following best describes this patient's diastolic function?

   A. Restrictive diastolic dysfunction

   B. Impaired relaxation

   C. Constrictive diastolic dysfunction

   D. Pseudonormal diastolic dysfunction

   E. Normal diastolic function

68. Given the transmitral flow velocities, which of the following statements concerning this patient's E/A ratio is most likely correct?

A. E/A will be increased with increasing heart rate.

B. E/A will be decreased after administration of nitroglycerin.

C. The E/A ratio is consistent with restrictive diastolic dysfunction.

D. The E/A ratio will be increased immediately after a valsalva.

E. None of the above.

NOTE: Use Figure 3.2C to answer the next question.

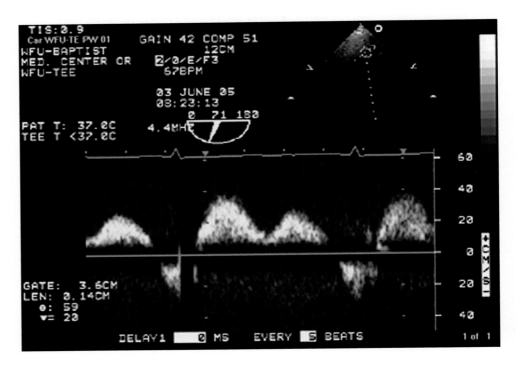

Fig. 3-2C

69. What valvular disorder would most likely be consistent with an abnormal enlargement of the hepatic venous flow wave indicated by the arrow in the figure?

A. Tricuspid regurgitation

B. Mitral regurgitation

C. Tricuspid stenosis

D. Pulmonic stenosis

E. Pulmonic regurgitation

NOTE: Use Figure 3.2D to answer the next five (5) questions.

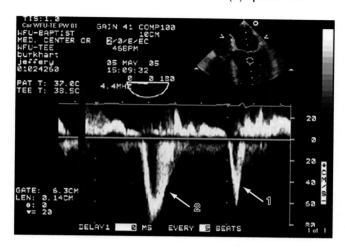

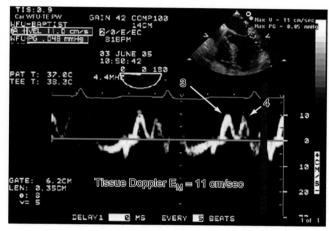

Fig. 3-2D

70. What name best describes the wave indicated by arrow 1 in the figure?

A. Transmitral pulsed-wave Doppler E wave

B. Transmitral pulsed-wave Doppler A wave

C. Transmitral pulsed-wave Doppler S wave

D. Transmitral pulsed-wave Doppler D wave

E. Transmitral pulsed-wave Doppler V wave

71. How would you describe this patient's diastolic function?

     A. Normal

     B. Restrictive

     C. Pseudonormal

     D. Impaired relaxation

     E. Constrictive

72. What name best describes the wave indicated by arrow 2 in the figure?

     A. Transmitral pulsed-wave Doppler E wave

     B. Transmitral pulsed-wave Doppler A wave

     C. Transmitral pulsed-wave Doppler S wave

     D. Transmitral pulsed-wave Doppler D wave

     E. Transmitral pulsed-wave Doppler V wave

73. What name best describes the wave indicated by arrow 3 in the figure?

     A. Lateral mitral annular tissue Doppler E_M wave

     B. Lateral mitral annular tissue Doppler A_M wave

     C. Lateral mitral annular tissue Doppler S wave

     D. Lateral mitral annular tissue Doppler D wave

     E. Lateral mitral annular tissue Doppler V wave

74. What name best describes the wave indicated by arrow 4 in the figure?

     A. Lateral mitral annular tissue Doppler E_M wave

     B. Lateral mitral annular tissue Doppler A_M wave

     C. Lateral mitral annular tissue Doppler S wave

     D. Lateral mitral annular tissue Doppler D wave

     E. Lateral mitral annular tissue Doppler V wave

NOTE: Use Figure 3.2E to answer the next question.

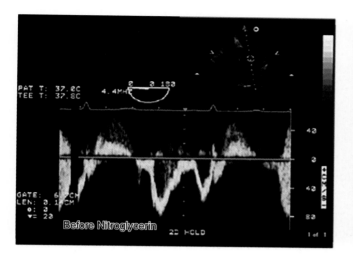

Fig. 3-2E1

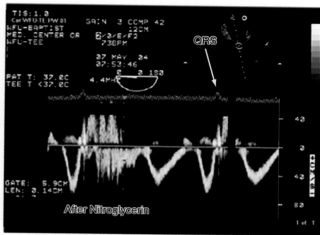

Fig. 3-2E2

75. The transmitral pulsed-wave Doppler velocity profiles were obtained from a patient before and after administration of nitroglycerin. Which of the following best describes this patient's diastolic function?

A. Normal

B. Pseudonormal

C. Restrictive

D. Impaired relaxation

E. Constrictive

NOTE: Use the pulmonary vein flow velocity profile shown in Figure 3.2F to answer the next three (3) questions.

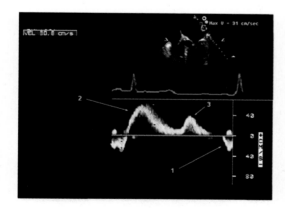

Fig. 3-2F

76. Which of the following best describes the wave labeled 1?

   A. PV$_{AR}$ wave

   B. S wave

   C. D wave

   D. V wave

   E. E wave

77. Which of the following best describes the wave labeled 2?

   A. PV$_{AR}$ wave

   B. S wave

   C. D wave

   D. V wave

   E. E wave

78. Which of the following best describes the wave labeled 3?

   A. PV$_{AR}$ wave

   B. S wave

   C. D wave

   D. V wave

   E. E wave

NOTE: Use the transmitral and pulmonary vein flow velocities shown in Figure 3.2G to answer the next five (5) questions.

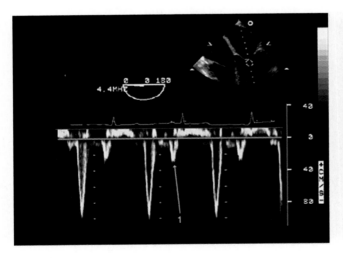
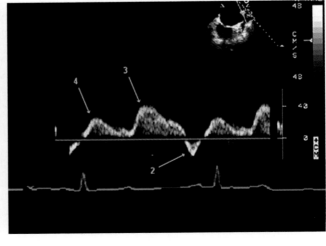

Fig. 3-2G

79. Given the transmitral and pulmonary vein pulsed-wave Doppler profiles, which of the following best describes this patient's diastolic function?

    A. Normal

    B. Pseudonormal

    C. Impaired relaxation

    D. Restrictive

    E. Constrictive

80. Arrow 1 indicates which of the following flow waves?

    A. E wave

    B. A wave

    C. S wave

    D. D wave

    E. PV_{AR} wave

81. Arrow 2 indicates which of the following flow waves?

    A. E wave

    B. A wave

    C. S wave

    D. D wave

    E. PV_{AR} wave

82. Arrow 3 indicates which of the following flow waves?

    A. E wave

    B. A wave

    C. S wave

    D. D wave

    E. PV$_{AR}$ wave

83. Arrow 4 indicates which of the following flow waves?

    A. E wave

    B. A wave

    C. S wave

    D. D wave

    E. PV$_{AR}$ wave

84. Which of the following is the range for a small pericardial effusion?

    A. < 0.1 cm

    B. < 0.5 cm

    C. < 1.0 cm

    D. < 1.5 cm

    E. < 2 cm

85. Which of the following would be expected to decrease with spontaneous expiration in constrictive pericarditis?

    A. Pulmonary venous D-wave peak velocity

    B. Pulmonary venous S-wave peak velocity

    C. Transmitral peak E-wave velocity

    D. Transtricuspid peak E-wave velocity

    E. Hepatic venous A wave

86. Which of the following is the most common location of a cardiac myxoma?

    A. Right atrium

    B. Left atrium

    C. Right ventricle

    D. Left ventricular apex

    E. Left ventricular outflow tract

87. Which of the following is the most common attachment site of an intracardiac myxoma?

    A. Interatrial septum on the right atrial side

    B. Interatrial septum on the left atrial side

    C. Near the internal vena cava of the right atrium

    D. Near the superior vena cava of the right atrium

    E. Posterior wall of the left ventricle

88. Which of the following is *not* a possible complication/finding associated with cardiac myxomas?

    A. Impaired left ventricular diastolic filling.

    B. Arrhythmias.

    C. Embolic events.

    D. Left ventricular outflow tract obstruction.

    E. All of the above are possible complications/findings associated with cardiac myxomas.

89. Which of the following is a benign primary cardiac tumor usually found within the left ventricular free wall?

    A. Myxoma

    B. Angiosarcoma

    C. Fibroma

    D. Thymoma

    E. Rhabdomyoma

90. Which of the following is the most common tumor in children?

   A. Angiosarcoma

   B. Malignant teratoma

   C. Rhabdomyosarcoma

   D. Rhabdomyoma

   E. Myxoma

91. Which of the following is most frequently affected by papillary fibroelastomas?

   A. Tricuspid valve

   B. Pulmonic valve

   C. Mitral valve

   D. Aortic valve

   E. Left atrium

92. Where do angiosarcomas most frequently occur?

   A. Right atrium

   B. Right ventricle

   C. Left atrium

   D. Left ventricle

   E. Aorta

93. Which of the following is a complication frequently associated with papillary fibroelastoma?

   A. Arrhythmias

   B. Impaired left ventricular diastolic filling

   C. Embolic events

   D. Heart failure

   E. Severe valvular insufficiency

94. Which of the following is associated with an increased incidence of a patent foramen ovale?

    A. Prominent thebesian valve

    B. Prominent eustachian valve

    C. Lipomatous interatrial septum

    D. Aneurysmal interatrial septum

    E. Crista teminalis

95. Which of the following is associated with an increased incidence of stroke?

    A. Chiari network

    B. Moderator band

    C. Aneurysmal interatrial septum

    D. Coumadin ridge

    E. Lipomatous interatrial septum

96. Which of the following will damage a TEE probe?

    A. Lodine

    B. Mineral oil

    C. Acetone

    D. Benzocaine spray

    E. All of the above

97. Which of the following is *not* a potential complication of intraoperative TEE?

    A. Thermal injury.

    B. Transient bacteremia.

    C. Cardiac arrhythmias.

    D. Splenic injury.

    E. All are potential complications of intraoperative TEE.

98. The ultrasound machine assumes that sound travels in a straight line. If sound bends, the ultrasound machine places objects in improper locations. What type of artifact is explained by this?

    A. Enhancement artifact

    B. Refraction artifact

    C. Acoustic warping

    D. Ring-down artifact

    E. Reverberation artifact

99. Which of the following artifacts places a second (artifactual) copy of a reflector to the side and very slightly deeper than the true (actual = anatomic) reflector?

    A. Reverberation artifact

    B. Refraction artifact

    C. Multipath artifact

    D. Comet tail artifact

    E. Acoustic speckle

100. Which of the following artifacts places a second copy (artifactual copy) of a reflector deeper and to the side of the true anatomy?

    A. Comet tail artifact

    B. Beam width artifact

    C. Mirror image artifact

    D. Grating lobe artifact

    E. Multipath artifact

101. Which of the following artifacts results in anatomic structures being placed at an improper depth?

    A. Side lobe artifact

    B. Enhancement artifact

    C. Propagation speed artifact

    D. Beam width artifact

    E. Acoustic speckle

102. Which of the following is an embryologic remnant of the sinus venosus?

    A. Coumadin ridge

    B. Moderator band

    C. Chiari network

    D. Cor triatriatum

    E. Transverse sinus

103. Which of the following best describes the frequency of audible sound?

    A. < 20 Hz

    B. 10 to 20 Hz

    C. 20 Hz to 20 KHz

    D. 20 KHz to 20 MHz

    E. > 20 MHz

104. Emission of an ultrasound pulse prior to the reception of all echoes generated by a previous pulse results in which of the following?

    A. Enhancement

    B. Range ambiguity

    C. Reverberation artifact

    D. Refraction artifact

    E. Beam width artifact

105. Which of the following is the function of the damping material?

    A. Decreases spatial pulse length

    B. Decreases beam width

    C. Decreases frequency

    D. Decreases wavelength

    E. Decreases pulse repetition period

106. Which of the following will improve lateral resolution?

   A. Decreasing beam width

   B. Decreasing pulse repetition frequency

   C. Decreasing pulse repetition period

   D. Increasing spatial pulse length

   E. Increasing wavelength

107. Which of the following will improve temporal resolution?

   A. Increasing imaging depth

   B. Increasing sector size

   C. Increasing pulse repetition frequency

   D. Increasing line density

   E. Increasing persistence

108. Which of the following provides selective depth-dependent amplification?

   A. Gain

   B. Time gain compensation

   C. Power

   D. Depth compression compensation

   E. Depth compensating amplification

109. Which of the following could result in a dilated coronary sinus?

   A. Persistent left superior vena cava

   B. Anomalous pulmonary venous return into the coronary sinus

   C. Tricuspid stenosis

   D. Carcinoid syndrome with severe tricuspid regurgitation

   E. All of the above

110. Following cardiopulmonary bypass for a mitral valve repair, a new left atrial mass is seen. The mass is located just superior to the mitral valve and inferior to the pulmonary veins. What is the most likely diagnosis?

    A. Left atrial myxoma

    B. Intracardiac thrombus

    C. Inverted left atrial appendage

    D. Cor triatriatum

    E. Accessory moderator band

111. What percentage of patients with an interatrial septal aneurysm have a patent foramen ovale?

    A. 20%

    B. 25%

    C. 35%

    D. 45%

    E. ≥ 50%

112. Which of the following is a prominent right ventricular trabeculum that runs from the interventricular septum to the base of the anterior papillary muscle?

    A. Pectinate muscle

    B. Christa terminalis

    C. Moderator band

    D. Thebesian band

    E. Transverse chordae

113. Which of the following is the best view for evaluating an apical left ventricular thrombus following a transmural myocardial infarction?

    A. Midesophageal four-chamber view

    B. Midesophageal two-chamber view

    C. Midesophageal long axis view

    D. Transgastric deep long axis view

    E. Transgastric long axis view

NOTE: Use Table 3.2F to answer the next five (5) questions.

Table 3.2F.

$V_{VSDPeak}$ = 350 cm/sec	HR = 100 beats/min	LVOT diameter = 2.0 cm
TVI_{PA} = 20 cm	BP = 100/60 mmHg	PA diameter = 2.4 cm
TVI_{LVOT} = 15 cm	CVP = 10 mmHg	Aortic valve side = 2.1 cm

Abbreviations: $V_{VSDPeak}$ = peak velocity of left to right flow across a ventricular septal defect, HR = heart rate, TVI_{PA} = time velocity integral of flow through the pulmonary artery, PA = pulmonary artery, TVI_{LVOT} = time velocity integral of flow through the left ventricular outflow tract, BP = blood pressure, CVP = central venous pressure, LVOT = left ventricular outflow tract.

114. Which of the following is the best estimate of the aortic valve area as calculated from the data?

 A. 1.9 cm²

 B. 2.5 cm²

 C. 3.1 cm²

 D. 3.6 cm²

 E. 4.3 cm²

115. Which of the following is the best estimate of the right ventricular stroke volume as calculated from the data?

 A. 50.4 cm³

 B. 60.4 cm³

 C. 70.4 cm³

 D. 80.4 cm³

 E. 90.4 cm³

116. Which of the following is the best estimate of the left ventricular stroke volume as calculated from the data?

 A. 47.1 cm³

 B. 57.1 cm³

 C. 67.1 cm³

 D. 77.1 cm³

 E. 87.1 cm³

117. Which of the following is the best estimate of the ratio of pulmonary to systemic flow (Q_p/Q_s) as calculated from the data?

   A. 1:1

   B. 1.5:1

   C. 2:1

   D. 2.5:1

   E. 3:1

118. Which of the following is the best estimate of the pulmonary artery systolic pressure (PASP)?

   A. 41 mmHg

   B. 51 mmHg

   C. 61 mmHg

   D. 71 mmHg

   E. 81 mmHg

119. Which of the following is a potential cause of dilated cardiomyopathy?

   A. Alcohol toxicity

   B. Cobalt toxicity

   C. Snake bite toxicity

   D. Postpartum (postpartum cardiomyopathy)

   E. All of the above

120. A parasternal long axis M-mode finding of increased E-point to septal separation (EPSS) is indicative of?

   A. Hypertrophic cardiomyopathy

   B. Restrictive cardiomyopathy

   C. Dilated cardiomyopathy

   D. Severe aortic stenosis

   E. Left ventricular hypertrophy

121. Which of the following would be expected in a patient with dilated cardiomyopathy?

    A. Increased aortic ejection velocity and time velocity integral

    B. Increased left ventricular dp/dt

    C. Mitral regurgitation color flow Doppler jet area = 5.3 cm^2

    D. Lateral mitral annular tissue Doppler E_M = 8.1 cm/sec

    E. Decreased right ventricular systolic pressure

122. Which of the following left ventricular wall thickness measurements is consistent with severe left ventricular hypertrophy in an adult?

    A. ≥16 mm

    B. ≥17 mm

    C. ≥18 mm

    D. ≥19 mm

    E. ≥20 mm

123. Which of the following would be expected in a patient with dilated cardiomyopathy?

    A. Fractional shortening (FS) = 33%

    B. Fractional area change (FAC) = 53%

    C. dp/dt = 600

    D. Left ventricular ejection fraction (LVEF) = 56%

    E. Cardiac index (CI) = 3.6 L/min/m^2

124. An increased septal wall thickness versus posterior wall thickness ratio would be expected in which of the following?

    A. Dilated cardiomyopathy

    B. Amyloidosis

    C. Hypertrophic cardiomyopathy

    D. Kartagener's syndrome

    E. Restrictive cardiomyopathy

125. Which of the following is most likely to cause dilated cardiomyopathy?

    A. Lead toxicity

    B. Mercury toxicity

    C. Barium toxicity

    D. Cobalt toxicity

    E. Fluoride toxicity

126. Which of the following best describes the genetics of hypertrophic cardiomyopathy?

    A. Autosomal recessive with variable penetrance

    B. Autosomal dominant with variable penetrance

    C. Autosomal dominant with 100% penetrance

    D. Autosomal recessive with 100% penetrance

    E. Sex linked

127. Which of the following is a difference between the left ventricular outflow obstruction seen in hypertrophic cardiomyopathy and aortic stenosis?

    A. Aortic stenosis creates a larger pressure gradient between the LV and the aorta.

    B. The outflow tract obstruction is influenced by loading conditions in hypertrophic cardiomyopathy.

    C. Systolic anterior motion of the anterior mitral valve leaflet is seen in aortic stenosis.

    D. The obstruction in aortic stenosis is dynamic.

    E. The obstruction in hypertrophic cardiomyopathy generates higher pressure gradients between the left ventricle and the aorta.

128. Which of the following is most affected by poor temporal resolution?

    A. Visualization of a bicuspid aortic valve in a neonate

    B. Visualization of a fibroelastoma in an adult

    C. Visualization of atherosclerosis in the descending aorta

    D. Visualization of rheumatic mitral valve stenosis

129. Which of the following is most likely true concerning pulse repetition frequency?

   A. Units = number of pulses per second

   B. Equal to frame rate * line density

   C. Increases as imaging depth increases

   D. Decreases as temporal resolution increases

130. A TEE probe emits a 6-MHz ultrasound pulse that strikes red blood cells. A returning echo/pulse has a frequency of 6 MHz. Given this information, which of the following is true concerning the direction of blood flow?

   A. Blood flow is away from the transducer.

   B. Blood flow is toward the transducer.

   C. The Doppler shift depends on the sine of the angle between the sound beam and the direction of red blood cell motion.

   D. The ultrasound beam is perpendicular to the direction of blood flow.

   NOTE: Use the data shown in Table 3.2G to answer the next two (2) questions.

Table 3.2G.

Dobutamine Dose	Inferior Wall	Anterior Wall	Lateral Wall	Posterior Wall	Septal Wall
0 mcg/kg/min	AK	Normal	Mildly HK	AK	Normal
5 mcg/kg/min	Severe HK	Normal	Moderately HK	AK	Normal
15 mcg/kg/min	Mild HK	Normal	Severely HK	AK	Mildly HK
30 mcg/kg/min	AK	Normal	Severely HK	AK	Mildly HK

Abbreviations: AK = akinesis, HK = hypokinesis, DK = dyskinesis.

131. Which of the following walls has hibernating myocardium?

   A. Lateral wall

   B. Inferior wall

   C. Septal wall

   D. Posterior wall

   E. Anterior wall

132. Which of the following walls has a region of fixed irreversible ischemia?

    A. Lateral wall

    B. Inferior wall

    C. Septal wall

    D. Posterior wall

    E. Anterior wall

133. What is the most common cause of tricuspid stenosis?

    A. Rheumatic heart disease

    B. Carcinoid syndrome

    C. Ebstein's anomaly

    D. Noonan's syndrome

    E. Kartagener's syndrome

134. A patient with metastatic ileal cancer presents with fibrotic sclerotic restrictive pulmonic and tricuspid valves. What is the most likely etiology?

    A. Rheumatic heart disease

    B. Carcinoid syndrome

    C. Ebstein's anomaly

    D. Noonan's syndrome

    E. Kartagener's syndrome

135. Which of the following best describes a valvular disorder in which one or more of the tricuspid valve (TV) leaflets are displaced from the TV annulus toward the ventricular apex?

    A. Rheumatic heart disease

    B. Carcinoid syndrome

    C. Ebstein's anomaly

    D. Noonan's syndrome

    E. Kartagener's syndrome

136. The interventricular septum flattens and is displaced toward the left ventricle at what point with right ventricular (RV) pressure overload?

   A. Early diastole.

   B. Late diastole.

   C. Early systole.

   D. Late systole.

   E. This does not occur with RV pressure overload.

Answers:

1. A	22. A	43. F
2. B	23. C	44. A
3. C	24. C	45. D
4. D	25. C	46. C
5. C	26. A	47. A
6. B	27. C	48. B
7. A	28. A	49. C
8. D	29. D	50. E
9. D	30. C	51. A
10. C	31. B	52. A
11. A	32. B	53. E
12. B	33. A	54. D
13. B	34. B	55. A
14. D	35. C	56. C
15. B	36. D	57. D
16. D	37. D	58. B
17. C	38. E	59. E
18. A	39. C	60. A
19. E	40. D	61. A
20. D	41. C	62. C
21. C	42. B	63. C

Answers:—continued

64. E	89. C	114. A
65. A	90. D	115. E
66. D	91. D	116. A
67. B	92. A	117. C
68. B	93. C	118. B
69. C	94. D	119. E
70. B	95. C	120. C
71. A	96. E	121. C
72. A	97. E	122. E
73. A	98. B	123. C
74. B	99. B	124. C
75. B	100. C	125. D
76. A	101. C	126. B
77. B	102. C	127. B
78. C	103. C	128. A
79. D	104. B	129. A
80. B	105. A	130. D
81. E	106. A	131. B
82. D	107. C	132. D
83. C	108. B	133. A
84. B	109. E	134. B
85. D	110. C	135. C
86. B	111. E	136. D
87. B	112. C	
88. E	113. B	

Explanations

1. **Answer = A, 100 mW/cm^2 is the maximum spatial peak temporal average intensity recommended for focused ultrasound beams.**

Reference: Sidebotham D, Merry A, Legget M (eds.). *Practical Perioperative Transoesophageal Echocardiography.* Burlington, MA: Butterworth Heinemann 2003:31.

2. **Answer = B, 0.31 mm is the numerical valve for the axial resolution.** *Axial resolution* has many synonyms, including *lateral resolution, axial resolution, radial resolution*, and *range resolution*. The numerical value for axial resolution is equal to half the spatial pulse length (SPL). The smaller the numerical value the better the axial resolution. The calculation in this case is as follows.

Axial resolution = 1/2 * SPL

Axial resolution = 1/2 * (2 cycles) (1540 m/s) / (5 × 10^6 cycles/sec)

Axial resolution = 0.31 × 10^{-6} m

Axial resolution = 0.31 mm

Reference: Sidebotham D, Merry A, Legget M (eds.). *Practical Perioperative Transoesophageal Echocardiography.* Burlington, MA: Butterworth Heinemann 2003:26.

3. **Answer = C, M mode has the best temporal resolution.** M-mode (motion mode) is essentially B-mode plotted versus time. M-mode allows visualization of the movement of cardiac structures. M-mode has outstanding temporal resolution because only one scan line of information is analyzed over time. Two-dimensional imaging involves analyzing multiple scan lines and therefore temporal resolution is not as great as with motion mode. This is why M-mode is useful for imaging rapidly moving structures such as neonatal cardiac valves. B-mode (brightness mode) does not image over time, and thus has no temporal resolution. B-mode is an older form of ultrasound in which returning echoes are plotted according to depth and amplitude, with stronger echoes appearing brighter and deeper echoes appearing deeper on the image. M-mode is essentially B-mode plotted versus time. Because of range ambiguity, continuous-wave Doppler cannot form images and thus does not have temporal resolution. A-mode (amplitude mode) is an antiquated form of obsolete ultrasound imaging in which amplitude is plotted on the Y axis versus depth on the X axis. A-mode does not image over time and therefore does not have temporal resolution.

References: Sidebotham D, Merry A, Legget M (eds.). *Practical Perioperative Transoesophageal Echocardiography.* Burlington, MA: Butterworth Heinemann 2003:24–25; Edelman SK. *Understanding Ultrasound Physics.* Woodlands, TX: ESP, Inc. 1994:96–97.

4. **Answer = D, Scenario D describes the findings typical of decreased systolic function.** The correct findings are found in Table 3.2H.

Table 3.2H.

Echo Parameter	Contractility	EDA	ESA	FAC	CO	E/E´
Hypovolemia	Normal	Decreased	Decreased	Normal	Decreased	< 15
Low LV compliance	Normal	Decreased	Decreased	Normal´	Decreased	> 15
Decreased SVR	Normal	Normal	Decreased	Increased	Increased	< 15
Decreased systolic function	Decreased	Increased	Increased	Decreased	Decreased	> 15
Nothing (trash)	Normal	Increased	Increased	Increased	Increased	< 15

Abbreviations: EDA = end diastolic area, ESA = end systolic area, FAC = fractional area change, CO = cardiac output, E/E´ = ratio of transmitral peak E-wave velocity to the early peak lateral mitral annular tissue velocity (E´ = E_M = E "prime").

References: Sidebotham D, Merry A, Legget M (eds.). *Practical Perioperative Transoesophageal Echocardiography.* Burlington, MA: Butterworth Heinemann 2003:90; Groban L, Dolinski SY. Transesophageal echocardiographic evaluation of diastolic function. *Chest* 2005;128:3652–3663.

5. **Answer = C, Scenario C describes the findings expected in a patient with low systemic vascular resistance.** This is sometimes difficult to distinguish from hypovolemia. However, usually the end diastolic area is normal and the cardiac output is increased with low SVR, and these findings are decreased with hypovolemia. The correct findings are found in Table 3.2I.

Table 3.2I.

Echo Parameter	Contractility	EDA	ESA	FAC	CO	E/E´
Hypovolemia	Normal	Decreased	Decreased	Normal	Decreased	< 15
Low LV compliance	Normal	Decreased	Decreased	Normal	Decreased	> 15
Decreased SVR	Normal	Normal	Decreased	Increased	Increased	< 15
Decreased systolic function	Decreased	Increased	Increased	Decreased	Decreased	> 15
Nothing (trash)	Normal	Increased	Increased	Increased	Increased	< 15

Abbreviations: EDA = end diastolic area, ESA = end systolic area, FAC = fractional area change, CO = cardiac output, E/E´ = ratio of transmitral peak E-wave velocity to the early peak lateral mitral annular tissue velocity (E´ = E_M = E "prime").

References: Sidebotham D, Merry A, Legget M (eds.). *Practical Perioperative Transoesophageal Echocardiography.* Burlington, MA: Butterworth Heinemann 2003:90; Groban L, Dolinski SY. Transesophageal echocardiographic evaluation of diastolic function. *Chest* 2005;128:3652–3663.

6. **Answer = B, Scenario B would be expected with reduced left ventricular compliance.** E/E´ > 15 is indicative of elevate left atrial pressures and this would be expected with decreased left ventricular compliance. The correct findings are found in Table 3.2J.

Table 3.2J.

Echo Parameter	Contractility	EDA	ESA	FAC	CO	E/E´
Hypovolemia	Normal	Decreased	Decreased	Normal	Decreased	< 15
Low LV compliance	Normal	Decreased	Decreased	Normal	Decreased	> 15
Decreased SVR	Normal	Normal	Decreased	Increased	Increased	< 15
Decreased systolic function	Decreased	Increased	Increased	Decreased	Decreased	> 15
Nothing (trash)	Normal	Increased	Increased	Increased	Increased	< 15

Abbreviations: EDA = end diastolic area, ESA = end systolic area, FAC = fractional area change, CO = cardiac output, E/E´ = ratio of transmitral peak E-wave velocity to the early peak lateral mitral annular tissue velocity (E´ = E_M = E "prime").

References: Sidebotham D, Merry A, Legget M (eds.). *Practical Perioperative Transoesophageal Echocardiography.* Burlington, MA: Butterworth Heinemann 2003:90; Groban L, Dolinski SY. Transesophageal echocardiographic evaluation of diastolic function. *Chest* 2005;128:3652–3663.

7. Answer = A, Scenario A is indicative of hypovolemia. The correct findings are found in Table 3.2K.

Table 3.2K.

Echo Parameter	Contractility	EDA	ESA	FAC	CO	E/E´
Hypovolemia	Normal	Decreased	Decreased	Normal	Decreased	< 15
Low LV compliance	Normal	Decreased	Decreased	Normal	Decreased	> 15
Decreased SVR	Normal	Normal	Decreased	Increased	Increased	< 15
Decreased systolic function	Decreased	Increased	Increased	Decreased	Decreased	> 15
Nothing (trash)	Normal	Increased	Increased	Increased	Increased	< 15

Abbreviations: EDA = end diastolic area, ESA = end systolic area, FAC = fractional area change, CO = cardiac output, E/E´ = ratio of transmitral peak E-wave velocity to the early peak lateral mitral annular tissue velocity (E´ = E_M = E "prime").

References: Sidebotham D, Merry A, Legget M (eds.). *Practical Perioperative Transoesophageal Echocardiography.* Burlington, MA: Butterworth Heinemann 2003:90; Groban L, Dolinski SY. Transesophageal echocardiographic evaluation of diastolic function. *Chest* 2005;128:3652–3663.

8. Answer = D, > 30% endocardial thickening is consistent with normal segmental wall motion (see Table 3.2L).

Table 3.2L.

Wall Motion	Grade	Endocardial Movement	Endocardial Thickening
Normal	1	Normal	> 30%
Mild HK	2	Slightly decreased	10–30%
Severe HK	3	Severely decreased	< 10%
AK	4	No movement	No thickening
DK	5	Outward during systole	Thins during systole

HK = hypokinesis, AK = akinesis, DK = dyskinesis.

Reference: Sidebotham D, Merry A, Legget M (eds.). *Practical Perioperative Transoesophageal Echocardiography.* Burlington, MA: Butterworth Heinemann 2003:110.

9. Answer = D, 10 to 30% endocardial thickening is consistent with mild hypokinesis.

Reference: Sidebotham D, Merry A, Legget M (eds.). *Practical Perioperative Transoesophageal Echocardiography.* Burlington, MA: Butterworth Heinemann 2003:110.

10. Answer = C, < 10% endocardial thickening is consistent with severe hypokinesis.

Reference: Sidebotham D, Merry A, Legget M (eds.). *Practical Perioperative Transoesophageal Echocardiography.* Burlington, MA: Butterworth Heinemann 2003:110.

11. **Answer = A, Grade 1 = normal wall motion** (see Table 3.2L).

Reference: Sidebotham D, Merry A, Legget M (eds.). *Practical Perioperative Transoesophageal Echocardiography.* Burlington, MA: Butterworth Heinemann 2003:110.

12. **Answer = B, Grade 2 = mild hypokinesis.**

13. **Answer = B, Second-order chordae arise from the papillary muscles and attach to the undersurface of the mitral valve leaflets.** First-order chordae tendinae arise from papillary muscles and attach to the mitral valve leaflet tips. Third-order chordae tendinae arise from the ventricular wall (not the papillary muscles) and are present only on the posterior mitral valve, where they attach to the base of the mitral leaflets.

Reference: Sidebotham D, Merry A, Legget M (eds.). *Practical Perioperative Transoesophageal Echocardiography.* Burlington, MA: Butterworth Heinemann 2003:133.

14. **Answer = D, P_1 is usually supported solely by the anterolateral papillary muscle.** The anterolateral papillary muscle supports A_1 and P_1 and part of A_2 and P_2. The posteromedial papillary muscle supports A_3 and P_3 and part of A_2 and P_2.

Reference: Sidebotham D, Merry A, Legget M (eds.). *Practical Perioperative Transoesophageal Echocardiography.* Burlington, MA: Butterworth Heinemann 2003:133.

15. **Answer = B, The right coronary artery supplies the posteromedial papillary muscle.** This papillary muscle is more likely to rupture secondarily to its single source of perfusion. The anterolateral papillary muscle is less likely to rupture given its dual blood supply (both the left anterior descending and circumflex coronary arteries).

Reference: Sidebotham D, Merry A, Legget M (eds.). *Practical Perioperative Transoesophageal Echocardiography.* Burlington, MA: Butterworth Heinemann 2003:138–141.

16. **Answer = D, A TR jet area to right atrial area of 63% is indicative of severe (grade IV) TR** (see Table 3.2M).

Table 3.2M.

Degree of TR	Trace (grade I)	Mild (grade II)	Moderate (grade III)	Severe (grade IV)
TR jet area/RA area	< 15%	16–30%	31–60%	> 60%

Reference: Konstadt SN, Shernon S, Oka Y (eds). *Clinical Transesophageal Echocardiography: A Problem-Oriented Approach, Second Edition.* Philadelphia: Lippincott Williams & Wilkins 2003:429.

17. **Answer = C, 42 ml is the left ventricular outflow tract valve stroke volume (SV_{LVOT}).** The calculation is as follows.

$$SV_{LVOT} = SV_{MV} = A_{MV} * TVI_{MV} = (759/DT_{MV}) * (59 \text{ cm}) = 42 \text{ ml}$$

This patient has no valvular regurgitation, and thus the stroke volume through all of the valves is equal (principle of continuity).

- SV_{LVOT} = stroke volume of blood flow through the left ventricular outflow tract
- SV_{MV} = stroke volume of blood flow through the mitral valve
- TVI_{MV} = time velocity integral of blood flow through the mitral valve
- DT_{MV} = mitral valve inflow deceleration time
- A_{MV} = area of the mitral valve

Reference: SCA/ASE Annual Comprehensive Review and Update of Perioperative Hemodynamics Workshop. 17 Feb. 2005, San Diego, CA; discussion lead by Stanton Shernon, et al.

18. **Answer = A, 0.81 cm² is the aortic valve area.** The calculation is as follows.

$$A_{AV} = SV/TVI_{AV} = 42 \text{ cm}^3 / 52 \text{ cm} = \underline{\textbf{0.8 cm}^2}$$

$$SV = SV_{AV} = SV_{LVOT} = SV_{MV} = A_{MV} * TVI_{MV} = (759/DT_{MV}) * (59 \text{ cm}) = 42 \text{ ml}$$

This patient has no valvular regurgitation, and thus the stroke volume through all of the valves is equal (principle of continuity).

- SV_{LVOT} = stroke volume of blood flow through the left ventricular outflow tract
- SV_{MV} = stroke volume of blood flow through the mitral valve
- TVI_{MV} = time velocity integral of blood flow through the mitral valve
- DT_{MV} = mitral valve inflow deceleration time
- A_{MV} = area of the mitral valve
- TVI_{AV} = time velocity integral of blood flow across the aortic valve
- A_{AV} = area of the aortic valve

Reference: SCA/ASE Annual Comprehensive Review and Update of Perioperative Hemodynamics Workshop. 17 Feb. 2005, San Diego, CA; discussion lead by Stanton Shernon, et al.

19. **Answer = E, 3.2 cm² is the tricuspid valve area.** The calculation is as follows.

$$A_{TV} = SV/TVI_{TV} = 42 \text{ cm}^3 / 13 \text{ cm} = 3.2 \text{ cm}^2$$

$$SV = SV_{TV} = SV_{LVOT} = SV_{MV} = A_{MV} * TVI_{MV} = (759/DT_{MV}) * (59 \text{ cm}) = 42 \text{ ml}$$

This patient has no valvular regurgitation, and thus the stroke volume through all of the valves is equal (principle of continuity).

- SV_{LVOT} = stroke volume of blood flow through the left ventricular outflow tract
- SV_{MV} = stroke volume of blood flow through the mitral valve
- TVI_{MV} = time velocity integral of blood flow through the mitral valve
- DT_{MV} = mitral valve inflow deceleration time
- A_{MV} = area of the mitral valve

- TVI_{TV} = time velocity integral of blood flow across the tricuspid valve
- A_{TV} = area of the tricuspid valve

Reference: SCA/ASE Annual Comprehensive Review and Update of Perioperative Hemodynamics Workshop. 17 Feb. 2005, San Diego, CA; discussion lead by Stanton Shernon, et al.

20. **Answer = D, Severe mitral stenosis is present.** A mitral valve area of 0.71 cm^2 is consistent with severe mitral stenosis (see Table 3.2N).

Table 3.2N.

Degree of Mitral Stenosis	Mild	Moderate	Severe
Mitral valve area	1.6–2.0 cm^2	1–1.5 cm^2	< 1.0 cm^2
Pressure half time	100 msec	200 msec	> 300 msec

Reference: Perrino AC, Reeves S. *A Practical Approach to TEE.* Philadelphia: Lippincott Williams & Wilkins 2003:150.

21. **Answer = C, Moderate aortic stenosis is present.** An aortic valve area of 0.81 cm^2 is consistent with moderate aortic stenosis (see Table 3.2O).

Table 3.2O.

Degree of AS:	Normal	Mild	Moderate	Severe
Aortic valve area (A_{AV})	> 2.5 cm^2	1–1.5 cm^2	0.8–1.0 cm^2	< 0.8 cm^2

Reference: Perrino AC, Reeves S. *A Practical Approach to TEE.* Philadelphia: Lippincott Williams & Wilkins 2003:189.

22. **Answer = A, No tricuspid valve stenosis is present.** The tricuspid valve area is normal (3.2 cm^3).

Reference: SCA/ASE Annual Comprehensive Review and Update of Perioperative Hemodynamics Workshop. 17 Feb. 2005, San Diego, CA; discussion lead by Stanton Shernon, et al.

23. **Answer = C, This is the definition of the duty factor.** The duty factor is a unitless number that describes the amount of time the ultrasound machine is producing sound (the percentage of "on" time). It is also known as the duty cycle. It has a value between 0 and 1 (0 to 100%). Duty factor can be calculated from the following relationship: Duty factor = PD / PRP, where PD = pulse duration and PRP = pulse repetition period. Continuous-wave ultrasound has a duty factor of 1 because it is producing ultrasound 100% of the time (continuously). If the ultrasound machine is off, no ultrasound is produced and the duty factor is 0. Quality factor = Q factor = RF/BW, where RF = resonant frequency and BW = bandwidth. Q factor is a unitless number, which describes the quality of an ultrasound pulse. The lower the Q factor the higher the quality of the pulse and the better the image quality. An imaging transducer tends to produce short ultrasound pulses with wide bandwidths, high resonant frequencies, and a small Q factor. The pulse repetition period (PRP) is the *time* from the start of one

pulse to the start of the next pulse. Pulse repetition frequency (PRF) is the inverse of the PRP. PRF is the number of pulses emitted per second. Power relates to the strength of the sound wave. Power is the amount of work (energy) transferred from the entire sound beam per unit of time. Power is measured in watts (1 watt = 1 joule/sec).

Reference: Edelman SK. *Understanding Ultrasound Physics.* Woodlands, TX: ESP, Inc. 1994:30.

24. **Answer = C, Amplitude: dB = 20 Log A_2/A_1.** The following are the correct formulas.

a. Pressure: dB = 20 Log p_2/p_1

b. Intensity: dB = 10 Log I_2/I_1

c. Amplitude: dB = 20 Log A_2/A_1

d. Power: dB = 10 Log P_2/P_1

Reference: http://www.phys.unsw.edu.au/~jw/dB.html.

25. **Answer = C, Attenuation is increased by increasing imaging depth, which increases the distance the sound travels.** It is also increased by increasing the frequency.

Reference: Edelman SK. *Understanding Ultrasound Physics.* Woodlands, TX: ESP, Inc. 1994:51.

26. **Answer = A, As the thickness of the piezoelectric crystal increases the frequency of the transducer decreases and attenuation decreases.** Pulse repetition period (PRP) is not related to attenuation. As wavelength (λ) increases attenuation decreases. Increasing spatial pulse length (SPL) may lead to an increases in attenuation if the wavelength is decreased. SPL = λ * (number of cycles per pulse). Bandwidth is not related to attenuation. Note that the symbol * refers to "times" (multiplication), as in (2 * 2) = (2 × 2) = 4.

Reference: Edelman SK. *Understanding Ultrasound Physics.* Woodlands, TX: ESP, Inc. 1994:51, 75.

27. **Answer = C** *Absorption* **is the primary component of attenuation in soft tissue.** It is responsible for ≥ 80% of the attenuation seen in soft tissue.

Reference: Edelman SK. *Understanding Ultrasound Physics.* Woodlands, TX: ESP, Inc. 1994:52.

28. **Answer = A, 3 dB of attenuation.** The *half-value layer thickness* is the thickness required to reduce the intensity of a sound beam by half. This represents 3 dB of attenuation. Note for ultrasound in soft tissue: intensity dB = 10 logI_2/I_1. When I_2 = 1/2 I_1, this represents 10 log 1/2 (or −3dB). Note that the negative sign (−3) implies a reduction in intensity. For the previous equation, I_1 = initial or reference intensity and I_2 = final intensity (or intensity at a given depth). I_2 is always less than I_1.

Reference: Edelman SK. *Understanding Ultrasound Physics.* Woodlands, TX: ESP, Inc. 1994:56.

29. **Answer = D, All of the above are true statements.**

Reference: Edelman SK. *Understanding Ultrasound Physics.* Woodlands, TX: ESP, Inc. 1994:62.

30. **Answer = C, When reflection occurs with oblique incidence the reflection angle equals the incident angle.**

Reference: Kremkau FW. *Diagnostic Ultrasound: Principles Instruments and Exercises, Third Edition.* Philadelphia: Saunders 1989:45.

31. **Answer = B, Refraction requires oblique incidence.** Refraction occurs at the interface between two media when the incidence is oblique and the velocity of sound in the two media is different. The greater the difference in the velocities the greater the refraction. If the velocity of sound in medium 2 is less than the velocity of medium 1, the transmission angle will be smaller than the incident angle.

Reference: Edelman SK. *Understanding Ultrasound Physics.* Woodlands, TX: ESP, Inc. 1994:67–68.

32. **Answer = B, The damping material is also known as the backing material.** The backing material decreases the transducer's sensitivity to reflected echoes. The backing material functions to improve the image quality. It does this by decreasing the spatial pulse length (SPL). Decreasing spatial pulse length improves axial resolution (as axial resolution = 1/2 * SPL), and the smaller the numerical value for axial resolution the better the image quality. Quality factor (Q factor) = resonant frequency / bandwidth. The backing material decreases the Q factor by decreasing the resonant frequency and increasing the bandwidth. Good imaging transducers have high frequencies, small spatial pulse lengths, and low Q factors.

Reference: Edelman SK. *Understanding Ultrasound Physics.* Woodlands, TX: ESP, Inc. 1994:73.

33. **Answer = A, Acoustic impedance: PZT > matching layer > gel > skin.**

Reference: Edelman SK. *Understanding Ultrasound Physics.* Woodlands, TX: ESP, Inc. 1994:74.

34. **Answer = B, Wavelength (frequency) is determined by the thickness of a TEE piezoelectric crystal.** The frequency of a continuous-wave Doppler beam is determined by the electrical frequency of the excitation voltage that stimulates the crystal. The pulse repetition period is the time from the beginning of one pulse to the beginning of another pulse. It is determined by the pulse duration and the listening time (depth). The velocity of an ultrasound beam is determined by the medium through which the beam travels. The velocity of a pulsed-wave Doppler beam and the velocity of a continuous-wave Doppler beam are identical if both beams are traveling through the same medium.

Reference: Edelman SK. *Understanding Ultrasound Physics.* Woodlands, TX: ESP, Inc. 1994:75.

35. **Answer = C, The electrical frequency of the excitation voltage applied to the active element determines the frequency of a continuous-wave ultrasound beam.** A pulsed-wave Doppler ultrasound beam frequency is determined by both the thickness of a piezoelectric crystal and the velocity of sound through the crystal. As velocity through the crystal increasesand thickness decreases, frequency increases. Very thin crystals with high velocities are utilized for clinical imaging purposes. The acoustic impedance of the damping material has nothing to do with the frequency of a continuous-wave ultrasound beam.

Reference: Edelman SK. *Understanding Ultrasound Physics.* Woodlands, TX: ESP, Inc. 1994:75.

36. **Answer = D, A pulsed-wave Doppler ultrasound beam frequency is determined by both the thickness of a piezoelectric crystal and the velocity of sound through the crystal.** As velocity through the crystal increases and thickness decreases, frequency increases. Very thin crystals with high velocities are utilized for clinical imaging purposes.

Reference: Edelman SK. *Understanding Ultrasound Physics.* Woodlands, TX: ESP, Inc. 1994:75.

37. **Answer = D, The resonant frequency (RF) is directly proportional to the velocity of ultrasound in the crystal.** $RF = V_{crystal} / 2(\text{Thickness})$ RF is inversely proportional to 2 times the crystal thickness. As the density of the crystal increases, the velocity decreases and therefore the RF decreases. The frequency of a continuous-wave Doppler beam (not pulsed-wave Doppler) is determined by the frequency of the excitation voltage applied to the crystal.

Reference: Edelman SK. *Understanding Ultrasound Physics.* Woodlands, TX: ESP, Inc. 1994:76.

38. **Answer = E, It cannot be determined from the given information.** The resonant frequency (RF) of a pulsed-wave ultrasound beam is determined by the thickness (T) of the ultrasound piezoelectric crystal and the velocity of sound in the crystal ($RF = V/2T$). We are not given enough information to determine the resonant frequency.

Reference: Edelman SK. *Understanding Ultrasound Physics.* Woodlands, TX: ESP, Inc. 1994:75.

39. **Answer = C, Short pulses contain sound with a broad range of frequencies and a low quality factor.** Quality factor (Q factor) = RF/bandwidth. The Q factor is a unitless number that describes the quality of an ultrasound pulse. The lower the Q factor the higher the quality of the pulse and the better the image quality. An imaging transducer tends to produce short ultrasound pulses with wide bandwidths, high resonant frequencies, and a small Q factor. The resonant frequency is directly related to the Q factor per the previous formula. Likewise, the bandwidth is inversely related to the bandwidth. Therapeutic ultrasound transducers tend to have lower Q factors than imaging transducers. RF = resonant frequency = operating frequency.

Reference: Kremkau FW. *Diagnostic Ultrasound: Principles Instruments and Exercises, Third Edition.* Philadelphia: Saunders 1989:70–73, 294.

40. **Answer = D, Bandwidth = 8 (14 − 6 = 8).** Bandwidth is the range of frequencies in a pulse.

Reference: Kremkau FW. *Diagnostic Ultrasound: Principles Instruments and Exercises, Third Edition.* Philadelphia: Saunders 1989:71.

41. **Answer = C, Quality factor = Q factor = RF/BW = 10/8. RF = resonant frequency, BW = bandwidth.** The Q factor is a unitless number that describes the quality of an ultrasound pulse. The lower the Q factor the higher the quality of the pulse and the better the image quality. An imaging transducer tends to produce short ultrasound pulses with wide bandwidths, high resonant frequencies, and a small Q factor. The resonant frequency is directly related to the Q factor per the previous formula. Likewise, the bandwidth is inversely related to the bandwidth. Therapeutic ultrasound transducers tend to have higher Q factors than imaging transducers. RF = resonant frequency = operating frequency.

Reference: Kremkau FW. *Diagnostic Ultrasound: Principles Instruments and Exercises, Third Edition.* Philadelphia: Saunders 1989:70–73, 294.

42. **Answer = B, Focal length is proportional to the radius of the transducer face squared.** Focal length = length of the near field = L_n = r^2/λ, where r = radius of the piezoelectric crystal and λ = wavelength. L_n *decreases* as frequency decreases. This is illustrated by the following relationships: $L_n = r^2/\lambda$ and $F = V / \lambda$, where *V* = velocity and λ = wavelength. As crystal diameter increases focal length increases. *Focal length* has several synonyms, including *near field length* (L_n), *focal zone,* and *Fresnel zone length.* *Fraunhofer zone length* is another name for the *far zone.*

Reference: Edelman SK. *Understanding Ultrasound Physics.* Woodlands, TX: ESP, Inc. 1994:75, 81, 82.

43. **Answer = F, None of the above.** All of the choices are synonyms of *longitudinal resolution.*

Reference: Edelman SK. *Understanding Ultrasound Physics.* Woodlands, TX: ESP, Inc. 1994:90.

44. **Answer = A, M-mode ultrasound provides excellent temporal resolution.** Temporal resolution reflects the ability to accurately locate the position of moving structures at particular instants in time. B-mode (brightness mode) is an older form of ultrasound imaging incapable of imaging moving structures. Therefore, B-mode has very poor temporal resolution. With continuous-wave ultrasound it is not possible to produce two-dimensional images. M-mode's temporal resolution is superior to the temporal resolution of a two-dimensional linear phased-array image.

Reference: Edelman SK. *Understanding Ultrasound Physics.* Woodlands, TX: ESP, Inc. 1994:96–100.

45. **Answer = D, All of the above are correct.** Electronic steering, electronic focusing, and the ability to change the focus are all properties of linear phased-array transducers.

Reference: Edelman SK. *Understanding Ultrasound Physics.* Woodlands, TX: ESP, Inc. 1994:107.

46. **Answer = C, Decreasing the imaging depth will increase the temporal resolution of a midesophageal four-chamber-view two-beat loop by decreasing the time required for the machine to listen for returning echoes (listening time).** *Temporal resolution* depends on the following two main factors.

   • How much the object being imaged moves.
   • The *frame rate* = frames/sec = images/sec.

The *frame rate* depends on the following factors.

   • Line density = scan lines per image.
   • Number of foci (focal points) per line = pulses per scan line.
   • Imaging depth (listening time).

Decreasing the imaging depth decreases the time the machine has to wait for echoes to return to the transducer (listening time) and thereby allows the machine to increase the number of images per second (frame rate). This improves the temporal resolution, which is the ability to accurately locate the position of moving structures at particular instants in time. An increase in heart rate will increase the movement of the heart and decrease temporal resolution. An increase in line density (scan lines per image) will decrease the frame rate (images/sec) and thereby decrease the temporal resolution. Increasing the number of foci per scan line increases the time required to image each scan line. This will decrease the frame rate and thereby decrease temporal resolution.

Reference: Edelman SK. *Understanding Ultrasound Physics.* Woodlands, TX: ESP, Inc. 1994:121–124.

47. **Answer = A, The listening time for returning echoes is increased as imaging depth is increased.** Pulse repetition period (PRP) is increased by an increase in depth. Pulse repetition frequency (PRF) is the reciprocal of PRP and is decreased by an increase in imaging depth. The time required to scan each line is increased by increasing the imaging depth. This decreases temporal resolution.

Reference: Edelman SK. *Understanding Ultrasound Physics.* Woodlands, TX: ESP, Inc. 1994:122.

48. **Answer = B, Turbulent flow moving toward the transducer with an incident angle of 30 degrees on a variance map will be represented by the letter/color on the top right of the variance map.** This is usually a yellow color.

Reference: Edelman SK. *Understanding Ultrasound Physics.* Woodlands, TX: ESP, Inc. 1994:155.

49. **Answer = C. Laminar flow away from the transducer at an angle of 60 degrees will be represented by the letter/color on the Bottom Left of the variance map.** This is usually represented by a blue color.

Reference: Edelman SK. *Understanding Ultrasound Physics.* Woodlands, TX: ESP, Inc. 1994:155.

50. **Answer = E. No flow will be observed when the angle between the transducer beam and the blood flow is 90 degrees.** This will be represented as black on the color flow Doppler display.

Reference: Edelman SK. *Understanding Ultrasound Physics.* Woodlands, TX: ESP, Inc. 1994:155.

51. **Answer = A, Perimembranous ventricular septal defects are sometimes associated with an aneurysm involving the membranous intraventricular septum composed of tricuspid valve tissue.** This pouch of tissue protrudes into the ventricle.

Reference: Perrino AC, Reeves S. *A Practical Approach to TEE.* Philadelphia: Lippincott Williams & Wilkins 2003:290.

52. **Answer = A, Perimembranous or membranous ventricular septal defects (VSDs) are the most common type, constituting about 70% of all VSDs.**

Reference: Otto C. *Textbook of Clinical Echocardiography, Third Edition.* Philadelphia: Elsevier 2004:473.

53. **Answer = E, Inlet ventricular septal defects when combined with ostium primum atrial septal defect create a complete atrioventricular (AV) canal defect (AV septal defect).**

Reference: Perrino AC, Reeves S. *A Practical Approach to TEE.* Philadelphia: Lippincott Williams & Wilkins 2003:290.

54. **Answer = D, Trabecular (muscular) ventricular septal defects occur in the muscular portion of the intraventricular septum.**

Reference: Otto C. *Textbook of Clinical Echocardiography, Third Edition.* Philadelphia: Elsevier 2004:473.

55. **Answer = A, 110 = the right ventricular systolic blood pressure (RVSP).** The calculation is as follows.

$\Delta P = 4V^2$

$(RVSP - RAP) = 4V_{TR}^2$

$(RVSP - CVP) = 4V^2$

$RVSP = 4V^2 + CVP$

$RVSP = 4(5m/s)^2 + 10$

$RVSP = 110 \text{ mmHg}$

- RVSP = right ventricular systolic pressure
- RAP = right atrial pressure
- CVP = central venous pressure
- V_{TR} = peak velocity of the tricuspid valve regurgitant jet

Reference: Otto C. *Textbook of Clinical Echocardiography, Third Edition.* Philadelphia: Elsevier 2004:463.

56. **Answer = C, 46 = the pulmonary artery systolic pressure (PASP).** The calculation is as follows.

$$PASP = (RVSP - \Delta P_{ps})$$

$$PASP = [RVSP - 4(V_{ps})^2]$$

$$PASP = [110 - 4(4m/s)^2] = 46 \text{ mmHg}$$

$\Delta P = 4V^2$

$(RVSP - RAP) = 4V_{TR}^2$

$(RVSP - CVP) = 4V^2$

$RVSP = 4V^2 + CVP$

$RVSP = 4(5m/s)^2 + 10$

$RVSP = 110 \text{ mmHg}$

- RVSP = right ventricular systolic pressure
- RAP = right atrial pressure
- CVP = central venous pressure
- PASP = pulmonary artery systolic pressure
- V_{ps} = pulmonic stenosis peak flow velocity by Doppler = Velocity of systolic flow across the pulmonic valve
- V_{TR} = peak velocity of the tricuspid valve regurgitant jet

Reference: Otto C. *Textbook of Clinical Echocardiography, Third Edition.* Philadelphia: Elsevier 2004:463.

57. **Answer = D, 26 mmHg = the left ventricular end diastolic pressure.** The calculation is as follows.

$\Delta P = 4V^2$

$DBP - LVEDP = 4(V_{Allate})^2$

$LVEDP = DBP - 4V^2$

$LVEDP = [90 - 4(4)^2] = 26 \text{mmHg}$

LVEDP = left ventricular end diastolic pressure, DBP = diastolic blood pressure

Reference: Otto C. *Textbook of Clinical Echocardiography, Third Edition.* Philadelphia: Elsevier 2004:463.

58. **Answer = B, 55 cm³ = the stroke volume of blood flow through the mitral valve.** The calculation is as follows.

$A_{MV} = 220/PHT_{MVinflow}$

$A_{MV} = 220/60$

$A_{MV} = 3.67 \text{ cm}^2$

$$SV_{MV} = A_{MV} * TVI_{MV}$$

$$SV_{MV} = 3.67 \text{ cm}^2 * 15 \text{ cm}$$

$$SV_{MV} = 55 \text{ cm}^3$$

- A_{MV} = mitral valve area
- TVI_{MV} = time velocity integral of diastolic flow through the mitral valve
- $PHT_{MVinflow}$ = pressure half time of diastolic mitral inflow

Reference: Perrino AC, Reeves S. *A Practical Approach to TEE.* Philadelphia: Lippincott Williams & Wilkins 2003:99.

59. **Answer = E, 94.2 cm³ = the left ventricular outflow tract stroke volume (SV$_{LVOT}$).** The calculation is as follows.

$SV_{LVOT} = A_{LVOT} * TVI_{LVOT}$

$SV_{LVOT} = \pi r^2 * TVI_{LVOT}$

$SV_{LVOT} = 3.14 \text{ cm}^2 * 30 \text{ cm}$

$SV_{LVOT} = 94.2 \text{ cm}^3$

- A_{LVOT} = area of the left ventricular outflow tract
- TVI_{LVOT} = time velocity integral of blood flow through the mitral valve
- SV_{LVOT} = the left ventricular outflow tract stroke volume

Reference: Perrino AC, Reeves S. *A Practical Approach to TEE.* Philadelphia: Lippincott Williams & Wilkins 2003:99.

60. **Answer = A, 39 cm³ = the aortic valve regurgitant volume (RVol$_{AV}$).** The calculation is as follows.

$RVol_{AV} = SV_{LVOT} - SV_{MV}$

$RVol_{AV} = 94.2 \text{ cm}^3 - 55 \text{ cm}^3$

$RVol_{AV} = 39 \text{ cm}^3$

$SV_{LVOT} = A_{LVOT} * TVI_{LVOT}$

$SV_{LVOT} = \pi r^2 * SV_{LVOT}$

$SV_{LVOT} = 3.14 \text{ cm}^2 * 30 \text{ cm}$

$SV_{LVOT} = 94.2 \text{ cm}^3$

$SV_{MV} = A_{MV} * TVI_{MV}$

$SV_{MV} = 3.67 \text{ cm}^2 * 15 \text{ cm}$

$SV_{MV} = 55 \text{ cm}^3$

Reference: SCA/ASE Annual Comprehensive Review and Update of Perioperative Hemodynamics Workshop. 17 Feb. 2005, San Diego, CA; discussion lead by Stanton Shernon, et al.

61. **Answer = A, 11 mmHg = LVEDP.** The calculation is as follows.

$\Delta P = 4V2$

$(DBP - LVEDP) = 4(V_{AIlate})^2$

$LVEDP = (DBP - 4(V_{AIlate})^2$

$LVEDP = (75 - 64)$

$LVEDP = 11 \text{ mmHg}$

- LVEDP = left ventricular end diastolic pressure
- DBP = diastolic blood pressure
- V_{AIlate} = late peak (max) velocity of the aortic insufficiency regurgitant jet (AI end diastolic V)

Reference: Perrino AC, Reeves S. *A Practical Approach to TEE.* Philadelphia: Lippincott Williams & Wilkins 2003:99.

62. **Answer = C, 41% = the aortic valve regurgitant fraction (AV Reg Fx).** The calculation is as follows.

AV Reg Fx = $RVol_{AV}$ / SV_{LVOT}

AV Reg Fx = 39 cm³ / 41.4 cm³

AV Reg Fx = 41.4%

- AV Reg Fx = aortic valve regurgitant fraction
- $RVol_{AV}$ = aortic insufficiency regurgitant volume
- SV_{LVOT} = left ventricular outflow tract stroke volume

Reference: Perrino AC, Reeves S. *A Practical Approach to TEE.* Philadelphia: Lippincott Williams & Wilkins 2003:99.

63. **Answer = C, A Crawford type III aortic aneurysm is described.** This thoracoabdominal aneurysm begins more distally than types I or II, but originates above the diaphragm (see Table 3.2P).

Table 3.2P.   CRAWFORD CLASSIFICATION FOR THORACOABDOMINAL ANEURYSMS

Type	Origin	Extends Distally:
I	Near left subclavian artery	Above renal arteries
II	Near left subclavian artery	Below renal arteries
III	More distal than types I or II but above the diaphragm	Below renal arteries
IV	Below the diaphragm (abdominal)	Below renal arteries

Reference: Perrino AC, Reeves S. *A Practical Approach to TEE.* Philadelphia: Lippincott Williams & Wilkins 2003:252.

64. **Answer = E, All of the above are correct.** Heart rate, atrial contractility, left ventricular compliance, and mitral valve disease can all affect the transmitral pulsed-wave Doppler flow velocity profile.

Reference: Perrino AC, Reeves S. *A Practical Approach to TEE.* Philadelphia: Lippincott Williams & Wilkins 2003:114.

65. **Answer = A, The isovolumic relaxation time (IVRT) is decreased in restrictive diastolic function.** It is decreased in patients with increased left atrial pressure, and increased in patients with impaired left ventricular relaxation. In normal and pseudonormal patients it is between 60 and 110 milliseconds.

Reference: Perrino AC, Reeves S. *A Practical Approach to TEE.* Philadelphia: Lippincott Williams & Wilkins 2003:115.

66. **Answer = D, The transmitral pulsed-wave Doppler E-wave deceleration time is prolonged in patients with impaired left ventricular relaxation.** With delayed relaxation the isovolumic relaxation time (IVRT) is prolonged, the E/A ratio is decreased, the lateral mitral annular tissue Doppler early-filling velocity (E′) is decreased (< 8 cm/sec), and the transmitral peak early-filling velocity (E wave) is decreased.

Reference: Perrino AC, Reeves S. *A Practical Approach to TEE.* Philadelphia: Lippincott Williams & Wilkins 2003:114.

67. **Answer = B, Impaired relaxation is shown.** The transmitral E-wave peak velocity is decreased, the E-wave deceleration time is prolonged, the transmitral A-wave peak velocity is increased, and the E/A is less than one. These findings are consistent with delayed (impaired) relaxation.

Reference: Perrino AC, Reeves S. *A Practical Approach to TEE.* Philadelphia: Lippincott Williams & Wilkins 2003:111–126.

68. **Answer = B, E/A will be decreased after the administration of nitroglycerin, as preload is decreased.** As heart rate increases, the A wave is superimposed on the E wave and the E/A ratio is decreased (not increased). The E/A ratio is indicative of delayed relaxation, because E is less than A. For restrictive diastolic dysfunction, E >> A. The E/A ratio will also decrease after a valsalva because preload will decrease.

Reference: Perrino AC, Reeves S. *A Practical Approach to TEE.* Philadelphia: Lippincott Williams & Wilkins 2003:111–126.

69. **Answer = C, A hepatic venous Doppler flow profile is shown.** This profile consists of four waves: S, V, D, and AR. The AR wave is illustrated. This wave results from right atrial contraction, which causes retrograde flow. In a patient with tricuspid stenosis there is obstruction of flow from the right atrium to the right ventricle, and therefore a prominent AR wave.

Reference: Perrino AC, Reeves S. *A Practical Approach to TEE.* Philadelphia: Lippincott Williams & Wilkins 2003:124.

70. **Answer = B, The arrow labeled 1 indicates the transmitral A-wave velocity.**

References: Otto C. *Textbook of Clinical Echocardiography, Third Edition.* Philadelphia: Elsevier 2004:179; Groban L, Dolinski SY. Transesophageal echocardiographic evaluation of diastolic function. *Chest* 2005;128:3652–3663.

71. **Answer = A, Normal transmitral flow velocities and normal lateral mitral annular tissue Doppler velocities are shown.**

References: Otto C. *Textbook of Clinical Echocardiography, Third Edition.* Philadelphia: Elsevier 2004:179; Groban L, Dolinski SY. Transesophageal echocardiographic evaluation of diastolic function. *Chest* 2005;128:3652–3663.

72. **Answer = A, The arrow labeled 2 indicates the transmitral E-wave velocity.**

References: Otto C. T*extbook of Clinical Echocardiography, Third Edition.* Philadelphia: Elsevier 2004:179; Groban L, Dolinski SY. Transesophageal echocardiographic evaluation of diastolic function. *Chest* 2005;128:3652–3663.

73. **Answer = A, The arrow labeled 3 indicates the lateral mitral annular tissue Doppler E$_M$ wave.**

References: Otto C. *Textbook of Clinical Echocardiography, Third Edition.* Philadelphia: Elsevier 2004:179; Groban L, Dolinski SY. Transesophageal echocardiographic evaluation of diastolic function. *Chest* 2005;128:3652–3663.

74. **Answer = B, The arrow labeled 4 indicates the lateral mitral annular tissue Doppler A$_M$ wave.**

References: Otto C. *Textbook of Clinical Echocardiography, Third Edition.* Philadelphia: Elsevier 2004:179; Groban L, Dolinski SY. Transesophageal echocardiographic evaluation of diastolic function. *Chest* 2005;128:3652–3663.

75. **Answer = B, Pseudonormal diastolic dysfunction is present.** The transmitral diastolic inflow velocities appear normal in the first figure obtained before administration of nitroglycerin, but with a decrease in preload an impaired relaxation pattern appears (indicating pseudonormal diastolic dysfunction). The decrease in early diastolic filling results from a decrease in the pressure gradient between the left atrium and the left ventricle in response to preload reduction.

As preload is decreased in patients with normal diastolic function both E and A will decrease to the same extent and the E/A ratio remains constant. Pseudonormal diastolic dysfunction will revert to an impaired relaxation wave form pattern with preload reduction. Note that the response of E and A waves to decreases in preload depends on the degree of diastolic dysfunction. As shown in Table 3.2Q, restrictive diastolic dysfunction will pseudonormalize if the diastolic dysfunction is reversible. Also note that in impaired relaxation E and A will both decrease, but E will decrease more than A (resulting in a decrease in the E/A ratio). E$_M$ and V$_P$ are not altered by decreases in loading conditions and this is one of their advantages over transmitral pulsed-wave Doppler flow velocities.

Table 3.2Q.   RESPONSE OF TRANSMITRAL FLOW VELOCITIES TO PRELOAD REDUCTION

Flow Pattern	E	A	E/A Ratio
Normal	Decreased	Decreased	No change
Impaired relaxation	Decreased	Decreased	Decreased
Pseudonormal	Decreased	Decreased	Decreased
Restrictive (reversible)	Decreased	Increased	Decreased
Restrictive (irreversible, end stage)	No change	No change	No change

Reference: Perrino AC, Reeves S. *A Practical Approach to TEE.* Philadelphia: Lippincott Williams & Wilkins 2003:117.

76. **Answer = A, The pulmonary vein atrial flow reversal wave (PV$_{AR}$ wave) is shown.**

Reference: Groban L, Dolinski SY. Transesophageal echocardiographic evaluation of diastolic function. *Chest* 2005;128:3652–3663.

77. **Answer = B, The pulmonary vein systolic wave (S wave) is shown.**

Reference: Groban L, Dolinski SY. Transesophageal echocardiographic evaluation of diastolic function. *Chest* 2005;128:3652–3663.

78. **Answer = C, The pulmonary vein diastolic wave (D wave) is shown.**

Reference: Groban L, Dolinski SY. Transesophageal echocardiographic evaluation of diastolic function. *Chest* 2005;128:3652–3663.

79. **Answer = D, Restrictive diastolic function is shown.** The transmitral pulsed-wave Doppler profile shows E >> A and decreased deceleration time (DT). The pulmonary vein pulsed-wave Doppler profile shows S < D.

Reference: Groban L, Dolinski SY. Transesophageal echocardiographic evaluation of diastolic function. *Chest* 2005;128:3652–3663.

80. **Answer = B, The transmitral pulsed wave Doppler A wave is indicated by the arrow.**

Reference: Groban L, Dolinski SY. Transesophageal echocardiographic evaluation of diastolic function. *Chest* 2005;128:3652–3663.

81. **Answer = E, Arrow 2 indicates pulmonary Doppler venous flow reversal wave (PV$_{AR}$ wave).**

Reference: Groban L, Dolinski SY. Transesophageal echocardiographic evaluation of diastolic function. *Chest* 2005;128:3652–3663.

82. **Answer = D, Arrow 3 indicates the pulmonary vein diastolic wave (D wave).**

Reference: Groban L, Dolinski SY. Transesophageal echocardiographic evaluation of diastolic function. *Chest* 2005;128:3652–3663.

83. **Answer = C, Arrow 4 indicates the pulmonary vein systolic wave (S wave).**

Reference: Groban L, Dolinski SY. Transesophageal echocardiographic evaluation of diastolic function. *Chest* 2005;128:3652–3663.

84. **Answer = B, A small pericardial effusion is < 0.5 cm (see Table 3.2R).**

Table 3.2R.	PERICARDIAL EFFUSION SEVERITY BY SIZE	
Mild	**Moderate**	**Severe**
< 0.5 cm	0.5–2.0 cm	> 2.0 cm

Reference: Otto C. *Textbook of Clinical Echocardiography, Third Edition.* Philadelphia: Elsevier 2004:262.

85. **Answer = D, A decrease in the transmitral peak E-wave velocity would be expected in constrictive pericarditis with spontaneous expiration.** With spontaneous expiration, intrathoracic pressure increases (compressing the thin-walled right ventricle, decreasing RV filling, and favoring LV filling and LV stroke volume).

Reference: Otto C. *Textbook of Clinical Echocardiography, Third Edition.* Philadelphia: Elsevier 2004:270–272.

86. **Answer = B, The left atrium is the most common location of a cardiac myxoma.** Myxoma, the most common primary cardiac tumor, accounts for 20 to 30% of intracardiac tumors and is most frequently located in the left atrium attached to the interatrial septum. This benign tumor can cause mechanical obstruction of left ventricular filling, embolic events, arrhythmias, and left ventricular outflow tract obstruction. It is recommended that these masses be removed if possible to prevent the complications listed.

Reference: Oh JK, Seward JB, Tajik AJ (eds). *The Echo Manual, Second Edition.* Philadelphia: Lippincott Williams & Wilkins 1999:205.

87. **Answer = B, The left atrial side of the interatrial septum is the most common location of a cardiac myxoma.** Myxoma, the most common primary cardiac tumor, accounts for 20 to 30% of intracardiac tumors and is most frequently located in the left atrium attached to the interatrial septum. This benign tumor can cause mechanical obstruction of left ventricular filling, embolic events, arrhythmias, and left ventricular outflow tract obstruction. It is recommended that these masses be removed if possible to prevent the complications listed.

Reference: Oh JK, Seward JB, Tajik AJ (eds). *The Echo Manual, Second Edition.* Philadelphia: Lippincott Williams & Wilkins 1999:205.

88. **Answer = E, All of the above are possible complications/findings associated with myxomas.** Myxoma, the most common primary cardiac tumor, accounts for 20 to 30% of intracardiac tumors and is most frequently located in the left atrium attached to the interatrial septum. This benign tumor can cause mechanical obstruction of left ventricular filling, embolic events, arrhythmias, and left ventricular outflow tract obstruction. It is recommended that these masses be removed if possible to prevent the complications listed.

Reference: Oh JK, Seward JB, Tajik AJ (eds). *The Echo Manual, Second Edition.* Philadelphia: Lippincott Williams & Wilkins 1999:205.

89. **Answer = C, A fibroma is a benign primary cardiac tumor usually found within the free wall of the left ventricle.** It must be distinguished from left ventricular wall thickening due to hypertrophic cardiomyopathy. It is generally well demarcated from the surrounding myocardium by multiple calcifications. Sometimes it grows into the left ventricular cavity and interferes with left ventricular filling. Rhabdomyoma

is the most common cardiac tumor seen in children. It is associated with tuberous sclerosis and is generally seen in the right ventricle. Myxoma, the most common primary cardiac tumor, accounts for 20 to 30% of intracardiac tumors and is most frequently located in the left atrium attached to the interatrial septum. Myxomas are benign tumors but they can cause mechanical obstruction of left ventricular filling, embolic events, arrhythmias, and left ventricular outflow tract obstruction. It is recommended that these masses be removed if possible to prevent the complications listed.

Reference: Oh JK, Seward JB, Tajik AJ (eds). *The Echo Manual, Second Edition.* Philadelphia: Lippincott Williams & Wilkins 1999:205.

90. **Answer = D, Rhabdomyoma is the most common cardiac tumor in children.** This malignant tumor is associated with tuberous sclerosis and is usually found in the right ventricle. Multiple tumors are frequently present.

Reference: Oh JK, Seward JB, Tajik AJ (eds). *The Echo Manual, Second Edition.* Philadelphia: Lippincott Williams & Wilkins 1999:209.

91. **Answer = D, The aortic valve is most frequently affected and the appearance is similar to that of lambl excrescences, but lambl excrescences are thinner and more broad based.** Embolic events can result from papillary fibroelastomas, and removal is recommended even in asymptomatic patients.

Reference: Oh JK, Seward JB, Tajik AJ (eds). *The Echo Manual, Second Edition.* Philadelphia: Lippincott Williams & Wilkins 1999:209–210.

92. **Answer = A, Angiosarcomas occur most frequently in the right atrium.** These are the most common malignant intracardiac tumors.

Reference: Oh JK, Seward JB, Tajik AJ (eds). *The Echo Manual, Second Edition.* Philadelphia: Lippincott Williams & Wilkins 1999:210.

93. **Answer = C, Embolic events are a complication frequently associated with papillary fibroelastomas, and removal is recommended even in asymptomatic patients.** Papillary fibroelastomas usually originate from the cardiac valves or adjacent endocardium. These benign tumors tend to originate on the atrial side of the atrioventricular valves and the ventricular surface of the similunar valves. The aortic valve is most frequently affected and the appearance is similar to that of lambl excrescences, but lambl excrescences are thinner and broader based.

Reference: Oh JK, Seward JB, Tajik AJ (eds). *The Echo Manual, Second Edition.* Philadelphia: Lippincott Williams & Wilkins 1999:209–210.

94. **Answer = D, An aneurysmal interatrial septum is associated with a patent foramen ovale.**

Reference: Mas J-L, Arquizan C, Lamy C, et al. Recurrent cerebrovascular events associated with patent foramen ovale, atrial septal aneurysm, or both. *N Engl J Med* 2001;345:1740–1746.

95. **Answer = C, An aneurysmal interatrial septum is associated with cerebrovascular accidents.**

Reference: Mas J-L, Arquizan C, Lamy C, et al. Recurrent cerebrovascular events associated with patent foramen ovale, atrial septal aneurysm, or both. *N Engl J Med* 2001;345:1740–1746.

96. **Answer = E, All of the above can damage a TEE probe.** Only glutaraldehyde-based solutions approved by the FDA and the manufacturer of the probe should be used.

Reference: Savage RM, Aronson S, Thomas JD, Shanewise JS, Shernan SK. *Comprehensive Textbook of Intraoperative Transesophageal Echocardiography.* Philadelphia: Lippincott Williams & Wilkins 2004:106.

97. **Answer = E, All of the above are possible complications of intraoperative TEE.**

Reference: Savage RM, Aronson S, Thomas JD, Shanewise JS, Shernan SK. *Comprehensive Textbook of Intraoperative Transesophageal Echocardiography.* Philadelphia: Lippincott Williams & Wilkins 2004:106.

98. **Answer = B, Refraction artifact results from the bending of sound.**

Reference: Edelman SK. *Understanding Ultrasound Physics.* Woodlands, TX: ESP, Inc. 1994:212.

99. **Answer = B, Refraction artifact places a second (artifactual) copy of a reflector to the side and slightly deeper than the true (actual = anatomic) reflector.**

Reference: Edelman SK. *Understanding Ultrasound Physics.* Woodlands, TX: ESP, Inc. 1994:212.

100. **Answer = C, Mirror image artifact places a second copy (artifactual copy) of a reflector deeper and to the side of the true anatomy.**

Reference: Edelman SK. *Understanding Ultrasound Physics.* Woodlands, TX: ESP, Inc. 1994:212.

101. **Answer = C, Propagation speed artifact results in the placement of objects at incorrect depth.** This occurs because the machine assumes that sound travels at exactly 1540 m/s through the body. If sound travels slower or faster than 1540 m/s, the machine will place an object too deep or too shallow (respectively).

Reference: Edelman SK. *Understanding Ultrasound Physics.* Woodlands, TX: ESP, Inc. 1994:210–212.

102. **Answer = C, A chiari network is an embryologic remnant of the sinus venosus.** It is a thin, mobile, web-like structure that can be seen in the bicaval view in about 2% of patients. It is associated with an aneurysmal interatrial septum and a patent foramen ovale.

Reference: Savage RM, Aronson S, Thomas JD, Shanewise JS, Shernan SK. *Comprehensive Textbook of Intraoperative Transesophageal Echocardiography.* Philadelphia: Lippincott Williams & Wilkins 2004:44.

103. **Answer = C, 20 Hz to 20 KHz is the frequency range of audible sound.**

Reference: Savage RM, Aronson S, Thomas JD, Shanewise JS, Shernan SK. *Comprehensive Textbook of Intraoperative Transesophageal Echocardiography.* Philadelphia: Lippincott Williams & Wilkins 2004:51.

104. Answer = B, Range ambiguity results when an ultrasound pulse is emitted prior to reception of all echoes generated from a previous pulse. The ultrasound machine cannot determine the correct depth of a reflector with range ambiguity.

Reference: Savage RM, Aronson S, Thomas JD, Shanewise JS, Shernan SK. *Comprehensive Textbook of Intraoperative Transesophageal Echocardiography.* Philadelphia: Lippincott Williams & Wilkins 2004:51.

105. Answer = A, The damping material decreases the piezoelectric crystal ringing and vibration, thereby producing a shorter spatial pulse length and improving axial resolution.

Reference: Savage RM, Aronson S, Thomas JD, Shanewise JS, Shernan SK. *Comprehensive Textbook of Intraoperative Transesophageal Echocardiography.* Philadelphia: Lippincott Williams & Wilkins 2004:53.

106. Answer = A, Decreasing beam width will improve lateral resolution.

Reference: Savage RM, Aronson S, Thomas JD, Shanewise JS, Shernan SK. *Comprehensive Textbook of Intraoperative Transesophageal Echocardiography.* Philadelphia: Lippincott Williams & Wilkins 2004:53.

107. Answer = C, Increasing the pulse repetition frequency will improve temporal resolution. The other options will all decrease temporal resolution.

Reference: Savage RM, Aronson S, Thomas JD, Shanewise JS, Shernan SK. *Comprehensive Textbook of Intraoperative Transesophageal Echocardiography.* Philadelphia: Lippincott Williams & Wilkins 2004:55.

108. Answer = B, The time gain compensation increases the receiver gain with increasing arrival time of echoes to compensate for ultrasound attenuation. Deeper structures have weaker echoes and require more gain for optimal visualization.

Reference: Savage RM, Aronson S, Thomas JD, Shanewise JS, Shernan SK. *Comprehensive Textbook of Intraoperative Transesophageal Echocardiography.* Philadelphia: Lippincott Williams & Wilkins 2004:55.

109. Answer = E, All of the above could result in a dilated coronary sinus. Anything that increases blood flow into the coronary sinus or pressure in the right atrium could dilate the coronary sinus.

Reference: Sidebotham D, Merry A, Legget M (eds.). *Practical Perioperative Transoesophageal Echocardiography.* Burlington, MA: Butterworth Heinemann 2003:72.

110. Answer = C, An inverted left atrial appendage is the most likely diagnosis.

Reference: Sidebotham D, Merry A, Legget M (eds.). *Practical Perioperative Transoesophageal Echocardiography.* Burlington, MA: Butterworth Heinemann 2003:74.

111. **Answer = E, > 50% of patients with an interatrial septum aneurysm have a patent foramen ovale.**

Reference: Sidebotham D, Merry A, Legget M (eds.). *Practical Perioperative Transoesophageal Echocardiography.* Burlington, MA: Butterworth Heinemann 2003:74.

112. **Answer = C, The moderator band is a prominent right ventricular trabeculum that runs from the interventricular septum to the base of the anterior papillary muscle.**

Reference: Sidebotham D, Merry A, Legget M (eds.). *Practical Perioperative Transoesophageal Echocardiography.* Burlington, MA: Butterworth Heinemann 2003:74.

113. **Answer = B, The midesophageal two-chamber view is the best view to rule out an apical left ventricular thrombus following a full thickness anterior myocardial infarction.** This is the best TEE view for visualizing the apex of the heart. Although the apex can sometimes be seen in some of the other views listed, the *best* view for imaging the apex is the midesophageal two-chamber view. The LV apex is usually better visualized with transthoracic echocardiography.

Reference: Sidebotham D, Merry A, Legget M (eds.). *Practical Perioperative Transoesophageal Echocardiography.* Burlington, MA: Butterworth Heinemann 2003:82.

114. **Answer = A, 1.9 cm^2 is the aortic valve area (AVA) (A_{AV}).** The calculation is as follows.

$$A_{AV} = (\text{aortic valve side})^2 * 0.433$$

$$A_{AV} = (2.1 \text{ cm})^2 * 0.433$$

$$A_{AV} = 1.9 \text{ cm}^2$$

Reference: Sidebotham D, Merry A, Legget M (eds.). *Practical Perioperative Transoesophageal Echocardiography.* Burlington, MA: Butterworth Heinemann 2003:232.

115. **Answer = E, 90.4 cm^3 is the right ventricular stroke volume.** The calculation is as follows.

$$SV_{PA} = A_{PA} * TVI_{PA}$$

$$SV_{PA} = \pi r^2 * TVI_{PA}$$

$$SV_{PA} = \pi (1.2 \text{ cm})^2 * 20 \text{ cm}$$

$$SV_{PA} = 90.4 \text{ cm}^3$$

Reference: SCA/ASE Annual Comprehensive Review and Update of Perioperative Hemodynamics Workshop. 17 Feb. 2005, San Diego, CA; discussion lead by Stanton Shernon, et al.

116. **Answer = A, 47.1 cm³ is the left ventricular stroke volume.** The calculation is as follows.

$$SV_{LVOT} = A_{LVOT} * TVI_{LVOT}$$

$$SV_{LVOT} = \pi r^2 * TVI_{LVOT}$$

$$SV_{LVOT} = \pi\ (1.0\ cm)^2 * 15\ cm$$

$$SV_{LVOT} = 47.1\ cm^3$$

Reference: SCA/ASE Annual Comprehensive Review and Update of Perioperative Hemodynamics Workshop. 17 Feb. 2005, San Diego, CA; discussion lead by Stanton Shernon, et al.

117. **Answer = C, 2:1 = Q$_p$/Q$_s$.** The calculation is as follows.

$$Q_p/Q_s = SV_{PA}/SV_{LVOT}$$

$$Q_p/Q_s = 90.4/47.1$$

$$Q_p/Q_s \cong 2{:}1$$

$$SV_{PA} = A_{PA} * TVI_{PA}$$

$$SV_{PA} = \pi r^2 * TVI_{PA}$$

$$SV_{PA} = \pi\ (1.2\ cm)^2 * 20\ cm$$

$$SV_{PA} = 90.4\ cm^3$$

$$SV_{LVOT} = A_{LVOT} * TVI_{LVOT}$$

$$SV_{LVOT} = \pi r^2 * TVI_{LVOT}$$

$$SV_{LVOT} = \pi\ (1.0\ cm)^2 * 15\ cm$$

$$SV_{LVOT} = 47.1\ cm^3$$

Reference: Sidebotham D, Merry A, Legget M (eds.). *Practical Perioperative Transoesophageal Echocardiography.* Burlington, MA: Butterworth Heinemann 2003:231.

118. **Answer = B, 51 mmHg = the pulmonary artery systolic pressure (PASP).** The calculation is as follows.

$$\Delta P = 4V^2$$

$$(LVSP - RVSP) = 4(V_{VSD})^2$$

$$RVSP = LVSP - 4(V_{VSD})^2$$

$$RVSP = SBP - 4(V_{VSD})^2$$

$$RVSP = 100 - 4(3.5)^2$$

$$RVSP = 51\ mmHg$$

$$PASP = RVSP = 51\ mmHg$$

LVSP = left ventricular systolic pressure

RVSP = right ventricular systolic pressure

V_{VSD} = peak velocity of the left-to-right flow across the ventricular septal defect

SBP = systemic systolic blood pressure

Reference: Perrino AC, Reeves S. *A Practical Approach to TEE.* Philadelphia: Lippincott Williams & Wilkins 2003:103.

119. **Answer = E, All of the choices listed are potential causes of dilated cardiomyopathy.**

Reference: Otto C. *Textbook of Clinical Echocardiography, Third Edition.* Philadelphia: Elsevier 2004:228.

120. **Answer = C, an increased E-point to septal separation (EPSS) is indicative of dilated cardiomyopathy.** The increased EPSS is due to a combo of left ventricular dilation and reduced mitral valve leaflet motion due to low transmitral flow rates.

Reference: Otto C. *Textbook of Clinical Echocardiography, Third Edition.* Philadelphia: Elsevier 2004:228.

121. **Answer = C, MR jet area = 5.3 cm^2 is consistent with moderate mitral regurgitation and this would be expected in a patient with dilated cardiomyopathy.** An increased aortic ejection velocity and TVI would be indicative of increased cardiac output, and this is not consistent with this disease. An increased dp/dt would indicate increased systolic function, and this would also not be expected. The lateral mitral annular tissue Doppler E_M would be expected to be less than 8 cm/sec.

Reference: Otto C. *Textbook of Clinical Echocardiography, Third Edition.* Philadelphia: Elsevier 2004:228.

122. **Answer = E, $\geq$ 20 mm is consistent with severe left ventricular hypertrophy** (see Table 3.2S).

Table 3.2S.

Degree of LVH	LV Free Wall Thickness
Normal	6–11 mm
Mild LVH	12–14 mm
Moderate LVH	15–19 mm
Severe LVH	$\geq$ 20 mm

Abbreviations: LV = left ventricle, LVH = left ventricle hypertrophy.

123. **Answer = C, A dp/dt of 600 is indicative of decreased systolic function, which would be expected in a patient with dilated cardiomyopathy.** The other choices list measures of systolic function indicative of normal systolic function.

Reference: Otto C. *Textbook of Clinical Echocardiography, Third Edition.* Philadelphia: Elsevier 2004:228.

124. **Answer = C, An increased septal wall thickness to posterior wall thickness ratio would be expected in a patient with hypertrophic cardiomyopathy.**

Reference: Otto C. *Textbook of Clinical Echocardiography, Third Edition.* Philadelphia: Elsevier 2004:228.

125. **Answer = D, Cobalt toxicity can result in dilated cardiomyopathy.**

Reference: Otto C. *Textbook of Clinical Echocardiography, Third Edition.* Philadelphia: Elsevier 2004:228.

126. **Answer = B, Hypertrophic cardiomyopathy is inherited and the genetics are best described as autosomal dominant with variable penetrance.** Penetrance is defined as the percentage of individuals with a given genotype who exhibit the phenotype associated with that genotype. With 100% penetrance every individual with the dominant gene will develop the disease. With variable penetrance, people with the gene for the disease may not develop the disease.

References: Otto C. *Textbook of Clinical Echocardiography, Third Edition.* Philadelphia: Elsevier 2004:228; Griffiths AJ. *An Introduction to Genetic Analysis, Fifth Edition.* New York: WH Freeman 1995:103.

127. **Answer = B, The outflow tract obstruction in hypertrophic cardiomyopathy is influenced by loading conditions.** Hemodynamic goals to decrease this dynamic obstruction are listed in Table 3.2T. Essentially, anything that keeps the heart full will help prevent SAM and decrease LVOT obstruction. SAM = systolic anterior motion of the anterior mitral valve leaflet, and LVOT = left ventricular outflow tract.

Table 3.2T. HEMODYNAMIC GOALS FOR HYPERTROPHIC CARDIOMYOPATHY

Preload	Afterload	Contractility	Heart Rate
Increase	Increase	Decrease	Decrease

Reference: Otto C. *Textbook of Clinical Echocardiography, Third Edition.* Philadelphia: Elsevier 2004:230–232.

128. **Answer = A, Visualization of a bicuspid aortic valve in a neonate will be adversely affected by poor temporal resolution more than the other choices.** Temporal resolution is the ability to accurately locate the position of moving structures at particular instants in time. *Temporal resolution* depends on the following two main factors.

- How much the object being imaged moves.
- The *frame rate* = frames/sec = images/sec.

The more an object moves the worse the temporal resolution. A neonatal heart moves faster than an adult heart. Therefore, temporal resolution of the neonatal valve will be worse than that of an adult valve. This is why M-mode is frequently used in neonatal imaging.

Reference: Edelman SK. *Understanding Ultrasound Physics.* Woodlands, TX: ESP, Inc. 1994:121.

129. **Answer = A, The units for pulse repetition frequency = pulses/sec.** Pulse repetition frequency (PRF) = (pulses/image) * (images/sec). Line density = scan lines per image. Frame rate = images/sec. Frame rate times line

density is *not* equal to PRF. PRF decreases as imaging depth increases. PRF increases as temporal resolution increases.

Reference: Edelman SK. *Understanding Ultrasound Physics.* Woodlands, TX: ESP, Inc. 1994:122.

130. **Answer = D, The ultrasound beam is perpendicular to the direction of blood flow.** Because the frequency returned is equal to the frequency emitted, there is no Doppler shift. Because there is no Doppler shift there is either no blood flow or the blood flow is perpendicular to the ultrasound beam. When blood flow is perpendicular to the ultrasound beam, the angle θ is equal to 90 degrees and the Doppler shift (Δf) is zero. The Doppler shift for ultrasound in soft tissue is determined by the following formula.

- $\Delta f = V \cos\theta\, 2 F_t / C$
- $\Delta f = (F_t - F_r)$
- F_t = transmitter frequency
- F_r = returning frequency
- V = velocity
- C = speed of sound in soft tissue (1,540 m/s)
- θ = angle between the sound beam and the red blood cell flow

Reference: Sidebotham D, Merry A, Legget M (eds.). *Practical Perioperative Transoesophageal Echocardiography.* Burlington, MA: Butterworth Heinemann 2003:34.

131. **Answer = B, The inferior wall has hibernating myocardium, as indicated by the wall motion seen.** The inferior wall is akinetic at rest, and then improves in response to low-dose dobutamine becoming mildly hypokinetic. The inferior wall then reverts to akinesis in response to high-dose dobutamine. This indicates hibernating myocardium, which is supplied by a nonfixed lesion in the right coronary artery.

Reference: Oh JK, Seward JB, Tajik AJ (eds). *The Echo Manual, Second Edition.* Philadelphia: Lippincott Williams & Wilkins 1999:96.

132. **Answer = D, The posterior wall remains akinetic in response to the administration of dobutamine, indicating dead nonviable myocardium.** This results from a fixed irreversible ischemic lesion.

Reference: Oh JK, Seward JB, Tajik AJ (eds). *The Echo Manual, Second Edition.* Philadelphia: Lippincott Williams & Wilkins 1999:96.

133. **Answer = A, Rheumatic heart disease is the most common cause of tricuspid stenosis (TS).** TS is rare because the tricuspid valve has a large area. Although rheumatic disease is the most common cause of TS, it usually causes tricuspid regurgitation. Rheumatic heart disease usually affects the mitral valve, but it can also affect the aortic and tricuspid valve (20 to 30% of cases). Carcinoid heart disease can also cause tricuspid stenosis, but this is less common than TS from rheumatic disease.

Reference: Perrino AC, Reeves S. *A Practical Approach to TEE.* Philadelphia: Lippincott Williams & Wilkins 2003:226.

134. **Answer = B, Carcinoid heart disease is the most likely cause of the tricuspid and pulmonic valve pathology in this patient.** Carcinoid tumors most commonly originate in the ileum. Carcinoid heart disease results from the release of active metabolites from carcinoid tumor cells. These metabolites (serotonin, bradykinin, histamine, and prostaglandins) damage the tricuspid and pulmonic valves. The left-sided valves are protected from these substances because they are degraded by monoamine oxidases in the lung. Carcinoid syndrome results in thickened fibrotic leaflets with restrictive mobility.

Reference: Perrino AC, Reeves S. *A Practical Approach to TEE.* Philadelphia: Lippincott Williams & Wilkins 2003:226.

135. **Answer = C, Ebstein's anomaly is a congenital disorder of the tricuspid valve (TV).** A malformed TV with one or more of the TV leaflets displaced from the TV annulus toward the ventricular apex is observed in this disorder.

Reference: Sidebotham D, Merry A, Legget M (eds.). *Practical Perioperative Transoesophageal Echocardiography.* Burlington, MA: Butterworth Heinemann 2003:210.

136. **Answer = D, Right ventricular pressure overload causes movement/displacement/flattening of the septum from the right to the left ventricle during late systole.** This occurs when the right ventricle pressure is highest, which is at end systole. Note that with right ventricular volume overload this movement occurs at late diastole because this is when right ventricular volume is highest.

Reference: Sidebotham D, Merry A, Legget M (eds.). *Practical Perioperative Transoesophageal Echocardiography.* Burlington, MA: Butterworth Heinemann 2003:206.

TEST IV PART 1

Video Test Booklet

This product is designed to prepare people for the PTEeXAM. This booklet is to be used with the CD-ROM to practice for the video portion of the PTEeXAM.

Preface

As stated previously, this part of this product is designed to prepare people for the video component of the PTEeXAM. Please do not open this test booklet until you have read the instructions. During the PTEeXAM, instructions similar to these will be written on the back of the test booklet. You will be asked to read these instructions by a proctor at the exam. After you have read these instructions you will be asked to break the seal on the test booklet and to remove an answer sheet, similar to the one included with this practice test.

After you have filled out your name, test number, and other identifying information on the answer sheet you will be instructed to open the test booklet and begin. This test will involve video images shown on a computer monitor. You will share this monitor with three other examinees. This portion of the PTEeXAM has about 50 questions. It consists of about 17 cases, with 2 to 5 questions for each case. It is timed. Good luck!

Instructions

This test will consist of several cases, accompanied by 3 to 5 questions per case. Each case will show one or more images. For each case, you are to utilize the information written in this booklet and the information shown in the images to answer questions concerning each case. An audible chime or tone will assist in timing the exam. This tone alerts you when the test advances to the next step.

The order of the exam is as follows.

Tone/chime

1. Read the questions for case 1.

Tone/chime

2. View the images for case 1.

Tone/chime

3. Answer the questions for case 1.

Tone/chime

4. View the images for case 1 again.

Tone/chime

5. Check your answers to the questions for case 1.

Tone/chime

6. Read the questions for case 2.

Tone/chime

The process continues in this manner. In summary: tone, read, tone, view, tone, answer, tone, view, tone, check answers, tone.

Cases

Case 1

1. Given the R-R interval and the time velocity integral proximal to the aortic valve (sample gate in the left ventricular outflow tract), what additional information is needed to calculate the cardiac output?

   A. Aortic valve area (AVA)

   B. Diameter of the left ventricular outflow tract (LVOT diameter)

   C. Time velocity integral of blood flow through the aortic valve obtained with continuous-wave Doppler

   D. None of the above

Case 2

2. What type of lesion is shown?

   A. Ostium primum atrial septal defect

   B. Ostium secundum atrial septal defect

   C. Sinus venosus atrial septal defect

   D. Coronary sinus atrial septal defect

3. Which of the following statements concerning the patient's condition is most likely true?

   A. It is associated with a cleft mitral valve.

   B. It is associated with anomalous pulmonary venous return.

   C. When combined with an inlet VSD this defect is part of an endocardial cushion defect.

   D. It is the most common type of atrial septal defect.

   E. It is associated with a persistent left superior vena cava.

Case 3

4. What walls are illustrated best in this image?

   A. Posterior and anterior

   B. Septal and lateral

   C. Anterior and inferior

   D. Anteroseptal and posterior

5. What coronary artery supplies the area shown to have a regional wall motion abnormality in this image?

   A. Left anterior descending coronary artery

   B. Right coronary artery

   C. Posterior descending coronary artery

   D. Circumflex coronary artery

6. What *other* TEE view could be used to evaluate the segmental wall motion abnormality shown?

A. Midesophageal four-chamber view

B. Transgastric two-chamber view

C. Midesophageal long axis view

D. Midesophageal two-chamber view

E. Transgastric RV outflow view

Case 4

A 67-year-old female has undergone mitral valve surgery. Use the information in the images to answer the following questions.

7. What type of surgery has the patient in case 4 undergone?

A. Mitral valve repair with a ring annuloplasty

B. Mitral valve replacement with a St. Jude mitral valve prosthesis

C. Mitral valve repair with a sliding annuloplasty and resection of the P2 scallop

D. Mitral valve replacement with a stented porcine heterograft (Carpentier/ Edwards valve)

E. Mitral valve replacement with stented bovine pericardial valve

8. Which of the following best describes the function of the valve shown in case 4?

A. Normal transvalvular regurgitation is present.

B. Moderate transvalvular regurgitation is present.

C. Severe stenosis is present.

D. Significant paravalvular regurgitation is present.

E. Systolic anterior motion of the anterior mitral valve leaflet is present.

9. The images were obtained immediately following separation from cardiopulmonary bypass (CPB). What treatment measures are indicated?

A. Return to CPB because one of the leaflets is not opening properly, resulting in a mitral stenosis.

B. Return to CPB to addresss significant paravalvular regurgitation.

C. Return to CPB to address significant transvalvular regurgitation.

D. Return to CPB to address systolic anterior motion of the anterior mitral valve leaflet.

E. The valve function is normal. If it is otherwise stable, administer protamine.

10. What structure is indicated by the arrow labeled C in image 6 for case 4?

A. Coronary sinus

B. Right coronary artery

C. Left coronary artery

D. Perivalvular abscess

E. No structure (this is echo dropout from acoustic shadowing)

Case 5

11. Which of the following best describes the severity of the mitral regurgitation (MR) shown in the images for case 5?

A. Trace.

B. Mild.

C. Moderate.

D. Severe.

E. Not enough information is given to determine the severity of MR.

12. In addition to mitral regurgitation, what other valvular disorder can be seen in the images shown for case 5?

   A. Mitral stenosis

   B. Aortic regurgitation

   C. Aortic stenosis

   D. Pulmonic regurgitation

   E. Tricuspid regurgitation

Case 6

13. What is the mechanism for the mitral regurgitation seen in image 1 for case 6?

   A. Systolic anterior motion of the anterior mitral valve leaflet with left ventricular outflow tract obstruction after mitral valve repair

   B. Paravalvular regurgitation

   C. Restricted mitral valve leaflet motion

   D. Annular dilation with incomplete coaptation

   E. Flail anterior mitral valve leaflet with a ruptured chord

14. What would be the most appropriate initial therapy for this patient?

   A. Stop inotropes, administer volume, direct vasoconstrictors (phenylephrine, vasopressin), and judicious doses of esmolol.

   B. Return to cardiopulmonary bypass and perform a mitral valve replacement.

   C. Increase contractility and afterload with drugs such as milrinone, epinephrine, and norepinephrine.

   D. Administer drugs that decrease afterload and increase contractility (such as milrinone and sodium nitroprusside).

   E. Administer drugs that help decrease pulmonary artery pressures and right heart failure (such as milrinone and inhaled nitric oxide).

Case 7

15. Which of the following best describes the severity of the mitral regurgitation seen in the patient for case 7?

    A. Trace to mild.

    B. Mild to moderate.

    C. Moderate to severe.

    D. Severe.

    E. Not enough information is provided to make this determination.

16. Using the Carpentier classification system for mitral valve leaflet motion in mitral regurgitation, describe the leaflet motion seen in case 7.

    A. Type I leaflet motion

    B. Type II leaflet motion

    C. Type III leaflet motion

    D. Type IV leaflet motion

    E. Type V leaflet motion

Case 8

17. What is the most likely diagnosis?

    A. Critical aortic stenosis with Stanford type B aortic dissection

    B. Stanford type A aortic dissection in a patient with Marfan's syndrome

    C. Aortic abscess cavity with a bicuspid aortic valve

    D. Stanford type B aortic dissection with a bicuspid aortic valve

    E. DeBakey type IIIa aortic dissection with bicuspid aortic valve

18. Which of the following is associated with the disorder seen in case 8?

    A. Aortic aneurysms

    B. Aortic coarctation

    C. Ventricular septal defects

    D. Aortic stenosis

    E. All of the above

Case 9

19. Which of the following is indicated by the arrow in image 1 for case 9?

    A. Christa terminalis

    B. Right atrial tumor

    C. Thrombus

    D. Eustachian valve

    E. Chiari network

20. Which of the following is true concerning location A versus location B in image 3 for case 9?

    A. Lateral resolution at location B is less than at location A.

    B. Temporal resolution at location B is greater than at location A.

    C. Beam width at location B is less than at location A.

    D. Azimuthal resolution at location B is greater than at location A.

    E. Transverse resolution at location B is greater than at location A.

21. Which mitral valve leaflet is indicated by arrow 1 in image 3 for case 9?

    A. Septal

    B. Medial

    C. Inferior

    D. Posterior

    E. Anterior

Case 10

22. Image 1 for case 10 shows which of the following?

    A. Interatrial septum tumor

    B. Right atrial thrombus

    C. Lipomatous interatrial septum

    D. Chiari network

    E. Infiltrative amyloidosis

23. What treatment is required for the patient shown in image 1 for case 10?

    A. Chemotherapy

    B. No treatment needed

    C. Heart transplantation

    D. Systemic anticoagulation

    E. Radiation therapy

Case 11

24. Which of the following is shown in image 1 for case 11?

    A. Right atrial tumor

    B. Left atrial tumor

    C. Thrombus

    D. Chiari network

    E. Christa terminalis

Case 12

25. Which of the following is indicated by the arrow in image 1 for case 12?

    A. Chiari network

    B. Christa terminalis

    C. Thrombus

    D. Right atrial tumor

    E. Eustachian valve

26. Arrow 1 in image 3 of case 12 shows which of the following?

    A. Left pulmonary artery

    B. Right pulmonary artery

    C. Coronary sinus

    D. Left atrial appendage

    E. Left main coronary artery

27. Arrow 2 in image 3 of case 12 shows which of the following?

    A. Right atrium

    B. Left atrium

    C. Superior vena cava

    D. Inferior vena cava

    E. Coronary sinus

28. Arrow 3 in image 3 of case 12 shows which of the following?

    A. Right pulmonary artery

    B. Left atrium

    C. Superior vena cava

    D. Inferior vena cava

    E. Coronary sinus

Case 13

29. What is the diagnosis?

    A. Normal St. Jude aortic valve prosthesis

    B. Infected carbomedic bileaflet valve prosthesis

    C. Medtronic Hall single tilting disc prosthesis

    D. Infected allograft prosthesis with perivalvular abscess

    E. Starr-Edwards® caged disc valve with perivalvular abscess

30. What artifact is indicated by the arrow shown in image 3, case 13?

A. Beam width artifact

B. Side lobe artifact

C. Reverberation artifact

D. Acoustic shadowing

E. Mirror image artifact

31. What view is shown in case 13?

A. Midesophageal long axis view

B. Midesophageal aortic outflow view

C. Midesophageal two-chamber view

D. Midesophageal aortic valve exit view

E. Midesophageal left ventricular inflow/outflow view

32. What other view could be used to evaluate the aortic valve?

A. Transgastric aortic valve short axis view

B. Deep transgastric long axis view

C. Transgastric aortic valve long axis view

D. Deep transgastric aortic outflow view

E. Transgastric left ventricular inflow/outflow view

Case 14

33. What is indicated by the arrow in image 1 for case 14?

A. Aorta

B. Azygos vein

C. Superior vena cava

D. Right pulmonary artery

E. Left pulmonary artery

34. What is indicated by the arrow in image 2 for case 14?

    A. Aorta

    B. Azygos vein

    C. Superior vena cava

    D. Right pulmonary artery

    E. Left pulmonary artery

35. What is indicated by the arrow in image 3 for case 14?

    A. Chiari network

    B. Aortic valve

    C. Eustachian valve

    D. Crista terminalis

    E. Pulmonic valve

36. What view is shown in case 14?

    A. Upper esophageal aortic arch short axis view

    B. Midesophageal ascending aortic short axis view

    C. Midesophageal aortic short axis view

    D. Midesophageal ascending aortic long axis view

    E. Upper esophageal aortic arch long axis view

Case 15

37. What is the diagnosis?

    A. Stanford type A dissection

    B. Stanford type B dissection

    C. DeBakey type I dissection

    D. DeBakey type IIa dissection

    E. DeBakey type IIb dissection

38. Which of the following is true concerning the disorder shown?

   A. Stanford type A dissections occur more frequently than Stanford type B.

   B. Medical and surgical treatments for this patient have similar mortality rates.

   C. Beta blockers are beneficial because they decrease the ejection velocity.

   D. Patients with Marfan's syndrome with an Ao ratio <1.3 are at decreased risk of developing this complication.

   E. All of the above are true.

Case 16

39. Arrow 1 indicates which of the following?

   A. Right atrium

   B. Left atrium

   C. Left pulmonary artery

   D. Right pulmonary artery

   E. Coronary sinus

40. Arrow 2 indicates which of the following?

   A. Sinotubular ridge

   B. Aortic valve annulus

   C. Pulmonic valve sulcus

   D. Sinus of valsalva

   E. Aortic root sulcus

41. Arrow 3 indicates which of the following?

   A. Sinotubular ridge

   B. Aortic valve annulus

   C. Pulmonic valve sulcus

   D. Sinus of valsalva

   E. Aortic root sulcus

42. Arrow 4 indicates which of the following?

    A. Right atrium

    B. Left atrium

    C. Left pulmonary artery

    D. Right pulmonary artery

    E. Coronary sinus

43. What view is shown in image 3 for case 16?

    A. Transgastric long axis view

    B. Deep transgastric long axis view

    C. Transgastric aortic valve long axis view

    D. Transgastric left ventricular inflow/outflow view

    E. Transgastric two-chamber view

44. Which of the following best describes the degree of regurgitation seen in case 16?

    A. Trace.

    B. Mild.

    C. Moderate.

    D. Severe.

    E. It cannot be determined from the information given.

Case 17

45. What is the diagnosis?

    A. Normally functioning Starr-Edwards valve

    B. Caged-disc Kay-Shiley valve with trace regurgitation

    C. Normally functioning St. Jude bileaflet prosthesis

    D. Normally functioning porcine bioprosthesis

    E. Medtronic Hall tilting disc valve with trace regurgitation

46. How many normal "cleansing jets" does the valve shown have when it is functioning normally?

    A. None

    B. 2

    C. 3

    D. 4

    E. 5

47. Which of the following is an advantage of the valve shown when compared to a mitral valve repair?

    A. Increased mitral valve orifice area

    B. Decreased need for anticoagulation

    C. Decreased risk of infection

    D. Decreased risk of the development of CHF

    E. None of the above

Case 18

48. According to the American Society of Echocardiography 16-segment model, what numerical segment of the left ventricle is described by arrow 1?

    A. 5

    B. 6

    C. 7

    D. 8

    E. 9

49. According to the American Society of Echocardiography 16-segment model, what numerical segment of the left ventricle is described by arrow 2?

    A. 9

    B. 10

    C. 11

    D. 12

    E. 13

50. According to the American Society of Echocardiography 16-segment model, what numerical segment of the left ventricle is described by arrow 3?

A. 12

B. 13

C. 14

D. 15

E. 16

51. According to the American Society of Echocardiography 16-segment model, what numerical segment of the left ventricle is described by arrow 4?

A. 12

B. 13

C. 14

D. 15

E. 16

52. According to the American Society of Echocardiography 16-segment model, what numerical segment of the left ventricle is described by arrow 5?

A. 8

B. 9

C. 10

D. 11

E. 12

53. According to the American Society of Echocardiography 16-segment model, what numerical segment of the left ventricle is described by arrow 6?

A. 1

B. 2

C. 3

D. 4

E. 5

Case 19

54. Given a right atrial pressure of 10 mmHg, what is the right ventricular systolic pressure?

    A. 26 mmHg

    B. 36 mmHg

    C. 46 mmHg

    D. 56 mmHg

    E. 66 mmHg

55. How would you describe the degree of tricuspid regurgitation?

    A. Trace.

    B. Mild.

    C. Moderate.

    D. Severe.

    E. It cannot be determined from the given data.

Case 20

56. Which of the following is indicated by arrow 1?

    A. Acoustic resonance artifact

    B. Comet tail artifact

    C. Refraction artifact

    D. Multipath artifact

    E. Acoustic speckle artifact

57. Which of the following is indicated by arrow 2?

    A. Posteromedial papillary muscle

    B. Anterolateral papillary muscle

    C. Anteromedial papillary muscle

    D. Posterolateral papillary muscle

    E. Inferior papillary muscle

58. Which of the following is indicated by arrow 3?

    A. Posteromedial papillary muscle

    B. Anterolateral papillary muscle

    C. Anteromedial papillary muscle

    D. Posterolateral papillary muscle

    E. Inferior papillary muscle

Case 21

59. Which of the following best describes the wall motion seen?

    A. Inferior wall dyskinesis

    B. Anterior wall hypokinesis

    C. Inferior wall hypokinesis

    D. Anterior wall dyskinesis

    E. Anterior wall akinesis

60. Which of the following findings would be expected on EKG?

    A. Q waves in leads II, III, and AVF

    B. Q waves in leads V1 and V2

    C. ST depression in I and AVF

    D. ST elevation in leads V2 through V6

    E. None of the above

61. Arrow 1 indicates which of the following?

    A. Comet tail artifact

    B. Acoustic shadowing artifact

    C. Acoustic streaking artifact

    D. Linear shadowing artifact

    E. Mirroring artifact

62. Arrow 2 indicates which of the following?

   A. Anterolateral papillary muscle

   B. Moderator band

   C. Anteromedial papillary muscle

   D. Posteromedial papillary muscle

   E. Posterolateral papillary muscle

63. According to the American Society of Echocardiography 16-segment model, what numerical segment of the left ventricle is shown to have a segmental wall motion abnormality?

   A. Segment 8

   B. Segment 9

   C. Segment 10

   D. Segment 11

   E. Segment 12

64. Arrow 3 indicates which of the following?

   A. A small pericardial effusion

   B. Acoustic shadowing artifact

   C. Reverberation artifact

   D. Refraction artifact

   E. A small pleural effusion

Case 22

65. Arrow 1 indicates which of the following?

   A. Ascites

   B. Pericardial effusion

   C. Pleural effusion

   D. Amniotic fluid

   E. Cerbrospinal fluid

66. Arrow 2 indicates which of the following?

   A. Superior vena cava

   B. Ascending aorta

   C. Descending aorta

   D. Main pulmonary artery

   E. Right pulmonary artery

67. Arrow 3 indicates which of the following?

   A. Ascites

   B. Pericardial effusion

   C. Pleural effusion

   D. Amniotic fluid

   E. Cerebrospinal fluid

Case 23

68. Arrow 1 indicates which of the following?

   A. Aorta

   B. Inferior vena cava

   C. Superior vena cava

   D. Coronary sinus

   E. Right upper pulmonary vein

69. Arrow 2 indicates which of the following?

   A. Right upper pulmonary vein

   B. Right lower pulmonary vein

   C. Left upper pulmonary vein

   D. Left lower pulmonary vein

   E. Superior vena cava

70. Arrow 3 indicates which of the following?

    A. Right upper pulmonary vein

    B. Right lower pulmonary vein

    C. Left upper pulmonary vein

    D. Left lower pulmonary vein

    E. Superior vena cava

Answers:

1. B	25. B	49. C
2. B	26. B	50. D
3. D	27. B	51. B
4. C	28. D	52. A
5. A	29. C	53. B
6. B	30. D	54. B
7. B	31. A	55. D
8. A	32. B	56. B
9. E	33. C	57. B
10. A	34. D	58. A
11. D	35. E	59. A
12. B	36. B	60. A
13. A	37. B	61. A
14. A	38. E	62. D
15. A	39. B	63. D
16. A	40. D	64. A
17. C	41. A	65. C
18. E	42. D	66. C
19. D	43. B	67. B
20. A	44. D	68. C
21. E	45. C	69. A
22. C	46. D	70. B
23. B	47. E	
24. A	48. A	

Explanations

Case 1

1. **Answer = B, The diameter of the left ventricular outflow tract.** The LVOT diameter is needed to calculate cardiac output in this case. Given the time velocity integral proximal to the aortic valve and the R-R interval, the only thing needed to calculate the cardiac output is the diameter of the left ventricular outflow tract.

Reference: Savage RM, Aronson S, Thomas JD, Shanewise JS, Shernan SK. *Comprehensive Textbook of Intraoperative Transesophageal Echocardiography.* Philadelphia: Lippincott Williams & Wilkins 2004:43.

Case 2

2. **Answer = B, An ostium secundum ASD is shown.** This is the most common type of ASD. It is located in the region of the fossa ovalis.

References: Perrino AC, Reeves S. *A Practical Approach to TEE.* Philadelphia: Lippincott Williams & Wilkins 2003:287; Savage RM, Aronson S, Thomas JD, Shanewise JS, Shernan SK. *Comprehensive Textbook of Intraoperative Transesophageal Echocardiography.* Philadelphia: Lippincott Williams & Wilkins 2004:43.

3. **Answer = D, An ostium secundum ASD is shown, and this is the most common type.** Sinus venosus defects are associated with anomalous pulmonary venous return. Mnemonic: Sinus **V**enosus defects → anomalous pulmonary **V**enous return. Ostium primum ASDs are associated with a cleft mitral valve. Ostium primum ASDs + inlet VSD = endocardial cushion defect = AV canal defect. Coronary sinus ASDs are very rare, and they are associated with a persistent left superior vena cava.

Reference: Otto C. *Textbook of Clinical Echocardiography, Third Edition.* Philadelphia: Elsevier 2004:466.

Case 3

4. **Answer = C, Anterior and inferior walls are shown in this midesophageal two-chamber view.** The arrow indicates the anterior wall.

Reference: Konstadt SN, Shernon S, Oka Y (eds). *Clinical Transesophageal Echocardiography: A Problem-Oriented Approach, Second Edition.* Philadelphia: Lippincott Williams & Wilkins 2003:45.

5. **Answer = A, The left anterior descending coronary artery supplies the apical anterior segment shown to be hypokinetic in this image.** This patient is undergoing an off-pump coronary artery bypass graft procedure and the anterior wall is prevented from contracting normally by an anterior wall stabilizing device (octopus).

Reference: Konstadt SN, Shernon S, Oka Y (eds). *Clinical Transesophageal Echocardiography: A Problem-Oriented Approach, Second Edition.* Philadelphia: Lippincott Williams & Wilkins 2003:44.

6. **Answer = B, The transgastric two-chamber view is another TEE view that could be used to image the anterior wall.** The transgastric two-chamber view also shows the anterior and inferior walls.

Reference: Konstadt SN, Shernon S, Oka Y (eds). *Clinical Transesophageal Echocardiography: A Problem-Oriented Approach, Second Edition.* Philadelphia: Lippincott Williams & Wilkins 2003:45.

Case 4

7. **Answer = B, A normal functioning St. Jude mitral valve is in place.** This bi-leaflet mechanical valve prosthesis is the most commonly implanted mechanical valve because of its durability and large orifice area.

Reference: Perrino AC, Reeves S. *A Practical Approach to TEE.* Philadelphia: Lippincott Williams & Wilkins 2003:202–205.

8. **Answer = A, Normal transvalvular regurgitation is present.** A normally functioning St. Jude valve prosthesis has four normal "cleansing jets" that originate from the hinge points of the mitral valve and serve to prevent the formation of thrombus within the hinge mechanism.

Reference: Perrino AC, Reeves S. *A Practical Approach to TEE.* Philadelphia: Lippincott Williams & Wilkins 2003:202–205.

9. **Answer = E, The valve function is normal. If it is otherwise stable, administer protamine.** This patient has a normally functioning St. Jude mitral valve prosthesis. Therefore, no treatment is needed.

Reference: Perrino AC, Reeves S. *A Practical Approach to TEE.* Philadelphia: Lippincott Williams & Wilkins 2003:202–205.

10. **Answer = A, The coronary sinus is shown.**

Case 5

11. **Answer = D, Severe mitral regurgitation is present.**

Reference: Sidebotham D, Merry A, Legget M (eds.). *Practical Perioperative Transoesophageal Echocardiography.* Burlington, MA: Butterworth Heinemann 2003:135.

12. **Answer = B, Aortic regurgitation is shown in image 1 for case 5.**

Case 6

13. **Answer = A, This patient clearly has systolic anterior motion of the anterior mitral valve leaflet (SAM) with left ventricular outflow tract (LVOT) obstruction after mitral valve repair, and this is causing the mitral regurgitation.**

Reference: Perrino AC, Reeves S. *A Practical Approach to TEE.* Philadelphia: Lippincott Williams & Wilkins 2003:165–166.

14. **Answer = A, Initial treatment should consist of stopping inotropes and administering volume, direct vasoconstrictors (phenylephrine, vasopressin), and judicious doses of esmolol.** This patient clearly has systolic anterior motion of the anterior mitral valve leaflet (SAM) with left ventricular outflow tract (LVOT) obstruction after mitral valve repair. Anything that increased the volume of the left ventricle should decrease SAM and thereby decrease the dynamic LVOT obstruction. Therefore, hemodynamic goals are listed in Table 4.1A.

Table 4.1A.

Hemodynamic Parameter	Goal
Heart rate	Slow
SVR	High
Preload	High
Contractility	Low

Often, manipulating the hemodynamic parameters cited previously will eliminate SAM, and this is the recommended initial management. However, if this is not successful return to cardiopulmonary bypass and valve repair performed (alternatively, replacement may be required).

Reference: Perrino AC, Reeves S. *A Practical Approach to TEE.* Philadelphia: Lippincott Williams & Wilkins 2003:165–166.

Case 7

15. **Answer = A, Trace to mild mitral regurgitation is present.**

Reference: Sidebotham D, Merry A, Legget M (eds.). *Practical Perioperative Transoesophageal Echocardiography.* Burlington, MA: Butterworth Heinemann 2003:135.

16. **Answer = A, Type I leaflet motion is present.** Using the Carpentier system of classification, normal leaflet motion is referred to as type I. The Carpentier classification system of leaflet motion for mitral regurgitation is outlined in Table 4.1B.

Table 4.1B.

Carpentier Class	Leaflet Motion
Type I	Normal
Type II	Excessive
Type III	Restrictive

Reference: Perrino AC, Reeves S. *A Practical Approach to TEE.* Philadelphia: Lippincott Williams & Wilkins 2003:162–163.

Case 8

17. **Answer = C, The patient has an aortic abscess cavity with a bicuspid aortic valve.**

Reference: Otto C. *Textbook of Clinical Echocardiography, Third Edition.* Philadelphia: Elsevier 2004:461.

18. **Answer = E, All of the above are correct.** The patient has a bicuspid aortic valve with increased risk for all of the listed problems: aortic stenosis, aortic aneurysms, and ventricular septal defects. Bicuspid aortic valve disease is the most common congenital heart defect, occurring in 1 to 2% of the population. It is the most common cause of symptomatic aortic stenosis in patients under the age of 65. Planimetry of a bicuspid valve is not accurate and valve area should be determined by the continuity equation. The bicuspid valve is often functional until age 50 to 60 years, when aortic stenosis from fibrocalcific changes occurs.

Reference: Otto C. *Textbook of Clinical Echocardiography, Third Edition.* Philadelphia: Elsevier 2004:461.

Case 9

19. **Answer = D, The arrow in image 1 of case 9 indicates a eustachian valve.**

20. **Answer = A, Lateral resolution at location B is less than at location A.** Location A is closer to the transducer and therefore beam width will be more narrow, resulting in improved lateral resolution. Temporal resolution would also be better at location A. There are many synonyms for *lateral resolution,* including: *lateral resolution, transverse resolution, azimuthal resolution,* and *angular resolution.*

Reference: Edelman SK. *Understanding Ultrasound Physics.* Woodlands, TX: ESP, Inc. 1994:92.

21. **Answer = E, The anterior mitral valve leaflet is shown.**

Reference: Sidebotham D, Merry A, Legget M (eds.). *Practical Perioperative Transoesophageal Echocardiography.* Burlington, MA: Butterworth Heinemann 2003:134.

Case 10

22. **Answer = C, A lipomatous interatrial septum is present.**

Reference: Sidebotham D, Merry A, Legget M (eds.). *Practical Perioperative Transoesophageal Echocardiography.* Burlington, MA: Butterworth Heinemann 2003:76.

23. **Answer = B, No treatment is required.**

Reference: Sidebotham D, Merry A, Legget M (eds.). *Practical Perioperative Transoesophageal Echocardiography.* Burlington, MA: Butterworth Heinemann 2003:76.

Case 11

24. **Answer = A, A right atrial tumor is present.**

Case 12

25. **Answer = B, The christa terminalis is shown.**

26. **Answer = B, The right pulmonary artery is shown.**

27. **Answer = B, The left atrium is shown.**

28. **Answer = D, The inferior vena cava is shown.**

Case 13

29. **Answer = C, A Medtronic Hall single tilting disc prosthesis is shown.**

30. **Answer = D, Acoustic shadowing artifact is shown.**

31. **Answer = A, The midesophageal long axis view is shown.**

32. **Answer = B, The deep transgastric long axis could also be utilized to evaluate this valve.**

Case 14

33. **Answer = C, The superior vena cava is shown.**

34. **Answer = D, The right pulmonary artery is shown.**

35. **Answer = E, The pulmonic valve is shown.**

36. **Answer = B, The midesophageal ascending aortic short axis view is shown.**

Case 15

37. **Answer = B, A Stanford type B aneurysm is shown.** The Stanford classification is simple and clinically relevant. Stanford class A includes all dissections involving the ascending aorta regardless of where the intimal tear is located and regardless of how far the dissection propagates. Remember that if the ascending aorta is involved it is type A. Stanford type B dissections involve the aorta distal to the origin of the left subclavian artery. Mortality rates for medical and surgical management are similar for type B dissections. The DeBakey classification system is outlined in Table 4.1C.

Table 4.1C.		DEBAKEY CLASSIFICATION FOR AORTIC DISSECTIONS	
Type	**Origin**	**Extends Distally to:**	**Stanford Classification**
I	Ascending thoracic aorta	Aortic bifurcation	A
II	Ascending thoracic aorta	Brachiocephalic trunk (ends before the arch)	A
IIIa	Near the left subclavian artery	Above the diaphragm	B
IIIb	Near the left subclavian artery	Aortic bifurcation	B

38. **Answer = E, All of the above are correct.** Type A dissections occur more frequently than type B dissections, comprising about 70%. A type B dissection is shown. Medical and surgical management of type B dissections have similar mortality rates. Beta blockers are beneficial in dissections because they decrease the ejection velocity. An Ao ratio <1.3 indicates a low-risk group in patients with Marfan's syndrome. The Ao ratio is the sinus of valsalva diameter divided by the predicted sinus diameter for a given age and BSA. An Ao ratio <1.3 or an annual rate of change < 5% indicates a low-risk group in patients with Marfan's syndrome. For adults (>40 years): predicted sinus dimension (cm) = 1.92 + [0.74 * BSA (m^2)].

References: Hensley HA, Martin DE, Gravlee GP. *A Practical Approach to Cardiac Anesthesia, Third Edition.* Philadelphia: Lippincott Williams & Wilkins 2002:621; Legget M, Unger TA, O'Sullivan CK, Zwink TR, Bennett RL, Byers PH, Otto CM. Aortic root complications in Marfan's syndrome: Identification of a lower risk group. *British Heart Journal* 1996;74(4):389–395.

Case 16

39. **Answer = B, The left atrium is shown.**

40. **Answer = D, The sinus of valsalva is shown.**

41. **Answer = A, The sinotubular ridge is shown.**

42. **Answer = D, The right pulmonary artery is shown.**

43. **Answer = B, The deep transgastric long axis view is shown.**

44. **Answer = D, Severe aortic insufficiency is present.** The ratio of the color flow jet height to LVOT diameter is greater than 2/3, indicating severe AI.

Case 17

45. **Answer = C, A normally functioning St. Jude mitral valve prosthesis is shown.** This bi-leaflet mechanical valve prosthesis is the most commonly implanted mechanical valve because of its durability and large orifice area. A normally functioning St. Jude valve prosthesis has four normal "cleansing jets" that originate from the hinge points of the mitral valve and serve to prevent the formation of thrombus within the hinge mechanism.

Reference: Perrino AC, Reeves S. *A Practical Approach to TEE.* Philadelphia: Lippincott Williams & Wilkins 2003:202–205.

46. **Answer = D, A normally functioning St. Jude valve prosthesis has four normal "cleansing jets" that originate from the hinge points of the mitral valve and serve to prevent the formation of thrombus within the hinge mechanism.**

Reference: Perrino AC, Reeves S. *A Practical Approach to TEE.* Philadelphia: Lippincott Williams & Wilkins 2003:202–205.

47. **Answer = E, None of the above.** Replacement with a St. Jude mitral prosthesis offers little advantage over repair. Repair is sometimes not possible, but when possible it has become the treatment of choice for mitral valve pathology. Replacement disrupts the mitral subvalvular apparatus and can lead to ventricular dilation and heart failure. Replacement also requires long-term anticoagulation with Coumadin. Replacement does not decrease the risk of infection, but does decrease the mitral valve inflow orifice area.

Reference: Perrino AC, Reeves S. *A Practical Approach to TEE.* Philadelphia: Lippincott Williams & Wilkins 2003:202–205.

Case 18

48. **Answer = A, Segment 5, the basal inferior wall segment, is indicated by arrow 1.**

Reference: ASE/SCA Guidelines for Performing a Comprehensive Intraoperative Multiplane Transesophageal Echocardiography Examination. *J Am Soc Echocardiog* 1999;12:884–900.

49. **Answer = C, Segment 11, the mid inferior wall segment, is indicated by arrow 2.**

Reference: ASE/SCA Guidelines for Performing a Comprehensive Intraoperative Multiplane Transesophageal Echocardiography Examination. *J Am Soc Echocardiog* 1999;12:884–900.

50. **Answer = D, Segment 15, the apical inferior wall segment, is indicated by arrow 3.**

Reference: ASE/SCA Guidelines for Performing a Comprehensive Intraoperative Multiplane Transesophageal Echocardiography Examination. *J Am Soc Echocardiog* 1999;12:884–900.

51. **Answer = B, Segment 13, the apical anterior wall segment, is indicated by arrow 4.**

Reference: ASE/SCA Guidelines for Performing a Comprehensive Intraoperative Multiplane Transesophageal Echocardiography Examination. *J Am Soc Echocardiog* 1999;12:884–900.

52. **Answer = A, Segment 8, the mid anterior wall segment, is indicated by arrow 5.**

Reference: ASE/SCA Guidelines for Performing a Comprehensive Intraoperative Multiplane Transesophageal Echocardiography Examination. *J Am Soc Echocardiog* 1999;12:884–900.

53. **Answer = B, Segment 2, the basal anterior wall segment, is indicated by arrow 6.**

Reference: ASE/SCA Guidelines for Performing a Comprehensive Intraoperative Multiplane Transesophageal Echocardiography Examination. *J Am Soc Echocardiog* 1999;12:884–900.

Case 19

54. **Answer = B, 36 mmHg is the right ventricular systolic pressure.** The calculation is as follows.

$$\Delta P = 4V^2$$

$$(RVSP - RAP) = 4V_{TR}^2$$

$$(RVSP - CVP) = 4V^2$$

$$RVSP = 4V^2 + CVP$$

$$RVSP = 4(2.55 \text{ m/s})^2 + 10$$

$$RVSP = 36 \text{ mmHg}$$

- RVSP = right ventricular systolic pressure
- RAP = right atrial pressure
- CVP = central venous pressure
- V_{TR} = peak velocity of the tricuspid valve regurgitant jet

Reference: Otto C. *Textbook of Clinical Echocardiography, Third Edition.* Philadelphia: Elsevier 2004:463.

55. **Answer = D, Severe tricuspid regurgitation is present (as indicated by systolic reversal of hepatic venous flow).**

Reference: Perrino AC, Reeves S. *A Practical Approach to TEE.* Philadelphia: Lippincott Williams & Wilkins 2003:225.

Case 20

56. **Answer = B, Comet tail artifact is present.** This type of reverberation artifact is also known as ring-down artifact and it occurs when two or more closely spaced strong reflectors reside in a medium with very high propagation speed. The ultrasound beam sound ricochets back and forth between the two strong reflectors before returning to the transducer.

References: Savage RM, Aronson S, Thomas JD, Shanewise JS, Shernan SK. *Comprehensive Textbook of Intraoperative Transesophageal Echocardiography.* Philadelphia: Lippincott Williams & Wilkins 2004:56.

57. **Answer = B, The anterolateral papillary muscle is shown.**

58. **Answer = A, The posteromedial papillary muscle is shown.**

Case 21

59. **Answer = A, Inferior wall dyskinesis is shown.**

60. **Answer = A, Q waves in leads II, III, and AVF would be expected.**

61. **Answer = A, Comet tail artifact is shown.** This is a form of reverberation artifact.

Reference: Edelman SK. *Understanding Ultrasound Physics.* Woodlands, TX: ESP, Inc. 1994:203.

62. **Answer = D, The posteromedial papillary muscle is shown.**

63. **Answer = D, Segment 11, the mid inferior wall, is shown.**

Reference: ASE/SCA Guidelines for Performing a Comprehensive Intraoperative Multiplane Transesophageal Echocardiography Examination. *J Am Soc Echocardiog* 1999;12:884–900.

64. **Answer = A, Arrow 3 indicates a small pericardial effusion. This may be due to Dressler's syndrome.**

Reference: Otto C. *Textbook of Clinical Echocardiography, Third Edition.* Philadelphia: Elsevier 2004:260.

Case 22

65. **Answer = C, Arrow 1 indicates a pleural effusion.**

66. **Answer = C, Arrow 2 indicates the descending thoracic aorta.**

67. **Answer = B, Arrow 3 indicates a pericardial effusion.**

Reference: Sidebotham D, Merry A, Legget M (eds.). Practical Perioperative Transoesophageal Echocardiography. Burlington, MA: Butterworth Heinemann 2003:2.

Case 23

68. **Answer = C, The superior vena cava is shown.**

69. **Answer = A, The right upper pulmonary vein is shown.**

70. **Answer = B, The left upper pulmonary vein is shown.**

TEST IV PART 2

Written Test Booklet

1. Which of the following is the processing method used for modern continuous-wave Doppler and pulsed-wave Doppler analysis?

   A. Autocorrelation.

   B. Fast Fourier transform.

   C. Time interval histograms.

   D. Chirp-Z transforms.

   E. Continuous-wave Doppler and pulsed-wave Doppler do *not* use the same processing method on modern echocardiography machines.

2. Which of the following utilizes two or more sample volumes along a scan line, which decreases aliasing artifact but introduces range ambiguity?

   A. Pulsed-wave Doppler

   B. High pulse repetition frequency pulsed-wave Doppler

   C. Continuous-wave Doppler

   D. High pulse repetition frequency continuous-wave Doppler

   E. B-mode imaging

3. With two-dimensional and M-mode imaging the true dimensions of a structure are obtained when measurements are made from which of the following?

   A. Trailing edge to leading edge.

   B. Leading edge to trailing edge.

   C. Trailing edge to trailing edge.

   D. Leading edge to leading edge.

   E. All of the above provide accurate measurements.

4. According to the American Society of Echocardiography, what numerical grade is given to akinesis?

   A. Grade 1

   B. Grade 2

   C. Grade 3

   D. Grade 4

   E. Grade 5

5. According to the American Society of Echocardiography, what numerical grade is given to dyskinesis?

   A. Grade 1

   B. Grade 2

   C. Grade 3

   D. Grade 4

   E. Grade 5

6. Which of the following is *not* a potential cause of a segmental wall motion abnormality?

   A. Myocardial ischemia

   B. Myocardial stunning

   C. Hypovolemia

   D. Epicardial pacing

   E. Severe left ventricular hypertrophy

7. Which of the following is *not* a potential cause of a segmental wall motion abnormality?

   A. Intracoronary air embolus.

   B. Hibernating myocardium.

   C. Left bundle branch block.

   D. Severe mitral stenosis.

   E. All of the above are potential causes.

8. Which of the following is a potential cause of a segmental wall motion abnormality?

    A. Sector scan passing through the membranous interventricular septum

    B. Hypovolemia

    C. Severe mitral stenosis

    D. Epicardial pacing

    E. All of the above

9. Which of the following mitral valve scallops is most likely to be supported solely by the posteromedial papillary muscle?

    A. A_1

    B. P_1

    C. A_3

    D. P_2

    E. None of the above

10. In the midesophageal five-chamber view, what tricuspid valve leaflets are seen?

    A. Septal and posterior.

    B. Septal and anterior.

    C. Anterior and posterior.

    D. Septal and lateral.

    E. It cannot be determined.

11. In which of the following views is the ultrasound beam the most perpendicular to the mitral valve regurgitant flow?

    A. Midesophageal four-chamber view

    B. Midesophageal long axis view

    C. Transgastric basal short axis view

    D. Deep transgastric long axis view

    E. Midesophageal commissural view

12. Which of the following views is the best for assessing the mitral valve papillary muscles and chordae?

    A. Transgastric mid papillary long axis view

    B. Midesophageal long axis view

    C. Transgastric two-chamber view

    D. Transgastric basal short axis view

    E. Midesophageal two-chamber view

13. Which of the following best describes the mitral regurgitation seen in hypertrophic obstructive cardiomyopathy?

    A. Anterior directed jet with anterior leaflet restriction.

    B. Posterior directed jet with posterior leaflet prolapse.

    C. Anterior directed jet with anterior leaflet prolapse.

    D. Anterior directed jet with posterior leaflet restriction.

    E. Mitral regurgitation is not usually seen in this disorder.

14. Which of the following best describes the most common perfusion of the anterolateral papillary muscle?

    A. Left anterior descending coronary artery

    B. Right coronary artery

    C. Circumflex coronary artery

    D. Circumflex and left anterior descending coronary arteries

    E. Circumflex and right coronary arteries

15. An increase in which of the following is <u>not</u> associated with an increase in the severity of mitral regurgitation?

    A. Vena contracta width

    B. Mitral valve regurgitant orifice area

    C. Color flow Doppler mitral regurgitant jet area

    D. Mean velocity of the mitral valve regurgitant jet

    E. Mitral valve regurgitant volume

16. Which of the following is the most common indication for mitral valve repair?

    A. Myxomatous degeneration

    B. Endocarditis

    C. Rheumatic heart disease

    D. Papillary muscle ischemia

    E. Dilated cardiomyopathy

17. Which of the following surgical maneuvers may help reduce the risk of systolic anterior motion following mitral valve repair?

    A. Reducing the base-to-tip length of the anterior mitral valve leaflet

    B. Reducing the base-to-tip length of the posterior mitral valve leaflet

    C. Using a sliding valvuloplasty repair technique

    D. Displacing the coaptation line posteriorly

    E. All of the above

18. Which of the following will increase the mean diastolic transmitral pressure gradient as determined by tracing the diastolic continuous-wave Doppler mitral inflow profile?

    A. Mitral stenosis

    B. Mitral regurgitation

    C. Infiltrative amyloidosis

    D. Constrictive pericarditis

    E. All of the above

19. Holodiastolic aortic flow reversal is most sensitive and specific for severe aortic insufficiency (AI) at what anatomic location?

    A. The abdominal aorta at the level of the renal arteries.

    B. The proximal aortic arch at the sinus of valsalva.

    C. Just distal to the aortic arch at the level of the left subclavian artery.

    D. The location of flow reversal does not reflect the significance of the AI.

    E. Holodiastolic flow reversal does not indicate severe AI.

20. What is the most common cause of aortic stenosis in adults?

   A. Congenitally bicuspid aortic valve

   B. Calcific aortic stenosis

   C. Rheumatic heart disease

   D. Carcinoid syndrome

   E. Noonan's syndrome

21. Autopsy studies have shown what percentage of the general population to have a patent foramen ovale?

   A. 5%

   B. 10%

   C. 15%

   D. 25%

   E. 35%

   F. 45%

22. Which of the following is the normal tricuspid annular plane systolic excursion?

   A. > 10 mm

   B. > 15 mm

   C. > 20 mm

   D. > 25 mm

   E. > 30 mm

NOTE: Use Table 4.2A to answer the next five (5) questions.

Table 4.2A.

$TVI_{LVOT} = 11$ cm	$V_{PIearly} = 300$ cm/sec	LA diameter = 34 mm
$TVI_{PI\,jet} = 50$ cm	$A_{TV} = 3.5$ cm^2	BP = 140/90 mmHg
$TVI_{main\,PA} = 14$ cm	$V_{PIend} = 200$ cm/sec	RAP = 10 mmHg
$TVI_{TV} = 15$ cm	BSA = 2 M^2	Main PA diameter = 2.4 cm

Abbreviations: TVI_{LVOT} = time velocity integral of blood flow through the left ventricular outflow tract, $TVI_{PI\,jet}$ = time velocity integral of the pulmonic insufficiency regurgitant jet, $TVI_{main\,PA}$ = time velocity integral of blood flow through the main pulmonary artery, TVI_{TV} = time velocity integral of blood flow through the tricuspid valve, $V_{PIearly}$ = peak early velocity of the pulmonic insufficiency jet, PA = pulmonary artery, A_{TV} = area of the tricuspid valve, V_{PIend} = late peak (end) velocity of the pulmonic insufficiency jet, BSA = body surface area, LA = left atrial, BP = blood pressure, RAP = right atrial pressure.

23. What is the pulmonary artery diastolic pressure?

A. 6 mmHg

B. 16 mmHg

C. 26 mmHg

D. 36 mmHg

E. 46 mmHg

24. What is the stroke volume of blood flow through the main pulmonary artery?

A. 53.3 ml

B. 63.3 ml

C. 73.3 ml

D. 83.3 ml

E. 93.3 ml

25. What is the pulmonic insufficiency regurgitant volume?

A. 5.8 ml

B. 10.8 ml

C. 15.8 ml

D. 20.8 ml

E. 25.8 ml

26. What is the pulmonic valve regurgitant orifice area?

    A. $8.6\,mm^2$

    B. $11.6\,mm^2$

    C. $21.6\,mm^2$

    D. $25.6\,mm^2$

    E. $31.6\,mm^2$

27. What is the mean pulmonary artery pressure?

    A. 6 mmHg

    B. 16 mmHg

    C. 26 mmHg

    D. 36 mmHg

    E. 46 mmHg

28. Which of the following is true concerning the indications for TEE, as stated in the ASE/SCA guidelines for performing a comprehensive intraoperative multiplane transesophageal echocardiography examination?

    A. Category V indications are supported by the strongest evidence.

    B. In category I indications, TEE is frequently useful in improving outcomes.

    C. Category III indications are supported by weaker evidence or expert opinion, but TEE may be useful in improving outcomes in these cases.

    D. In category II indications, TEE is infrequently useful in improving clinical outcomes.

    E. None of the above.

29. Which of the following types of ultrasound imaging essentially plots a B-mode image versus time?

    A. A-mode

    B. B-mode

    C. C-mode

    D. M-mode

    E. Two-dimensional grayscale imaging

30. Which of the following will increase the duty factor?

   A. Increasing the pulse repetition frequency

   B. Increasing the imaging depth

   C. Increasing the pulse repetition period

   D. Decreasing the pulse duration

   E. None of the above

31. Which of the following is true concerning the spatial pulse length?

   A. It is directly related (proportional) to the frequency.

   B. It is inversely related (inversely proportional) to the number of cycles in the pulse.

   C. It is determined by both the ultrasound source and the medium.

   D. As it decreases transverse resolution increases.

   E. None of the above.

32. Which of the following is determined by the ultrasound source and by the medium through which the ultrasound travels?

   A. Pulse duration

   B. Pulse repetition period

   C. Pulse repetition frequency

   D. Spatial pulse length

   E. Duty factor

33. Why do high-frequency transducers produce higher-quality images than low-frequency transducers?

   A. Duty factor is increased

   B. Wavelength is increased

   C. Spatial pulse length is lower

   D. Pulse duration is greater

   E. Pulse repetition period is lower

34. Which of the following are inversely related?

    A. Spatial pulse length and image quality

    B. Spatial pulse length and lateral resolution

    C. Wavelength and spatial pulse length

    D. Wavelength and pulse duration

    E. Imaging depth and spatial pulse length

35. Which of the following is true concerning Rayleigh scattering?

    A. It occurs when the ultrasound beam wavelength is much smaller than the reflector it strikes.

    B. It is responsible for Doppler determinations of blood flow velocities.

    C. It is the major form of attenuation in soft tissues.

    D. None of the above.

36. What percentage of attenuation in soft tissues is caused by absorption?

    A. 10%

    B. 20%

    C. 40%

    D. 80%

    E. 100%

37. Which of the following is true concerning reflection?

    A. Reflection can occur at the interface of two tissues with different reflection coefficients.

    B. Specular reflection allows the lateral and septal walls to be visualized in the mid esophageal four-chamber view.

    C. Reflection is the primary form of attenuation in soft tissue.

    D. Echoes from scattering are stronger (higher amplitude) than echoes produced by specular reflection.

38. In TEE imaging of soft tissue, which of the following is true concerning the attenuation coefficient (AC)?

A. AC = 1/2 (wavelength)

B. AC = 2 (period)

C. AC = 2 (pulse repetition frequency)

D. AC = 2 (spatial pulse length)

E. None of the above

NOTE: Use Table 4.2B to answer question 39.

Table 4.2B.

Initial intensity = 16 mWatts/cm^2
Frequency = 20 MHz
Velocity = 1540 M/S
Density of soft tissue = 1.2 g/ml

39. A mid-esophageal four-chamber view is obtained with a TEE probe. Given the information in the table, determine the intensity of the ultrasound beam at a depth of 1 cm.

A. 8 mWatts/cm^2

B. 1.6 mWatts/cm^2

C. 2 mWatts/cm^2

D. 4 mWatts/cm^2

E. 0.16 mWatts/cm^2

40. What is the thickness of tissue required to reduce the amplitude of a 12-MHz TEE transducer by half?

A. 1 cm

B. 3 cm

C. 6 cm

D. 12 cm

E. 18 cm

NOTE: Use Table 4.2C to answer the next three (3) questions.

Table 4.2C.

	Medium 1	Medium 2	Medium 3	Medium 4
Acoustic impedance (Z, rayls):	1	1	1	2
Attenuation coefficient (AC, dB/cm):	3	3	3	3
Velocity (V, m/s):	1,540	1,600	1,540	1,540

41. A TEE ultrasound beam travels from left to right through mediums 1 through 4. If the angle of incidence between medium 1 and medium 2 is oblique, what can occur at the interface of these two media?

    A. Transmission

    B. Reflection and transmission

    C. Refraction

    D. All of the above

42. If the angle of incidence between mediums 2 and 3 is orthogonal, what can occur at this interface?

    A. Transmission

    B. Reflection and transmission

    C. Refraction

    D. All of the above

43. If the angle of incidence between mediums 3 and 4 is normal, what can occur at this interface?

    A. Transmission

    B. Reflection and transmission

    C. Refraction

    D. All of the above

44. Which of the following is true concerning the damping material?

   A. It improves depth resolution.

   B. It has acoustic impedance between that of the skin and the active element in the transducer (acoustic impedance: active element > damping material > skin).

   C. It increases the Q factor.

   D. It increases the transducer's sensitivity to reflected echoes.

45. Which of the following is true concerning resolution?

   A. Longitudinal resolution is determined by beam width.

   B. Lateral resolution = 1/2 (spatial pulse length).

   C. For axial resolution the smaller the numerical value the better the picture quality.

   D. As pulse repetition frequency (PRF) decreases temporal resolution increases.

46. *Azimuthal resolution* is also known as which of the following terms?

   A. *Temporal resolution*

   B. *Range resolution*

   C. *Axial resolution*

   D. *Lateral resolution*

   E. None of the above

47. Which of the following types of resolution is determined by the beam diameter?

   A. Lateral resolution

   B. Depth resolution

   C. Temporal resolution

   D. Range resolution

48. With respect to resolution, which of the following typically has the highest numerical value?

    A. Axial resolution

    B. Lateral resolution

    C. Range resolution

    D. None of the above (they are identical)

49. Which of the following describes how spectral analysis for pulsed-wave Doppler is achieved with modern ultrasound transducers?

    A. Chirp-Z transforms

    B. Fast Fourier transform

    C. Time interval histograms

    D. Zero crossing detection

    E. Autocorrelation

50. A 10-MHz TEE probe is used to perform a pulsed-wave Doppler examination. The pulse repetition frequency is 400 Hz. What is the Nyquist limit?

    A. 5 Hz

    B. 10 Hz

    C. 20 Hz

    D. 100 Hz

    E. 200 Hz

51. Which of the following ventricular septal defect terminology is incorrect?

    A. Subarterial defect = doubly committed outlet defect

    B. Subartierial defect = supracristal defect

    C. Trabecular defect = muscular defect

    D. Membranous defect = sinus venosus defect

    E. Inlet defect + ostium primum ASD = AV canal defect

52. Which type of ventricular septal defect is a component of tetralogy of fallot?

   A. Perimembranous

   B. Aortic outflow

   C. Subarterial

   D. Trabecular

   E. Inlet

53. Which type of atrial septal defect is associated with mitral regurgitation due to mitral valve prolapse, without a cleft anterior mitral valve leaflet?

   A. Ostium secundum

   B. Ostium primum

   C. Sinus venosus

   D. Coronary sinus

   E. Perimembranous

54. Which of the following ventricular septal defects (VSDs) is also known as a conal VSD?

   A. Perimembranous

   B. Aortic outflow

   C. Subarterial

   D. Trabecular

   E. Inlet

55. With congenitally corrected transposition of the great vessels (ventricular inversion), which of the following statements is true concerning the tricuspid valve?

   A. It is located on the right side of the heart.

   B. It separates the left atrium from the right ventricle.

   C. It is attached to the left ventricle.

   D. It often has a cleft septal leaflet in this disorder.

   E. It separates the right atrium from the right ventricle but these structures are located on the left side of the heart.

56. With congenitally corrected transposition of the great vessels (ventricular inversion), which of the following correctly describes a possible path/route for a red blood cell (SVC = superior vena cava, RA = right atrium, TV = tricuspid valve, ASD = atrial septal defect, PFO = patent foramen ovale, LA = left atrium, LV = left ventricle, RV = right ventricle, L = lungs, Ao = aorta, PDA = patent ductus arteriosus, MV = mitral valve, PA = pulmonary artery, PV = pulmonary vein, VSD = ventricular septal defect)?

A. SVC → RA → TV → LV → PA → L → PV → LA → MV → RV → Ao

B. SVC → RA → MV → LV → PA → L → PV → LA → TV → RV → Ao

C. SVC → RA → TV → RV → Ao → PDA → PA → L → PV → LA → MV → LV → VSD → RV → Ao

D. SVC → RA → PFO → LA → MV → LV → PA → L → PV → LA → MV → LV → VSD → RV → Ao

E. SVC → RA → ASD → LA → TV → RV → PA → L → PV → RA → RV → Ao

NOTE: Use Table 4.2D to answer question 57.

Table 4.2D.

Patient A	Patient B	Patient C	Patient D	Patient E
Tricuspid atresia	Epstein's anomaly	Ventricular inversion	VSD	Aortic coarctation
ASD	ASD	ASD	ASD	ASD
PDA	PDA	PDA	PDA	PDA

57. Which of the patients in the table would most likely benefit from a Blalock-Taussig shunt or Glenn shunt?

A. Patient A

B. Patient B

C. Patient C

D. Patient D

E. Patient E

NOTE: Use Table 4.2E to answer the next five (5) questions.

Table 4.2E.

$V_{PIearly} = 200$ cm/sec	HR = 100 mmHg	MV annular diameter = 35 mm
$V_{PIlate} = 100$ cm/sec	BP = 150/80 mmHg	LVOT diameter = 20 mm
$V_{TRpeak} = 300$ cm/sec	CVP = 11 mmHg	Main PA diameter = 21 mm
$V_{PVpeak\ systolic} = 80$ cm/sec	$TVI_{LVOT} = 18$ cm	Sinus of valsalva diameter = 32 mm

58. Which of the following is the best estimate of the pulmonary artery mean pressure (PAMP) as calculated from the data in the table?

A. 17 mmHg

B. 27 mmHg

C. 37 mmHg

D. 47 mmHg

E. 57 mmHg

59. Which of the following is the best estimate of the pulmonary artery diastolic pressure as calculated from the data in the table?

A. 15 mmHg

B. 18 mmHg

C. 21 mmHg

D. 24 mmHg

E. 27 mmHg

60. Which of the following is the best estimate of the right ventricular systolic pressure as calculated from the data in the table?

A. 27 mmHg

B. 37 mmHg

C. 47 mmHg

D. 57 mmHg

E. 67 mmHg

61. Which of the following is the best estimate of the systolic pressure gradient across the pulmonic valve as calculated from the data in the table?

    A. 2.6 mmHg

    B. 3.6 mmHg

    C. 4.6 mmHg

    D. 5.6 mmHg

    E. 6.6 mmHg

62. Which of the following is the best estimate of the pulmonary artery systolic pressure as calculated from the data in the table?

    A. 27 mmHg

    B. 37 mmHg

    C. 47 mmHg

    D. 57 mmHg

    E. 67 mmHg

63. An aortic aneurysm starts just below the diaphragm and extends distally to the aortic bifurcation. How would this aneurysm be best described according to the Crawford classification system?

    A. Crawford type I

    B. Crawford type II

    C. Crawford type III

    D. Crawford type IV

    E. Crawford type V

64. Which of the following is true concerning restrictive diastolic dysfunction?

    A. E/A is decreased.

    B. Lateral mitral annular tissue Doppler E' < 8 cm/sec.

    C. Pulmonary vein S wave > D wave.

    D. Isovolumetric relaxation time (IVRT) >110 msec.

    E. Decreased transmitral pulsed-wave Doppler E-wave peak velocity.

65. Which of the following is true concerning normal aging and diastolic left ventricular (LV) function?

  A. Early left ventricular filling increases with age.

  B. Transmitral A-wave velocity increases with age.

  C. IVRT decreases as age increases.

  D. E-wave deceleration time shortens (becomes smaller) as age increases.

  E. Lateral mitral annular tissue Doppler E_M increases with age.

NOTE: Use Table 4.2F to answer the next two (2) questions.

Table 4.2F.

E = 180 cm/sec	Pulm vein S wave = 38 cm/sec
A = 20 cm/sec	Pulm vein D wave = 49 cm/sec
DT = 80 cm/sec	Pulm vein A wave = 20 cm/sec
IVRT = 42 msec	Tissue Doppler E_M = 6.3 cm/sec

Abbreviations: E = pulsed-wave Doppler transmitral early filling velocity,
A = pulsed-wave Doppler transmitral peak A-wave velocity,
E_M = lateral mitral annular tissue Doppler E wave (E_M = E' = E prime),
IVRT = isovolumic relaxation time, DT = deceleration time, S wave = pulmonary vein systolic flow wave,
D wave = pulmonary vein diastolic flow wave.

66. Given the data in the table, which of the following best describes this patient's diastolic function?

  A. Normal

  B. Pseudonormal

  C. Restrictive

  D. Impaired relaxation

  E. Constrictive

67. Which of the following is true concerning this patient's left atrial filling pressures?

  A. Increased filling pressures.

  B. Decreased filling pressures.

  C. Normal filling pressures.

  D. It cannot be determined from the given information.

68. A patient with a 35-mm pericardial effusion has late diastolic right atrial inversion and early diastolic right ventricular collapse. Which of the following will most likely be increased during spontaneous inspiration?

A. Transtricuspid peak E-wave velocity

B. Transmitral peak E-wave velocity

C. Pulmonary vein diastolic flow peak velocity

D. Hepatic vein A-wave peak velocity

E. Hepatic vein V-wave peak velocity

69. Nitroglycerin administration to a patient with reversible restrictive diastolic dysfunction may convert the pulsed-wave Doppler transmitral flow velocity profile from a restrictive pattern to a profile resembling which of the following?

A. Constrictive diastolic dysfunction

B. Restrictive diastolic dysfunction

C. Impaired relaxation

D. Pseudonormal diastolic dysfunction

E. Normal diastolic function

NOTE: Use Figure 4.2A to answer the next three (3) questions.

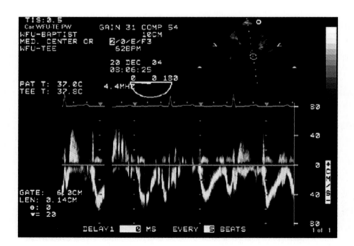

Fig. 4-2AI

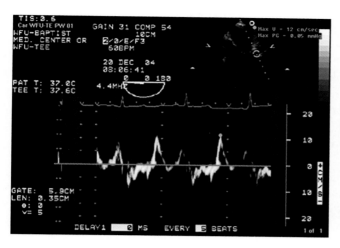

Fig. 4-2A2

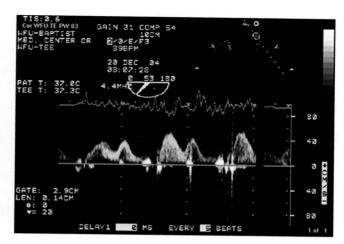

Fig. 4-2A3

70. How would you describe this patient's diastolic function?

    A. Normal

    B. Delayed relaxation (impaired relaxation)

    C. Pseudonormal

    D. Restrictive

    E. Constrictive

71. Pulsed-wave Doppler measurement of which of the following is most likely
    to be a load-independent predictor of diastolic function?

    A. Transmitral Doppler flow velocities

    B. Pulmonary vein Doppler flow velocities

    C. Hepatic vein Doppler flow velocities

    D. Tissue Doppler velocities of the lateral mitral annular

    E. Transtricupid Doppler flow velocities

72. Which of the following is most likely true concerning restrictive diastolic dysfunction?

   A. PV_{AR} may be prolonged secondarily to decreased left ventricular compliance.

   B. PV_{AR} may be increased secondarily to atrial mechanical failure.

   C. Typically pulmonary vein waves show an S/D ratio > 1.

   D. Tissue Doppler E_M > 8 cm/sec.

   E. Transmitral E-wave deceleration time (DT) is prolonged.

   [PV_{AR} = atrial reversal flow velocity (late diastolic pulmonary vein flow reversal velocity), E_M = lateral mitral annular tissue Doppler peak E-wave velocity, DT = transmitral early-filling E-wave deceleration time, S/D = ratio of the pulmonary vein peak S-wave velocity to pulmonary vein peak D wave velocity]

NOTE: Use Figure 4.2B to answer the next question.

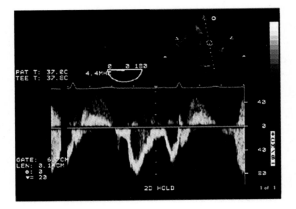

Fig. 4-2B1

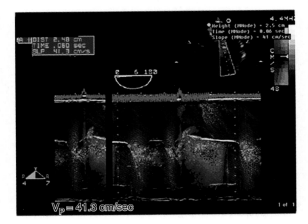

Fig. 4-2B2

73. Given the transmitral pulsed-wave Doppler flow velocities and the transmitral color M-mode Doppler flow propagation velocity (V$_P$), which of the following best describes this patient's diastolic function?

A. Normal

B. Pseudonormal

C. Impaired relaxation

D. Constrictive

E. Restrictive

NOTE: Use the transmitral pulsed-wave Doppler and lateral mitral annular velocity profiles shown in Figure 4.2C to answer the next three (3) questions.

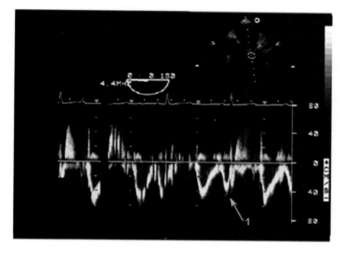

Fig. 4-2C1

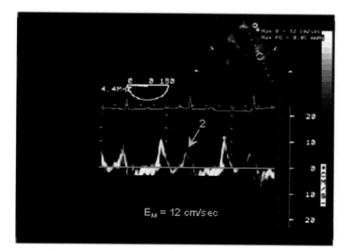

Fig. 4-2C2

74. Which of the following best describes this patient's diastolic function?

    A. Normal

    B. Pseudonormal

    C. Restrictive

    D. Constrictive

    E. Impaired relaxation

75. Which of the following best describes the wave labeled 1?

    A. PV_{AR} wave

    B. S wave

    C. D wave

    D. V wave

    E. A wave

76. Which of the following best describes the wave labeled 2?

    A. A_M wave

    B. E_M wave

    C. S wave

    D. A wave

    E. E wave

NOTE: Use the pulmonary vein pulsed-wave Doppler flow velocity profile shown in Figure 4.2D to answer the next four (4) questions.

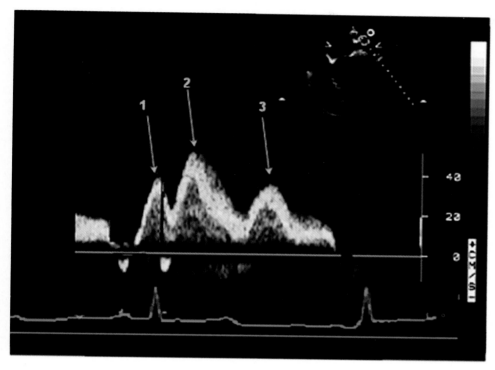

Fig. 4-2D

77. Which of the following best describes the wave labeled 1?

    A. PV$_{AR}$ wave

    B. S$_1$ wave

    C. S$_2$ wave

    D. D$_1$ wave

    E. V wave

78. Which of the following best describes the wave labeled 2?

    A. PV$_{AR}$ wave

    B. S$_1$ wave

    C. S$_2$ wave

    D. D$_1$ wave

    E. V wave

79. Which of the following best describes the wave labeled 3?

   A. PV$_{AR}$ wave

   B. S$_2$ wave

   C. E wave

   D. D wave

   E. V wave

80. Which of the following is true concerning the wave indicated by arrow 2?

   A. It is influenced by right ventricular stroke volume.

   B. It is influenced by left atrial relaxation and the subsequent decrease in left atrial pressure.

   C. It is influenced by left atrial contractility.

   D. It is influenced by aortic regurgitation.

   E. It is influenced by aortic stenosis.

81. Which of the following would be consistent with moderate pericardial effusion?

   A. 0.4 cm

   B. 0.7 cm

   C. 2.1 cm

   D. 2.5 cm

   E. 3 cm

82. Right atrial inversion for greater than 1/3 of systole is indicative of which of the following?

   A. Constrictive pericarditis

   B. Pericardial tamponade

   C. Restrictive cardiomyopathy

   D. Hypertrophic cardiomyopathy

   E. Dilated cardiomyopathy

83. Which of the following is *not* seen in pericardial tamponade?

    A. Right atrial diastolic collapse

    B. Right ventricular diastolic collapse

    C. Reciprocal changes in right ventricular and left ventricular volumes

    D. Reciprocal respiratory changes in right ventricular and left ventricular filling

    E. Inferior vena cava plethora

84. Which of the following is important in determining the hemodynamic severity of a pericardial effusion?

    A. Size of the pericardial effusion

    B. Speed at which the fluid accumulation occurs

    C. Location of the pericardial effusion

    D. Presence or absence of loculation

    E. All of the above

85. Which of the following would be expected to increase with spontaneous inspiration in constrictive pericarditis?

    A. Left ventricular isovolumic (isovolumetric) relaxation time

    B. Transmitral peak E-wave velocity

    C. Pulmonary venous S-wave peak velocity

    D. Pulmonary venous D-wave peak velocity

    E. Hepatic venous A wave

86. Which of the following is a characteristic of a left ventricular pseudoaneurysm that facilitates distinguishing pseudoaneurysms from true LV aneurysms?

    A. Abrupt transition from normal myocardium to the aneurysm with a true aneurysm.

    B. Acute angles between the myocardium and aneurysm are more likely with a true aneurysm.

    C. Ratio of neck diameter to aneurysm diameter < 0.5 is more likely with a pseudoaneurysm.

    D. Thrombus formation is more likely with true aneurysms.

    E. Regional wall motion abnormalities are more likely with a true aneurysm.

87. Which of the following is the most common primary intracardiac tumor?

   A. Lipoma

   B. Myxoma

   C. Rhabdomyosarcoma

   D. Fibroma

   E. Papillary fibroelastoma

88. Which of the following is the most common benign cardiac tumor?

   A. Neurofibroma

   B. Papillary fibroelastoma

   C. Lipoma

   D. Myxoma

   E. Fibroma

89. Which of the following is the most common primary malignant cardiac tumor?

   A. Angiosarcoma

   B. Rhabdomyosarcoma

   C. Fibrosarcoma

   D. Leiomyosarcoma

   E. Malignant lymphoma

90. Which of the following is *not* a potential complication of intraoperative TEE?

   A. Dysphagia.

   B. Vocal cord paralysis.

   C. Odynophagia.

   D. Tracheal compression.

   E. All are potential complications of intraoperative TEE.

91. What is the maximum leakage current recommended for an electrically safe TEE probe?

    A. 40 microamperes

    B. 50 microamperes

    C. 40 milliamperes

    D. 50 milliamperes

    E. 100 milliamperes

92. Which of the following is an absolute contraindication to perioperative TEE?

    A. Esophageal stricture

    B. Esophageal diverticulum

    C. Large hiatal hernia

    D. Recent esophageal or gastric surgery

    E. History of mediastinal radiation

NOTE: Use Figure 4.2E to answer the next five (5) questions.

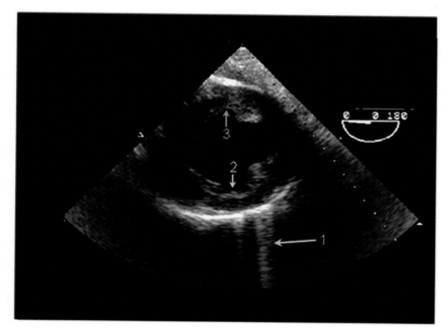

Fig. 4-2E

93. Arrow 1 could be classified as which of the following?

   A. Comet tail artifact

   B. Ring-down artifact

   C. Reverberation artifact

   D. All of the above

   E. None of the above

94. According to the American Society of Echocardiography 16-segment model, what numerical segment of the left ventricle is described by arrow 2?

   A. 7

   B. 8

   C. 9

   D. 10

   E. 11

95. Which of the following supplies perfusion to the myocardium, indicated by arrow 2?

   A. Right coronary artery

   B. Left anterior descending coronary artery

   C. Circumflex coronary artery

   D. Posterior descending coronary artery

   E. Marginal coronary artery

96. According to the American Society of Echocardiography 16-segment model, what numerical segment of the left ventricle is described by arrow 3?

   A. 7

   B. 8

   C. 9

   D. 10

   E. 11

97. Which of the following supplies perfusion to the myocardium, indicated by arrow 3?

    A. Right coronary artery

    B. Left anterior descending coronary artery

    C. Circumflex coronary artery

    D. Marginal coronary artery

    E. Anterior coronary artery

98. Why does the wall indicated by arrow 2 appear brighter than the wall indicated by arrow 3?

    A. Ring-down artifact

    B. Acoustic brightening

    C. Reverberation artifact

    D. Enhancement artifact

    E. Acoustic resonance

99. Which of the following are small mobile connective tissue densities that protrude out linearly from the coaptation point of the aortic valve? These thin flexible filamentous structures are *not* associated with embolic events.

    A. Moderator bands

    B. Lambls' excrescences

    C. Nodules of Arantius

    D. Papillary fibroelastomas

    E. Chiari networks

100. Which of the following are best described as normal leaflet thickenings seen at the central portion of the aortic valve leaflets?

    A. Moderator bands

    B. Lambls' excrescences

    C. Nodules of Arantius

    D. Papillary fibroelastomas

    E. Chiari networks

101. Which of the following is/are associated with thromboembolic events?

A. Lipomatous interatrial septum

B. Moderator bands

C. Nodules of Arantius

D. Lambls' excrescences

E. Papillary fibroelastomas

102. Which of the following best describes the motion of particles in a medium as sound passes through it?

A. Compression and rarefaction

B. Compaction and expansion

C. Compression and expansion

D. Compaction and rarefaction

E. None of the above

103. Which of the following best describes the frequency of ultrasound?

A. > 10 Hz

B. > 20 Hz

C. > 10 KHz

D. > 20 KHz

E. > 20 MHz

104. Which of the following will decrease aliasing artifact?

A. Decreasing the emitted frequency of the transducer

B. Increasing the depth of the sample volume

C. Increasing the velocity of blood flow in the sample gate

D. Decreasing the Nyquist limit

E. Decreasing the pulse repetition frequency

105. Which of the following is a difference between optimum two-dimensional imaging conditions and optimum conditions for pulsed-wave Doppler analysis?

   A. Imaging is best with an incident angle of 0 degrees.

   B. Doppler is best with an incident angle of 90 degrees.

   C. Imaging is best with a low-frequency transducer.

   D. Doppler is best with high-frequency transducers.

   E. Both imaging and Doppler analysis are improved with a decrease in depth.

106. A 12-MHz transducer interrogates blood flow using pulsed-wave Doppler in a vessel with a blood flow velocity of 100 cm/sec and a pulse repetition frequency of 6,000 Hz. Which of the following is the highest Doppler shift that can be accurately measured?

   A. 1,000 Hz

   B. 2,000 Hz

   C. 3,000 Hz

   D. 4,000 Hz

   E. 6,000 Hz

107. Which of the following views can be used to estimate the pulmonary artery systolic pressure?

   A. Midesophageal right ventricular inflow/outflow view

   B. Midesophageal two-chamber view

   C. Transgastric two-chamber view

   D. Transgastric pulmonic valve outflow view

   E. Upper esophageal aortic arch short axis view

NOTE: Use Table 4.2G to answer the next five (5) questions.

Table 4.2G.

TVI $_{Mrjet}$ = 180 cm	Peak E wave = 200 cm/sec	α = 160	PISA radius = 0.8 cm
TVI $_{LVOT}$ = 15 cm	V$_{MRpeak}$ = 500 cm/sec	BP = 120/80	LA diameter = 48 mm
TVI$_{MVinflow}$ = 11 cm	LAP = 18 mmHg	CVP = 10 mmHg	PISA alias velocity = 30 cm/sec
C-sept = 3.1 cm	AL/PL = 0.8	BSA = 2 m²	LVOT diameter = 2.0 cm

Abbreviations: TVI $_{Mrjet}$ = time velocity integral of the mitral regurgitant jet, peak E wave = peak transmitral E-wave velocity, α = angle correction factor, PISA radius = distance from the mitral valve leaflets to first aliasing velocity shell, TVI $_{LVOT}$ = time velocity integral of flow through the left ventricular outflow tract, V$_{MRpeak}$ = peak velocity of transmitral inflow, BP = blood pressure, TVI$_{MVinflow}$ = time velocity integral of diastolic mitral inflow, LAP = left atrial pressure, PISA = proximal isovelocity surface area, C-sept = distance from the mitral valve coaptation point to the septum, AL/PL = mitral valve anterior leaflet to posterior leaflet ratio, CVP = central venous pressure, BSA = body surface area, LVOT = left ventricular outflow tract.

108. Which of the following is the best estimate of the regurgitant flow rate?

A. 87.2 ml/sec

B. 97.2 ml/sec

C. 107.2 ml/sec

D. 117.2 ml/sec

E. 127.2 ml/sec

109. Which of the following is the best estimate of the regurgitant orifice area?

A. 0.114 cm²

B. 0.214 cm²

C. 0.314 cm²

D. 0.414 cm²

E. 0.514 cm²

110. Which of the following is the best estimate of the regurgitant volume?

A. 38.6 ml

B. 48.6 ml

C. 58.6 ml

D. 68.6 ml

E. 78.6 ml

111. Which of the following best describes the degree of mitral regurgitation?

    A. Trace.

    B. Mild.

    C. Moderate.

    D. Severe.

    E. It cannot be determined from the given data.

112. Which of the following will increase this patient's risk for post mitral valve repair systolic anterior motion of the anterior mitral valve leaflet with left ventricular outflow tract obstruction?

    A. C-sept = 3.1 cm

    B. AL/PL = 0.8

    C. LA diameter = 48 mm

    D. LVOT diameter = 2.0 cm

    E. LAP = 18 mmHg

113. Which of the following would be expected in a patient with dilated cardiomyopathy?

    A. dp/dt = 1,600

    B. Color flow Doppler mitral regurgitant area = $1.2\,cm^2$

    C. Left atrial diameter = 52 mm

    D. Left ventricular end diastolic diameter = 50 mm

    E. Right ventricular end diastolic diameter = 30 mm

114. A dagger-shaped continuous-wave Doppler left ventricular outflow pattern with the peak velocity occurring in late systole is indicative of which of the following?

    A. Aortic stenosis due to a congenitally bicuspid valve

    B. Hypertrophic obstructive cardiomyopathy

    C. Aortic stenosis due to senile degenerative calcification

    D. Aortic stenosis due to rheumatic heart disease

    E. LVOT obstruction due to a subaortic membrane

115. Which of the following is true concerning hypertrophic cardiomyopathy?

   A. It is divided into five types based on the location of the left ventricular hypertrophy.

   B. Dynamic LVOT obstruction can occur.

   C. It is caused by a defect in the beta-myosin light chain gene.

   D. It has autosomal recessive inheritance.

   E. All of the above.

116. Which of the following is *not* a synonym of *hypertrophic cardiomyopathy?*

   A. *Idiopathic hypertrophic subaortic stenosis* (IHSS)

   B. *Hypertrophic obstructive cardiomyopathy* (HOCOM)

   C. *Asymmetric septal hypertrophy*

   D. *Hypertrophic cardiomyopathy*

   E. *Dynamically occlusive septal hypertrophy*

NOTE: Use Table 4.2H to answer question 117.

Table 4.2H.

Scenario	Preload	Afterload	Contractility	Heart Rate
A	Increase	Increase	Decrease	Decrease
B	Decrease	Decrease	Increase	Increase
C	Increase	Increase	Increase	Increase
D	Decrease	Increase	Increase	Decrease
E	Increase	Decrease	Increase	Increase

117. Which of the following hemodynamic scenarios is least likely to result in LVOT obstruction in a hypertrophic cardiomyopathy patient?

   A. Scenario A

   B. Scenario B

   C. Scenario C

   D. Scenario D

   E. Scenario E

118. Which of the following would be expected in a patient with chronic hypertension?

　　A. Elevated pulsed-wave Doppler transmitral peak E-wave velocity

　　B. Transmitral pulsed-wave Doppler E/A > 1

　　C. Lateral mitral annular tissue Doppler E_M < 8 cm/sec

　　D. Color M-mode transmitral propagation velocity (V_P) > 50 cm/sec

　　E. Short transmitral E-wave deceleration time (DT)

119. Which of the following would be expected in a patient with chronic hypertension?

　　A. Left ventricular end diastolic diameter = 63 mm

　　B. Left atrial diameter = 52 mm

　　C. Left ventricular free wall thickness = 11 mm

　　D. Transmitral pulsed-wave Doppler E/A > 1

　　E. Lateral mitral annular tissue Doppler E_M = 8.2 cm/sec

120. Which of the following will increase left ventricular wall stress?

　　A. Decreasing left ventricular end diastolic dimension

　　B. Decreasing left ventricular pressure (LVEDP)

　　C. Decreasing left ventricular free wall thickness

　　D. Decreasing wall tension

　　E. Increasing heart rate

NOTE: Use Table 4.21 to answer the next three (3) questions.

Table 4.21.

LVED diameter = 52 mm	LA diameter = 40 mm	LV free wall thickness = 12 mm
LVES diameter = 33 mm	RA diameter = 30 mm	BP = 110/60
V_{AIlate} = 350 cm/sec	LVOT diameter = 2 cm	CVP = 10
$V_{AIearly}$ = 300 cm/sec	TVI_{LVOT} = 15 cm	V_{TRjet} = 200 cm/sec

Abbreviations: $V_{AIearly}$ = early peak aortic regurgitant velocity, V_{AIlate} = late peak aortic regurgitant velocity, LVED = left ventricular end diastolic, LVES = left ventricular end systolic, RA = right atrial, LVOT = left ventricular outflow tract, TVI = time velocity integral, CVP = central venous pressure, BP = blood pressure, LV = left ventricular, V_{TRjet} = peak tricuspid regurgitant velocity.

121. Using the data in the table, calculate the left ventricular end diastolic pressure (LVEDP).

    A. LVEDP = 4

    B. LVEDP = 7

    C. LVEDP = 11

    D. LVEDP = 13

    E. LVEDP = 15

122. Given the data in the table, what is the left ventricular wall tension?

    A. 215 mmHg mm

    B. 286 mmHg mm

    C. 350 mmHg mm

    D. 572 mmHg mm

    E. 623 mmHg mm

123. Given the data in the table, what is the left ventricular wall stress?

    A. 8.9 mmHg

    B. 10.9 mmHg

    C. 11.9 mmHg

    D. 12.9 mmHg

    E. 13.9 mmHg

124. Which of the following is most likely to be true concerning the number of pulses per scan line?

    A. As this increases the numerical value for lateral resolution is decreased.

    B. This is referred to as the line density.

    C. As this increases temporal resolution increases.

    D. As this increases the frame rate increases.

125. Which of the following is most likely to be associated with multiple pulses per scan line?

    A. Multifocus systems.

    B. Phased-array transducers.

    C. Improved lateral resolution.

    D. Decreased temporal resolution.

    E. All of the above are correct.

126. Which of the following is *not* a side effect observed after the administration of dobutamine during dobutamine stress echocardiography?

    A. Paradoxical bradycardia.

    B. Ventricular tachycardia.

    C. Light-headedness.

    D. Shortness of breath.

    E. All of the above are side effects of dobutamine.

NOTE: Use the data in Table 4.2J to answer the next two (2) questions.

Table 4.2J.

Dobutamine Dose	Inferior Wall	Anterior Wall	Lateral Wall	Posterior Wall
0 mcg/kg/min	AK	Normal	Normal	AK
5 mcg/kg/min	Severe HK	Normal	Normal	Mild HK
15 mcg/kg/min	Mild HK	Mild HK	Normal	Mild HK
30 mcg/kg/min	AK	Severe HK	Normal	AK

Abbreviations: AK = akinesis, HK = hypokinesis, DK = dyskinesis, RCA = right coronary artery, LAD = left anterior descending coronary artery.

127. Given the stress echo results, which of the following is true?

    A. The myocardium supplied by the RCA is nonviable.

    B. There is a fixed lesion in the LAD, resulting in nonviable myocardium.

    C. The LAD is supplying stunned myocardium.

    D. The anterior wall contains hibernating myocardium, which may benefit from revascularization.

    E. The circumflex coronary artery is supplying hibernating myocardium.

128. Which of the following vessels are likely to show lesions?

    A. LAD

    B. Circumflex

    C. RCA and circumflex

    D. LAD and circumflex

    E. LAD, circumflex, and RCA

129. The interventricular septum flattens and is displaced toward the left ventricle at what point with right ventricular (RV) volume overload?

    A. Early diastole.

    B. Late diastole.

    C. Early systole.

    D. Late systole.

    E. This does not occur with RV pressure overload.

130. Which of the following views allows accurate determination of the instantaneous peak pressure gradient across the pulmonic valve by continuous-wave Doppler?

    A. Midesophageal right ventricular inflow/outflow view

    B. Transgastric right ventricular inflow view

    C. Midesophageal right ventricular outflow view

    D. Midesophageal pulmonic outflow view

    E. Upper esophageal aortic arch short axis view

131. Which of the following structures is located in the left atrium?

    A. Eustachian valve

    B. Crista terminalis

    C. Cor triatriatum

    D. Chiari network

    E. Moderator band

132. Which of the following structures is located in the right ventricle?

    A. Cor triatriatum

    B. Coumadin ridge

    C. Crista terminalis

    D. Moderator band

133. Which of the following will decrease the apparent severity of mitral regurgitation by color flow Doppler TEE examination?

    A. Increasing the systemic vascular resistance

    B. Increasing the color gain

    C. Increasing the Nyquist limit of the color flow Doppler map

    D. Increasing the size of the regurgitant orifice

    E. Increasing the mean arterial pressure

134. Which TEE view is correctly matched with the mitral valve scallops shown?

    A. ME commissural view to $A_1P_2A_3$.

    B. ME long axis view to A_2P_2.

    C. ME 4 chamber view to A_1P_1.

    D. ME 5 chamber view to A_3P_3.

    E. None of the above is correct.

135. Which of the following statements concerning the use of the pressure half time method (PHT) to determine mitral valve area (MVA) is correct?

    A. Severe aortic insufficiency (AI) can result in an underestimation of MVA by the PHT method.

    B. Decreased LV compliance can result in an overestimate of MVA by the PHT method.

    C. Severe mitral regurgitation (MR) can result in an underestimate of MVA by the PHT method.

    D. Delayed left ventricular relaxation can result in an overestimation of the mitral valve area by the PHT method.

136. The pressure half time for the transmitral inflow velocity spectrum by continuous-wave Doppler is 110 ms. What is the mitral valve area?

A. $1.0\,cm^2$

B. $1.5\,cm^2$

C. $1.75\,cm^2$

D. $2\,cm^2$

E. $2.5\,cm^2$

Answers:

1. B	22. D	43. B
2. B	23. C	44. A
3. D	24. B	45. C
4. D	25. B	46. D
5. E	26. C	47. A
6. E	27. E	48. B
7. E	28. B	49. B
8. E	29. D	50. E
9. C	30. A	51. D
10. B	31. C	52. A
11. C	32. D	53. A
12. C	33. C	54. C
13. A	34. A	55. B
14. D	35. A	56. B
15. D	36. D	57. A
16. A	37. A	58. B
17. E	38. B	59. A
18. E	39. B	60. C
19. A	40. A	61. A
20. B	41. D	62. C
21. D	42. A	63. D

Answers:—continued

64. B	89. A	114. B
65. B	90. E	115. B
66. C	91. B	116. E
67. A	92. A	117. A
68. A	93. D	118. C
69. D	94. B	119. B
70. A	95. B	120. C
71. D	96. E	121. C
72. A	97. A	122. B
73. B	98. D	123. C
74. A	99. B	124. A
75. E	100. C	125. E
76. A	101. E	126. E
77. B	102. A	127. E
78. C	103. D	128. E
79. D	104. A	129. B
80. A	105. E	130. E
81. B	106. C	131. C
82. B	107. A	132. D
83. A	108. C	133. C
84. E	109. B	134. B
85. A	110. A	135. B
86. C	111. C	136. D
87. B	112. B	
88. D	113. C	

Explanations

1. **Answer = B, Fast Fourier transformation is a processing method used for continuous-wave Doppler and pulsed-wave Doppler analysis.**

References: Sidebotham D, Merry A, Legget M (eds.). *Practical Perioperative Transoesophageal Echocardiography.* Burlington, MA: Butterworth Heinemann 2003:141; Edelman SK. *Understanding Ultrasound Physics.* Woodlands, TX: ESP, Inc. 1994:30–31.

2. **Answer = B, High pulse repetition frequency pulsed-wave Doppler utilizes two or more sample volumes along a scan line, which decreases aliasing artifact but introduces range ambiguity.**

Reference: Sidebotham D, Merry A, Legget M (eds.). *Practical Perioperative Transoesophageal Echocardiography.* Burlington, MA: Butterworth Heinemann 2003:39.

3. **Answer = D, With two-dimensional imaging the true dimensions of a structure are obtained when measurements are made from leading edge to leading edge.**

Reference: Sidebotham D, Merry A, Legget M (eds.). *Practical Perioperative Transoesophageal Echocardiography.* Burlington, MA: Butterworth Heinemann 2003:26–28 (Figure 2.12).

4. **Answer = D, Grade 4 = akinesis (AK).** (See Table 4.2K.)

Table 4.2K.

Wall Motion	Grade	Endocardial Movement	Endocardial Thickening
Normal	1	Normal	> 30%
Mild HK	2	Slightly decreased	10 to 30%
Severe HK	3	Severely decreased	< 10%
AK	4	No movement	No thickening
DK	5	Outward during systole	Thins during systole

Abbreviations: HK = hypokinesis, AK = akinesis, DK = dyskinesis.

Reference: Sidebotham D, Merry A, Legget M (eds.). *Practical Perioperative Transoesophageal Echocardiography.* Burlington, MA: Butterworth Heinemann 2003:110.

5. **Answer = E, Grade 5 = dyskinesis (DK).**

Reference: Sidebotham D, Merry A, Legget M (eds.). *Practical Perioperative Transoesophageal Echocardiography.* Burlington, MA: Butterworth Heinemann 2003:110.

6. **Answer = E, Severe left ventricular hypertrophy is not a potential cause of a segmental wall motion abnormality.** Potential causes of segmental wall motion abnormalities include the following.

- Myocardial ischemia
  - Myocardial infarction
  - Intracoronary air embolus
  - Occlusion of coronary ostia during root replacement
  - Occlusion of coronary ostia during type A dissection
  - Inadequate cardioplegia

- Myocardial stunning
- Hibernating myocardium
- Hypovolemia
- Conduction abnormalities
  - Bundle branch blocks
  - RV epicardial pacing
- Sector scan passing through the membranous ventricular septum
- Severe mitral stenosis (basal segments)

Reference: Sidebotham D, Merry A, Legget M (eds.). *Practical Perioperative Transoesophageal Echocardiography.* Burlington, MA: Butterworth Heinemann 2003:111.

7. **Answer = E, All of the choices are potential causes of segmental wall motion abnormalities.** Potential causes of segmental wall motion abnormalities include the following.

- Myocardial ischemia
  - Myocardial infarction
  - Intracoronary air embolus
  - Occlusion of coronary ostia during root replacement
  - Occlusion of coronary ostia during type A dissection
  - Inadequate cardioplegia
- Myocardial stunning
- Hibernating myocardium
- Hypovolemia
- Conduction abnormalities
  - Bundle branch blocks
  - RV epicardial pacing
- Sector scan passing through the membranous ventricular septum
- Severe mitral stenosis (basal segments)

Reference: Sidebotham D, Merry A, Legget M (eds.). *Practical Perioperative Transoesophageal Echocardiography.* Burlington, MA: Butterworth Heinemann 2003:111.

8. **Answer = E, All of the choices listed are potential causes of segmental wall motion abnormalities.** Potential causes of segmental wall motion abnormalities include the following.
- Myocardial ischemia
  - Myocardial infarction
  - Intracoronary air embolus
  - Occlusion of coronary ostia during root replacement
  - Occlusion of coronary ostia during type A dissection
  - Inadequate cardioplegia
- Myocardial stunning
- Hibernating myocardium
- Hypovolemia
- Conduction abnormalities
  - Bundle branch blocks
  - RV epicardial pacing

• Sector scan passing through the membranous ventricular septum
• Severe mitral stenosis (basal segments)

Reference: Sidebotham D, Merry A, Legget M (eds.). *Practical Perioperative Transoesophageal Echocardiography.* Burlington, MA: Butterworth Heinemann 2003:111.

9. **Answer = C, A$_3$ is usually supported solely by the posteromedial papillary muscle.** The anterolateral papillary muscle supports A$_1$ and P$_1$ and part of A$_2$ and P$_2$; the posteromedial papillary muscle supports A$_3$ and P$_3$ and part of A$_2$ and P$_2$.

Reference: Sidebotham D, Merry A, Legget M (eds.). *Practical Perioperative Transoesophageal Echocardiography.* Burlington, MA: Butterworth Heinemann 2003:133.

10. **Answer = B, The septal and anterior leaflets of the tricuspid valve are seen in the midesophageal five-chamber view.**

Reference: Sidebotham D, Merry A, Legget M (eds.). *Practical Perioperative Transoesophageal Echocardiography.* Burlington, MA: Butterworth Heinemann 2003:135 (Figure 9.6).

11. **Answer = C, In the transgastric basal short axis view the ultrasound beam is the most perpendicular to the mitral valve regurgitant flow.** This may make evaluation of mitral regurgitation by color flow Doppler more difficult to interpret in this view.

Reference: Sidebotham D, Merry A, Legget M (eds.). *Practical Perioperative Transoesophageal Echocardiography.* Burlington, MA: Butterworth Heinemann 2003:138.

12. **Answer = C, The transgastric two-chamber view is the best view listed for assessing the mitral valve papillary muscles and chordae.**

Reference: Sidebotham D, Merry A, Legget M (eds.). *Practical Perioperative Transoesophageal Echocardiography.* Burlington, MA: Butterworth Heinemann 2003:139.

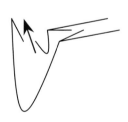

13. **Answer = A, a posterior directed jet with anterior mitral valve leaflet restriction describes the mitral regurgitation seen in hypertrophic obstructive cardiomyopathy with systolic anterior motion of the anterior mitral valve leaflet.** Although anterior leaflet restriction usually results in an anterior directed jet, with systolic anterior motion of the anterior mitral valve leaflet a posterior directed jet occurs. See the figure to the left:

Reference: Sidebotham D, Merry A, Legget M (eds.). *Practical Perioperative Transoesophageal Echocardiography.* Burlington, MA: Butterworth Heinemann 2003:140.

14. **Answer = D, The anterolateral papillary muscle is supplied by both the left anterior descending and circumflex coronary arteries.** This dual blood supply makes the anterolateral papillary less likely to rupture than the posteromedial papillary muscle, which is supplied solely by the right coronary artery.

Reference: Sidebotham D, Merry A, Legget M (eds.). *Practical Perioperative Transoesophageal Echocardiography.* Burlington, MA: Butterworth Heinemann 2003:138–141.

15. **Answer = D, An increase in the mean velocity of the mitral regurgitant jet is not associated with an increase in the severity of the mitral regurgitant jet.** The velocity of the mitral regurgitant jet

reflects the pressure gradient between the left atrium and the left ventricle and is not directly related to the degree of mitral regurgitation. In fact, the velocity may be lower with the elevated left atrial pressures seen in significant mitral regurgitation.

Reference: Sidebotham D, Merry A, Legget M (eds.). *Practical Perioperative Transoesophageal Echocardiography.* Burlington, MA: Butterworth Heinemann 2003:146.

16. **Answer = A, Myxomatous degeneration is the most common indication for mitral valve repair.**

Reference: Sidebotham D, Merry A, Legget M (eds.). *Practical Perioperative Transoesophageal Echocardiography.* Burlington, MA: Butterworth Heinemann 2003:147.

17. **Answer = E, All are surgical maneuvers that may help reduce the risk of systolic anterior motion (SAM) of the anterior mitral valve leaflet following mitral valve repair.** Reducing the base-to-tip length of the posterior mitral valve leaflet, and using a sliding valvuloplasty technique both displace the coaptation line posteriorly and thus increase the distance from the coaptation point to the septum. Reducing the base-to-tip length of the anterior leaflet also appears to reduce the risk of SAM, possibly by reducing the redundant anterior leaflet tissue distal to the coaptation point.

Reference: Sidebotham D, Merry A, Legget M (eds.). *Practical Perioperative Transoesophageal Echocardiography.* Burlington, MA: Butterworth Heinemann 2003:149–150.

18. **Answer = E, All will increase the mean diastolic transmitral pressure gradient as determined by tracing the diastolic continuous-wave Doppler mitral valve flow profile.**

Reference: Sidebotham D, Merry A, Legget M (eds.). *Practical Perioperative Transoesophageal Echocardiography.* Burlington, MA: Butterworth Heinemann 2003:152.

19. **Answer = A, Holodiastolic flow reversal in the abdominal aorta is sensitive and specific for severe aortic insufficiency.** Holodiastolic flow reversal in the descending thoracic aorta may also indicate severe AI, but this is not as sensitive or specific as flow reversal in the abdominal aorta.

Reference: Sidebotham D, Merry A, Legget M (eds.). *Practical Perioperative Transoesophageal Echocardiography.* Burlington, MA: Butterworth Heinemann 2003:167.

20. **Answer = B, Calcific aortic stenosis is the most common cause of aortic stenosis in adults.** Bicuspid aortic stenosis is the most common cause in younger patients, and 2% of the general population has a bicuspid aortic valve. Rheumatic heart disease is the most common cause of mitral stenosis. Carcinoid syndrome usually only affects the right-sided heart valves, because monoamine oxidases in the lungs protect the left-sided heart valves from the offending metabolites. Noonan's syndrome usually

affects the pulmonic valve. Clinical features of Noonan's syndrome include short stature, low-set ears, skeletal deformities (of which the commonest are pectus excavatum and cubitus valgus), and cardiac abnormalities. Cardiac abnormalities occur in 50% of patients. These include pulmonary valve stenosis, thick and dysplastic pulmonary valves, right heart anomalies, and left ventricular cardiomyopathy.

References: Sidebotham D, Merry A, Legget M (eds.). *Practical Perioperative Transoesophageal Echocardiography.* Burlington, MA: Butterworth Heinemann 2003:158; www.whonamedit.com/synd.cfm/1920.html.

21. **Answer = D, Autopsy studies have shown that 25% of the general population has a probe patent foramen ovale.**

Reference: Konstadt SN, Shernon S, Oka Y (eds). *Clinical Transesophageal Echocardiography: A Problem-Oriented Approach, Second Edition.* Philadelphia: Lippincott Williams & Wilkins 2003:429.

22. **Answer = D, ≥25 mm is considered normal tricuspid annular plane systolic excursion.**

References: Perrino AC, Reeves S. *A Practical Approach to TEE.* Philadelphia: Lippincott Williams & Wilkins 2003:220; Sidebotham D, Merry A, Legget M (eds.). *Practical Perioperative Transoesophageal Echocardiography.* Burlington, MA: Butterworth Heinemann 2003:206.

23. **Answer = C, 26 mmHg is the pulmonary artery diastolic pressure.**
The calculation is as follows.

$\Delta P = 4V^2$

$(PADP - RVDP) = 4 (V_{PIlate})^2$

$(PADP - CVP) = 4 (V_{PIlate})^2$

$PADP = 4(V_{PIlate})^2 + CVP$

$PADP = 4(V_{PIlate})^2 + CVP$

$PADP = 4(2 \text{ m/s})^2 + 10$

$PADP = 26 \text{ mmHg}$

- ΔP = change in pressure (pressure gradient)
- PADP = pulmonary artery diastolic pressure
- CVP = central venous pressure
- VPIlate = the late peak velocity of the pulmonic insufficiency jet obtained with CWD
- CWD = continuous-wave Doppler

Reference: Perrino AC, Reeves S. *A Practical Approach to TEE.* Philadelphia: Lippincott Williams & Wilkins 2003:104.

24. **Answer = B, 63.3 ml is the stroke volume of blood flow through the pulmonary artery. The calculation is as follows.**

$SV_{PA} = A_{PA} * TVI_{PA}$

$SV_{PA} = \pi r^2 * TVI_{PA}$

$SV_{PA} = \pi (1.2 cm)^2 * 14 cm$

$SV_{PA} = 63.3 cm^3$

- SV_{PA} = stroke volume of blood flow through the pulmonary artery
- TVI_{PA} = time velocity integral of blood flow through the pulmonary artery
- A_{PA} = area of the pulmonary artery

Reference: SCA/ASE Annual Comprehensive Review and Update of Perioperative Hemodynamics Workshop. 17 Feb. 2005, San Diego, CA; discussion lead by Stanton Shernon, et al.

25. **Answer = B, 10.8 ml is the pulmonic valve regurgitant volume (PV_{RVol}). The calculation is as follows.**

$PV_{RVol} = SV_{PA} - SV_{TV} = SV_{PA} - (A_{TV} * TVI_{TV}) = 63.3 ml - (3.5 cm^2 * 13 cm) = \underline{\mathbf{10.8 cm^3}}$

$SV_{PA} = A_{PA} * TVI_{PA}$

$SV_{PA} = \pi r^2 * TVI_{PA}$

$SV_{PA} = \pi (1.2 cm)^2 * 14 cm$

$SV_{PA} = 63.3 cm^3$

- SV_{PA} = stroke volume of blood flow through the pulmonary artery
- TVI_{PA} = time velocity integral of blood flow through the pulmonary artery
- A_{PA} = area of the pulmonary artery
- SV_{TV} = stroke volume of blood flow through the TV
- TV = tricuspid valve
- A_{TV} = tricuspid valve area
- PV_{RVol} = pulmonic valve regurgitant orifice area
- TVI_{TV} = time velocity integral of blood flow through the tricuspid valve

Reference: SCA/ASE Annual Comprehensive Review and Update of Perioperative Hemodynamics Workshop. 17 Feb. 2005, San Diego, CA; discussion lead by Stanton Shernon, et al.

26. **Answer = C, 21.6 mm² = 0.216 cm² is the pulmonic valve regurgitant orifice area (PV ROA). The calculation is as follows.**

$PV\ ROA = PV_{RVol} / TVI_{PI} = 10.8 cm^3 / 50 cm = \underline{\mathbf{0.216 cm^2}}$

$PV_{RVol} = SV_{PA} - SV_{TV} = SV_{PA} - (A_{TV} * TVI_{TV}) = 63.3 ml - (3.5 cm^2 * 13 cm) = 10.8 cm^3$

$SV_{PA} = A_{PA} * TVI_{PA}$

$SV_{PA} = \pi r^2 * TVI_{PA}$

$SV_{PA} = \pi (1.2 cm)^2 * 14 cm$

$SV_{PA} = 63.3 cm^3$

- SV_{PA} = stroke volume of blood flow through the pulmonary artery
- TVI_{PA} = time velocity integral of blood flow through the pulmonary artery
- A_{PA} = area of the pulmonary artery
- SV_{TV} = stroke volume of blood flow through the TV
- TV = tricuspid valve
- A_{TV} = tricuspid valve area
- PV_{RVol} = pulmonic valve regurgitant orifice area
- TVI_{TV} = time velocity integral of blood flow through the tricuspid valve

Reference: SCA/ASE Annual Comprehensive Review and Update of Perioperative Hemodynamics Workshop. 17 Feb. 2005, San Diego, CA; discussion lead by Stanton Shernon, et al.

27. **Answer = E, 46 mmHg is the pulmonary artery mean pressure. The calculation is as follows.**

$\Delta P = 4V^2$

$(PAMP - RVDP) = 4\,(V_{Plearly})^2$

$(PAMP - CVP) = 4\,(V_{Plearly})^2$

$PAMP = 4\,(V_{Plearly})^2 + CVP$

$PAMP = 4\,(3\ m/s)^2 + 10$

$PAMP = 46\ mmHg$

- ΔP = change in pressure (pressure gradient)
- PAMP = pulmonary artery mean pressure
- CVP = central venous pressure
- RVDP = right ventricular diastolic pressure
- $V_{Plearly}$ = the early peak velocity of the pulmonic insufficiency jet obtained with CWD
- CWD = continuous-wave Doppler

Reference: Perrino AC, Reeves S. *A Practical Approach to TEE.* Philadelphia: Lippincott Williams & Wilkins 2003:104.

28. **Answer = B, In category I indications TEE is frequently useful in improving outcomes.** These cases are supported by the strongest evidence or by expert opinion. These indications were first published in 1996 by the American Society of Anesthesiologists (ASA) and the Society of Cardiovascular Anesthesiologists (SCA). They are likely somewhat outdated, and are not listed in the content outline for the PTEeXAM (*http://www. echoboards.org/pte/outline.html*). You should not waste time memorizing these lists, but you should read them and be familiar with them. The important thing to consider when performing a TEE is the risk/benefit ratio. If the information gained by doing the exam will potentially change management and improve patient care, and the patient is at low risk for complications, the exam should be performed. This has to be determined on a case-by-case basis.

Category I indications:

- Evaluation of acute, persistent, and life-threatening hemodynamic instability in the operating room, or of ICU in which ventricular function and its determinants are uncertain and have not responded to treatment
- Intraoperative use in valve repair
- Intraoperative use in congenital heart disease for most lesions requiring cardiopulmonary bypass
- Intraoperative use during repair of hypertrophic obstructive cardiomyopathy
- Intraoperative use for endocarditis when preoperative testing was inadequate or extension of infection to perivalvular tissue is suspected
- Intraoperative assessment of aortic valve function in repair of aortic dissections
- Intraoperative evaluation of pericardial window procedures

Category II indications are supported by weaker evidence or by expert opinion. TEE may be useful in improving outcomes in these cases.

Category II indications:

- Perioperative use in patients at increased risk of myocardial ischemia or infarction
- Perioperative use in patients at increased risk of hemodynamic disturbances
- Intraoperative assessment of valve replacement
- Intraoperative assessment of repair of cardiac aneurysms
- Intraoperative evaluation of removal of cardiac tumors
- Intraoperative detection of foreign bodies
- Intraoperative detection of air emboli during cardiotomy for heart transplantation and during upright neurological procedures
- Intraoperative use during intracardiac thrombectomy or pulmonary emobolectomy
- Intraoperative use for suspected cardiac trauma
- Preoperative assessment of patients with suspected acute thoracic aortic dissections, aneurysms, or disruptions
- Intraoperative use during repair of thoracic aortic dissections without suspected aortic valve involvement
- Intraoperative evaluation of pericardectomy, pericardial effusion, or evaluation of pericardial surgery (note pericardial window is a class I indication)
- Intraoperative evaluation of anastomotic sites during heart and/or lung transplantation
- Monitoring placement and function of assist devices

Category III indications are supported by little current scientific evidence or expert opinion. TEE is infrequently useful in improving outcomes.

Category III indications:

- Intraoperative evaluation of myocardial perfusion, coronary artery anatomy, graft patency, or cardioplegia administration

- Intraoperative use during cardiomyopathies other than hypertrophic cardiomyopathy
- Intraoperative use for uncomplicated endocarditis during non-cardiac surgery
- Intraoperative assessment of repair of thoracic aortic injuries
- Intraoperative use for uncomplicated pericariditis
- Intraoperative evaluation of pleuropulmonary diseases
- Monitoring placement of intra-aortic balloon pump, automatic implantable cardiac defibrillators, or pulmonary artery catheters

Reference: Sidebotham D, Merry A, Legget M (eds.). *Practical Perioperative Transoesophageal Echocardiography.* Burlington, MA: Butterworth Heinemann 2003:2.

29. Answer = D, M-mode is essentially a B-mode image plotted against time.

References: Sidebotham D, Merry A, Legget M (eds.). *Practical Perioperative Transoesophageal Echocardiography.* Burlington, MA: Butterworth Heinemann 2003:25; Edelman SK. *Understanding Ultrasound Physics*, Woodlands, TX: ESP, Inc. 1994:1997

30. Answer = A, Increasing the pulse repetition frequency (PRF) will increase the duty factor. PRF is the number of pulses per second. The more pulses per second the greater the percentage of "on" time and thus the greater the duty factor. The duty factor is a unitless number that describes the amount of time the ultrasound machine is producing sound (the percentage of "on" time). The other choices listed will decrease the duty factor.

Reference: Edelman SK. *Understanding Ultrasound Physics.* Woodlands, TX: ESP, Inc. 1994:30–31.

31. Answer = C, Spatial pulse length (SPL) is determined by both the sound source and the medium through which it travels. SPL is *inversely* related (inversely proportional) to the frequency. SPL is *directly* proportional to the number of cycles in the pulse. SPL = (number of cycles) *λ, where λ = wavelength = length of one cycle. As SPL decreases longitudinal resolution increases, but transverse resolution (lateral resolution) is not necessarily changed. Transverse resolution is determined by the width of the ultrasound beam, not the SPL. *Lateral resolution has several synonyms,* including *angular resolution, azimuthal resolution,* and *transverse resolution.*

Reference: Edelman SK. *Understanding Ultrasound Physics.* Woodlands, TX: ESP, Inc. 1994:32.

32. Answer = D, The spatial pulse length (SPL) is determined by both the ultrasound source and the medium through which the sound travels. All other choices listed are determined solely by the ultrasound source. Pulse repetition period (PRP), pulse repetition frequency (PRF), spatial pulse length (SPL), and duty factor are all determined by the sound source.

Reference: Edelman SK. *Understanding Ultrasound Physics.* Woodlands, TX: ESP, Inc. 1994:32.

33. **Answer = C, Spatial pulse length is lower with high-frequency transducers and this improves axial resolution.**

Reference: Kremkau FW. *Diagnostic Ultrasound: Principles Instruments and Exercises, Third Edition.* Philadelphia: Saunders 1989:89.

34. **Answer = A, Spatial pulse length (SPL) and image quality are inversely related.** The smaller the spatial pulse length the higher the longitudinal resolution and therefore the higher the image quality. Spatial pulse length and lateral resolution are not related, as lateral resolution is determined by beam width. Wavelength (λ) and SPL are inversely related. Wavelength and pulse duration are inversely related. Imaging depth and SPL are not related.

References: Edelman SK. *Understanding Ultrasound Physics.* Woodlands, TX: ESP, Inc. 1994:32; Kremkau FW. *Diagnostic Ultrasound: Principles Instruments and Exercises, Third Edition.* Philadelphia: Saunders 1989:89.

35. **Answer = A, Rayleigh scattering is responsible for the Doppler determinations of blood flow velocities.** Rayleigh scattering occurs when the wavelength (λ) is much *larger* than the reflector it strikes (e.g., red blood cells produce Rayleigh scattering). Absorption is the primary component of attenuation in soft tissue.

Reference: Edelman SK. *Understanding Ultrasound Physics.* Woodlands, TX: ESP, Inc. 1994:52.

36. **Answer = D, Absorption is responsible for $\geq$ 80% of the attenuation seen in soft tissue.**

Reference: Edelman SK. *Understanding Ultrasound Physics.* Woodlands, TX: ESP, Inc. 1994:52.

37. **Answer = A, Reflection can occur at the interface of two tissues with different reflection coefficients.** *Scattering* (not specular reflection) allows the lateral and septal walls to be visualized in the ME four-chamber view. Echoes from scattering are *weaker* (not stronger) than echoes produced by specular reflection.

Reference: Edelman SK. *Understanding Ultrasound Physics.* Woodlands, TX: ESP, Inc. 1994:52–53.

38. **Answer = B, AC is equal to 1/2 frequency or 2 * (period).**

Reference: Edelman SK. *Understanding Ultrasound Physics.* Woodlands, TX: ESP, Inc. 1994:54.

39. **Answer = B, 1.6 mWatts/cm^2 = the intensity of the ultrasound beam at a depth of 1 cm.** The attenuation coefficient is 1/2 * frequency = 10 dB/cm. The path length is 1 cm. Therefore, the attenuation will be 1 cm * 10 dB/cm = 10 dB of attenuation. Given that for intensity dB = 10 Log I_2/I_1 this correlates to a decrease in the new intensity to 1/10 the initial intensity or 1.6 mWatts/cm^2. *Alternative detailed explanation*: The attenuation coefficient is AC = 1/2 * frequency = 10 dB/cm. Because the path length is 1 cm there will be 1 cm * 10 dB/cm = 10 dB of attenuation. This is a change

of -10 dB (negative because the intensity is decreasing). For intensity, dB = $10 \log I_2/I_1$. Thus, if there are 10 dB of attenuation -10dB = $10 \log I_2/I_1 \rightarrow$ $\log I_2/I_1 = -10/10 = -1 \rightarrow I_2/I_1 = 10^{-1} \rightarrow I_2$ (the new intensity) is 1/10 the old intensity I_1. Therefore, $I_2 = 1/10\ I_1 = 1.6$ mWatts/cm^2.

Reference: Edelman SK. *Understanding Ultrasound Physics.* Woodlands, TX: ESP, Inc. 1994:55.

40. **Answer = A, 1 cm = the thickness of tissue required to reduce the amplitude of a 12-MHz TEE transducer by half.** For ultrasound in soft tissue: amplitude dB = $20 \log A_2/_{A1}$. When $A_2 = 1/2\ A_1$ then $20 \log 2 = 6$ dB (thus, every 6 dB represents a halving of the amplitude). Therefore, for amplitude the *half value layer thickness* is equal to 6 dB/AC = 1 cm. AC = the attenuation coefficient = 1/2 frequency. Thus, for every 1 cm the amplitude will decrease by 1/2.

Reference: Edelman SK. *Understanding Ultrasound Physics.* Woodlands, TX: ESP, Inc. 1994:56.

41. **Answer = D, All are correct.** The two media have different velocities and the beam has oblique incidence and therefore refraction can occur. Reflection and transmission can also occur with oblique incidence.

Reference: Edelman SK. *Understanding Ultrasound Physics.* Woodlands, TX: ESP, Inc. 1994:67–68.

42. **Answer = A, Transmission.** The incidence of ultrasound is orthogonal = perpendicular, and thus refraction cannot occur. With normal incidence and the same acoustic impedance, reflection cannot occur. Thus, all of the ultrasound will be transmitted and none will be reflected.

Reference: Edelman SK. *Understanding Ultrasound Physics.* Woodlands, TX: ESP, Inc. 1994:67–68.

43. **Answer = B, Reflection and transmission.** Media 3 and 4 have different acoustic impedance. Therefore, with normal incidence reflection and transmission can occur.

Reference: Edelman SK. *Understanding Ultrasound Physics.* Woodlands, TX: ESP, Inc. 1994:67–68.

44. **Answer = A, Depth resolution is improved by the damping material.** The matching layer is described by the statement in answer B. The damping material decreases the Q factor (quality factor) by increasing the bandwidth and decreasing the resonant frequency. The damping material decreases the sensitivity of the transducer to reflected echoes. Longitudinal = axial = radial = range = depth resolution. This is somewhat confusing because range resolution is also used to describe the ability of pulsed-wave Doppler to determine the depth of a Doppler shift using a sample volume.

Reference: Edelman SK. *Understanding Ultrasound Physics.* Woodlands, TX: ESP, Inc. 1994:74.

45. **Answer = C, For axial resolution the smaller the numerical value the better the picture quality.** Choice A is incorrect because lateral

resolution (not longitudinal resolution) is determined by beam width. Choice B is wrong because longitudinal resolution (not lateral resolution) = 1/2 spatial pulse length (SPL). Choice D is incorrect because as pulse repetition frequency (PRF) decreases temporal resolution *decreases*.

Reference: Edelman SK. *Understanding Ultrasound Physics.* Woodlands, TX: ESP, Inc. 1994:90.

46. **Answer = D, Azimuthal resolution is also know as lateral resolution.** The other choices listed are synonyms of *longitudinal resolution*. In addition to being a synonym of *longitudinal resolution*, *range resolution* is also used to describe the ability of pulsed-wave Doppler (PWD) to evaluate velocities at a specific depth/location (the sample gate or sample volume).

Reference: Edelman SK. *Understanding Ultrasound Physics.* Woodlands, TX: ESP, Inc. 1994:92.

47. **Answer = A, Lateral resolution is determined by the beam diameter.** Depth resolution, temporal resolution, and range resolution are not determined by the beam width. Depth resolution (also known as longitudinal resolution, axial resolution, radial resolution, and range resolution) is determined by the spatial pulse length (SPL) according to the following relationship: depth resolution = 1/2 SPL. Range resolution is also used to describe the ability of pulsed-wave Doppler (PWD) to evaluate velocities at a specific location (the sample gate or sample volume). Temporal resolution is determined by the frame rate (frames/sec or images/sec). The higher the frame rate the "smoother" the image appears to move, and the better the temporal resolution. Temporal resolution is not related to beam width.

Reference: Edelman SK. *Understanding Ultrasound Physics.* Woodlands, TX: ESP, Inc. 1994:92.

48. **Answer = B, Lateral resolution has the highest numerical value.** Axial resolution, the ability to distinguish two objects located in series (one in front of the other, or one deeper than the other), has a lower numerical value than lateral resolution and is therefore superior to lateral resolution. The lower the numerical value the better the image quality and thus the higher the resolution. *Range resolution* has two definitions: It is a synonym of *axial resolution* and it is used to describe the ability of pulsed-wave Doppler (PWD) to evaluate velocities at a specific location (the sample gate or sample volume).

Reference: Edelman SK. *Understanding Ultrasound Physics.* Woodlands, TX: ESP, Inc. 1994:92, 134.

49. **Answer = B, Fast Fourier transformation is the current method of spectral analysis for pulsed-wave Doppler.** Zero crossing detection, use of time interval histogram, and use of Chirp-z transforms are older methods of spectral analysis no longer widely used. Autocorrelation is used to analyze color flow Doppler.

Reference: Edelman SK. *Understanding Ultrasound Physics.* Woodlands, TX: ESP, Inc. 1994:138, 141.

50. **Answer = E, 200 Hz = the Nyquist limit.** The Nyquist limit (Nyquist frequency) is equal to 1/2 the pulse repetition frequency.

Reference: Perrino AC, Reeves S. *A Practical Approach to TEE.* Philadelphia: Lippincott Williams & Wilkins 2003:79.

51. **Answer = D, Membranous defect = sinus venosus defect is incorrect because sinus venosus defects are a type of atrial septal defect.**

Reference: Otto C. *Textbook of Clinical Echocardiography, Third Edition.* Philadelphia: Elsevier 2004:474.

52. **Answer = A, A large nonrestrictive perimembranous ventricular septal defect, right ventricular outflow tract obstruction, overriding aorta, and right ventricular hypertrophy are the four classic components of tetralogy of fallot (TOF).** The ventricular septal defect in TOF is usually perimembranous (> 80%).

Reference: Perrino AC, Reeves S. *A Practical Approach to TEE.* Philadelphia: Lippincott Williams & Wilkins 2003:294.

53. **Answer = A, Ostium secundum atrial septal defects are associated with mitral regurgitation due to mitral valve prolapse without a cleft anterior mitral valve leaflet.**

Reference: Sidebotham D, Merry A, Legget M (eds.). *Practical Perioperative Transoesophageal Echocardiography.* Burlington, MA: Butterworth Heinemann 2003:223.

54. **Answer = C, Subarterial = conal = subpulmonic = supracristal = doubly committed outlet ventricular septal defect.** This defect is located in the right ventricular outflow tract above the crista supraventricularis. It is the most likely VSD to be associated with aortic cusp herniation. Note that a membranous (perimembranous) VSD is located below the ridge of the supraventricularis in the membranous portion of the septum near the tricuspid valve, close to the junction of the septal and anterior tricuspid valve leaflets. Both of these defects can cause aortic cusp herniation, and both can be seen in the right ventricular inflow/outflow view. In this view a subpulmonic defect is seen just below the pulmonic valve, and a membranous defect is seen closer to the tricuspid valve.

Reference: Sidebotham D, Merry A, Legget M (eds.). *Practical Perioperative Transoesophageal Echocardiography.* Burlington, MA: Butterworth Heinemann 2003:222, 225.

55. **Answer = B, The tricuspid valve separates the left atrium from the right ventricle in congenitally corrected transposition of the great vessels (ventricular inversion).** In this disorder the ventricles are essentially switched (ventricular inversion). The right ventricle is located on the left side of the heart and the left ventricle is located on the right

side of the heart. The atrioventricular valves are attached normally to correct ventricles. Therefore, the tricuspid valve is attached to the right ventricle and the mitral valve is attached to the left ventricle. However, the location of the ventricles is switched. The right side of the heart has a right atrium attached to the left ventricle and the left side of the heart has a left atrium attached to the right ventricle. The right atrium connects to the left ventricle by the tricuspid valve and the left atrium connects to the right ventricle by the mitral valve. Blood flows as follows: SVC→RA→MV→LV→PA →L →PV →LA →TV →RV →Ao

Reference: Otto C. *Textbook of Clinical Echocardiography, Third Edition.* Philadelphia: Elsevier 2004:477.

56. **Answer = B, SVC →RA →MV →LV →PA →L →PV →LA →TV →RV →Ao describes the correct path of blood flow in a patient with congenitally corrected transposition of the great vessels, which is also known as ventricular inversion.**

Reference: Otto C. *Textbook of Clinical Echocardiography, Third Edition.* Philadelphia: Elsevier 2004:477.

57. **Answer = A, Patient A would benefit most from a procedure (such as a Blalock-Taussig shunt or a Glenn shunt) that increases pulmonary blood flow because this patient has tricuspid atresia and decreased pulmonary blood flow.** A Blalock-Taussig shunt increases pulmonary blood flow by establishing communication between the arterial circulation and the pulmonary artery (usually via a subclavian-to-PA shunt). A Glenn shunt increases pulmonary blood flow by connecting the superior vena cava directly to the right pulmonary artery.

Reference: Otto C. *Textbook of Clinical Echocardiography, Third Edition.* Philadelphia: Elsevier 2004:482.

58. **Answer = B, 27 mmHg is the pulmonary artery mean pressure (PAMP).** The calculation is as follows.

$\Delta P = 4V^2$

$(PAMP - RVDP) = 4\,(V_{Plearly})^2$

$(PAMP - CVP) = 4\,(V_{Plearly})^2$

$PAMP = 4\,(V_{Plearly})^2 + CVP$

$PAMP = 4(2 \text{ m/s})^2 + 11$

$PAMP = 27 \text{ mmHg}$

- ΔP = change in pressure (pressure gradient)
- PAMP = pulmonary artery mean pressure
- CVP = central venous pressure
- RVDP = right ventricular diastolic pressure

- $V_{PIearly}$ = the early peak velocity of the pulmonic insufficiency jet obtained with CWD
- CWD = continuous-wave Doppler

Reference: Perrino AC, Reeves S. *A Practical Approach to TEE.* Philadelphia: Lippincott Williams & Wilkins 2003:104.

59. **Answer = A, 15 mmHg = the pulmonary artery diastolic pressure.** This is calculated as follows.

$$\Delta P = 4V^2$$

$$(PADP - RVDP) = 4\,(V_{PIlate})^2$$

$$(PADP - CVP) = 4\,(V_{PIlate})^2$$

$$PADP = 4\,(V_{PIlate})^2 + CVP$$

$$PADP = 4(1\ m/s)^2 + 11$$

$$PADP = 15\ mmHg$$

- ΔP = change in pressure (pressure gradient)
- PADP = pulmonary artery diastolic pressure
- CVP = central venous pressure
- V_{PIlate} = the late peak velocity of the pulmonic insufficiency jet obtained with CWD
- CWD = continuous-wave Doppler

Reference: Perrino AC, Reeves S. *A Practical Approach to TEE.* Philadelphia: Lippincott Williams & Wilkins 2003:104.

60. **Answer = C, 47 mmHg = the right ventricular systolic blood pressure (RVSP).** The calculation is as follows.

$$\Delta P = 4V^2$$

$$(RVSP - RAP) = 4V_{TR}^{\ 2}$$

$$(RVSP - CVP) = 4V^2$$

$$RVSP = 4V^2 + CVP$$

$$RVSP = 4(3\ m/s)^2 + 11$$

$$RVSP = 47\ mmHg$$

- ΔP = change in pressure (pressure gradient)
- RVSP = right ventricular systolic pressure
- RAP = right atrial pressure
- CVP = central venous pressure
- V_{TR} = peak velocity of the tricuspid valve regurgitant jet

Reference: Otto C. *Textbook of Clinical Echocardiography, Third Edition.* Philadelphia: Elsevier 2004:463.

61. **Answer = A, 2.6 mmHg is the peak instantaneous systolic pressure gradient across the pulmonic valve (ΔP_{PV}).** The calculation is as follows.

$$\Delta P = 4V^2$$

$$\Delta P_{PV} = 4(V_{PVsystolic\ peak})^2$$

$$\Delta P_{PV} = 4\ (0.8\ m/s)^2$$

$$\Delta P_{PV} = 2.6\ mmHg$$

- $V_{PVsystolic\ peak}$ = peak velocity of systolic flow across the pulmonic valve
- ΔP_{PV} = the peak instantaneous systolic pressure gradient across the pulmonic valve

Reference: Otto C. *Textbook of Clinical Echocardiography, Third Edition.* Philadelphia: Elsevier 2004:463.

62. **Answer = C, 47 mmHg.** The pulmonary artery systolic pressure (PASP) is equal to the right ventricular systolic blood pressure (RVSP) if no pulmonic stenosis is present. We know that pulmonic stenosis is not present given the low systolic pressure gradient across the pulmonic valve. The calculation is as follows.

$$\Delta P = 4V^2$$

$$(RVSP - RAP) = 4V_{TR}^2$$

$$(RVSP - CVP) = 4V^2$$

$$RVSP = 4V^2 + CVP$$

$$RVSP = 4(3\ m/s)^2 + 11$$

$$RVSP = 47\ mmHg$$

$$PASP = RVSP = 47\ mmHg$$

- PASP = pulmonary artery systolic pressure
- RVSP = right ventricular systolic pressure
- RAP = right atrial pressure
- CVP = central venous pressure
- V_{TR} = peak velocity of the tricuspid valve regurgitant jet

Reference: Otto C. *Textbook of Clinical Echocardiography, Third Edition.* Philadelphia: Elsevier 2004:463.

63. **Answer = D, A Crawford type IV aortic aneurysm is described.** This is an abdominal aneurysm that begins below the diaphragm and extends distally to below the renal arteries. (See also Table 4.2L.)

Table 4.2L.	CRAWFORD CLASSIFICATION FOR THORACOABDOMINAL ANEURYSMS	
Type	**Origin**	**Extends Distally to:**
I	Near left subclavian artery	Above renal arteries
II	Near left subclavian artery	Below renal arteries
III	More distal than types I or II but above the diaphragm	Below renal arteries
IV	Below the diaphragm (abdominal)	Below renal arteries

Reference: Perrino AC, Reeves S. *A Practical Approach to TEE.* Philadelphia: Lippincott Williams & Wilkins 2003:252.

64. **Answer = B, In restrictive diastolic dysfunction the lateral mitral annular tissue Doppler (E' = E$_M$) < 8 cm/sec.** In restrictive disease the E/A ratio is increased, the isovolumic relaxation time (IVRT) is decreased (< 110 msec), and the pulmonary vein S wave < D wave.

Reference: Otto C. *Textbook of Clinical Echocardiography, Third Edition.* Philadelphia: Elsevier 2004:174.

65. **Answer = B, The transmitral A-wave velocity increases with aging.** Atrial contraction contributes more to left ventricular filling as patients get older and left ventricular relaxation becomes impaired. Early left ventricular filling decreases, isovolumic relaxation time increases, and transmitral E-wave deceleration time increases with increased age.

Reference: Sidebotham D, Merry A, Legget M (eds.). *Practical Perioperative Transoesophageal Echocardiography.* Burlington, MA: Butterworth Heinemann 2003:123–128.

66. **Answer = C, Restrictive diastolic dysfunction is present.** This patient has decreased left ventricular compliance with elevated left atrial filling pressures. E >> A, E$_M$ < 8 cm/sec, S < D, decreased IVRT, and DT are all characteristics of restrictive diastolic dysfunction.

  • E = pulsed-wave Doppler transmitral early-filling velocity
  • A = pulsed-wave Doppler transmitral peak A-wave velocity
  • E$_M$ = lateral mitral annular tissue Doppler E wave (E$_M$ = E' = E prime)
  • IVRT = isovolumic relaxation time
  • DT = deceleration time

Reference: Groban L, Dolinski SY. Transesophageal echocardiographic evaluation of diastolic function. *Chest* 2005;128:3652–3663.

67. **Answer = A, Increased filling pressures.** The E/E$_M$ > 15 is indicative of elevated left atrial filling pressures.

  • E = pulsed-wave Doppler transmitral early-filling velocity
  • E$_M$ = lateral mitral annular tissue Doppler E wave (E$_M$ = E' = E prime)

Reference: Perrino AC, Reeves S. *A Practical Approach to TEE.* Philadelphia: Lippincott Williams & Wilkins 2003:117.

68. **Answer = A, The transtricuspid peak A-wave velocity will be increased during spontaneous inspiration in a patient with a hemodynamically significant pericardial effusion.** With spontaneous inspiration intrathoracic pressure is decreased, resulting in dilation of the thin-walled right ventricle and thus increasing right ventricular forward flow. This increased right ventricular inflow dilates the RV and causes the intraventricular septum to bulge into the left ventricle, impeding LV filling. Thus, right-sided filling is increased and left-sided filling is decreased. The increased right ventricular filling will increase the transtricuspid peak E-wave velocity as early diastolic transtricuspid flow is increased. Forward RV flow is increased at the expense of reverse flow in the hepatic veins, and thus spontaneous inspiration results in decreased hepatic A and V waves.

The decreased left-sided filling results in a decreased transmitral E-wave peak velocity and a decreased pulmonary vein D-wave peak velocity.

References: Otto C. *Textbook of Clinical Echocardiography, Third Edition.* Philadelphia: Elsevier 2004:179; Groban L, Dolinski SY. Transesophageal echocardiographic evaluation of diastolic function. *Chest* 2005;128:3652–3663.

69. **Answer = D, A pseudonormal profile will be seen when nitroglycerin is administered to a patient with reversible restrictive diastolic dysfunction.** Nitroglycerin decreases preload and this facilitates the reversion to a pseudonormal pattern. If the restrictive pattern does not pseudonormalize in response to preload reduction, this indicates end-stage irreversible restrictive diastolic dysfunction.

Reference: Perrino AC, Reeves S. *A Practical Approach to TEE.* Philadelphia: Lippincott Williams & Wilkins 2003:117.

70. **Answer = A, Normal transmitral flow, tissue Doppler, and pulmonary vein flow velocities are shown.**

Reference: Konstadt SN, Shernon S, Oka Y (eds). *Clinical Transesophageal Echocardiography: A Problem-Oriented Approach, Second Edition.* Philadelphia: Lippincott Williams & Wilkins 2003:74–77.

71. **Answer = D, Tissue Doppler velocities of the lateral mitral annulus are not affected by loading conditions to the same extent as the other parameters of diastolic function listed.** As diastolic function deteriorates tissue Doppler velocities decrease, with less than 8 cm/sec considered significant.

Reference: Oh JK, Seward JB, Tajik AJ (eds). *The Echo Manual, Second Edition.* Philadelphia: Lippincott Williams & Wilkins 1999:55.

72. **Answer = A, PV_{AR} may be prolonged secondarily to decreased left ventricular compliance and increased retrograde flow.** The late diastolic pulmonary vein atrial flow reversal wave (PV_{AR}) results from retrograde flow into the pulmonary veins during atrial contraction. In restrictive diastolic dysfunction, PV_{AR} can be prolonged due to decreased left ventricular compliance or PV_{AR} can be decreased due to left atrial mechanical failure. Pulmonary systolic (S) and diastolic (D) waves are also affected by diastolic dysfunction. With restrictive disease S is typically less than D because left atrial pressures are elevated due to decreased LV compliance. These elevated LA pressures blunt systolic pulmonary flow into the LA and favor diastolic filling of the LA, resulting in an S/D ratio of < 1. Lateral mitral annular tissue Doppler E_M is decreased in restrictive diastolic function (< 8 cm/sec). Transmitral E-wave deceleration time (DT) is decreased in restrictive diastolic dysfunction.

- PV_{AR} = atrial reversal flow velocity (late diastolic pulmonary vein flow reversal velocity)
- E_M = lateral mitral annular tissue Doppler peak E-wave velocity

- DT = transmitral early-filling wave (E-wave) deceleration time
- S/D = ratio of the pulmonary vein peak S-wave velocity to pulmonary vein peak D-wave velocity

Reference: Perrino AC, Reeves S. *A Practical Approach to TEE.* Philadelphia: Lippincott Williams & Wilkins 2003:117.

73. **Answer = B, Pseudonormal diastolic dysfunction is present.** A normal transmitral pulsed-wave Doppler diastolic velocity profile is shown. This normal E- and A-wave profile could result from normal or pseudonormal diastolic function. The transmitral color M-mode propagation velocity (V_P) shown is decreased (< 50 cm/sec), indicating diastolic dysfunction. Therefore, this patient's transmitral inflow velocities are pseudonormal.

Reference: Groban L, Dolinski SY. Transesophageal echocardiographic evaluation of diastolic function. *Chest* 2005;128:3652–3663.

74. **Answer = A, Normal diastolic function is present.** A normal-appearing transmitral pulsed-wave Doppler diastolic velocity profile is shown. This normal-appearing E- and A-wave profile could result from normal or pseudonormal diastolic function. A normal lateral mitral annular tissue Doppler E_M peak velocity is also present and this confirms the diagnosis of normal diastolic function. If pseudonormal diastolic function were present the lateral mitral annular tissue Doppler E_M peak velocity would be decreased (< 8 cm/sec).

Reference: Groban L, Dolinski SY. Transesophageal echocardiographic evaluation of diastolic function. *Chest* 2005;128:3652–3663.

75. **Answer = E, The arrow labeled 1 indicates the transmitral pulsed-wave Doppler A wave.**

Reference: Groban L, Dolinski SY. Transesophageal echocardiographic evaluation of diastolic function. *Chest* 2005;128:3652–3663.

76. **Answer = A, The arrow indicates the lateral mitral annular tissue Doppler A_M wave.**

Reference: Groban L, Dolinski SY. Transesophageal echocardiographic evaluation of diastolic function. *Chest* 2005;128:3652–3663.

77. **Answer = B, Arrow 1 indicates pulmonary vein S_1 wave.**

Reference: Groban L, Dolinski SY. Transesophageal echocardiographic evaluation of diastolic function. *Chest* 2005;128:3652–3663.

78. **Answer = C, Arrow 2 indicates the pulmonary vein S_2 wave.**

Reference: Groban L, Dolinski SY. Transesophageal echocardiographic evaluation of diastolic function. *Chest* 2005;128:3652–3663.

79. **Answer = D, Arrow 3 indicates the pulmonary vein diastolic flow wave (D wave).**

Reference: Groban L, Dolinski SY. Transesophageal echocardiographic evaluation of diastolic function. *Chest* 2005;128:3652–3663.

80. **Answer = A, Arrow 2 indicates the pulmonary vein S_2 wave.** This wave is influenced by right ventricular stroke volume. The S_1 wave is influenced by left atrial relaxation. Both waves are subject to systolic suppression or reversal with mitral regurgitation.

Reference: Groban L, Dolinski SY. Transesophageal echocardiographic evaluation of diastolic function. *Chest* 2005;128:3652–3663.

81. **Answer = B, 0.7 cm would be considered a moderate pericardial effusion** (see Table 4.2M).

Table 4.2M.   PERICARDIAL EFFUSION SEVERITY BY SIZE

Mild	Moderate	Severe
< 0.5 cm	0.5 to 2.0 cm	> 2.0 cm

Reference: Otto C. *Textbook of Clinical Echocardiography, Third Edition.* Philadelphia: Elsevier 2004:262.

82. **Answer = B, Right atrial inversion for greater than 1/3 of systole has 94% sensitivity and 100% specificity for pericardial tamponade physiology.** During ventricular systole the ventricular pressure is high, preventing ventricular collapse and favoring collapse of the low-pressure right atria. During diastole the ventricular pressure falls and right ventricular diastolic collapse occurs.

Reference: Otto C. *Textbook of Clinical Echocardiography, Third Edition.* Philadelphia: Elsevier 2004:264.

83. **Answer = A, Right atrial systolic (*not* diastolic) collapse is seen in pericardial tamponade.** The other findings: right ventricular diastolic collapse, reciprocal changes in right ventricular and left ventricular volumes, reciprocal respiratory changes in right ventricular and left ventricular filling, and inferior vena cava plethora are classic findings. During ventricular systole the ventricular pressure is high, preventing ventricular collapse and favoring collapse of the low-pressure right atria. During diastole the ventricular pressure falls and right ventricular diastolic collapse occurs. Reciprocal changes can be explained as follows: fluid is not compressible and with pericardial tamponade the total pericardial volume (heart chambers plus pericardial fluid) is fixed. If right ventricular volume is high, left ventricular volume will be low (and vice versa). During spontaneous inspiration intrathoracic pressure decreases and the thin-walled right ventricle dilates, increasing venous return. This increases right

ventricular filling and transmitral flow velocities. As the right ventricle fills, right ventricular pressure exceeds left ventricular pressure and the interventricular septum shifts to the left (compressing the left ventricle). This LV compression decreases transmitral inflow and decreases left ventricular stroke volume (TVI_{LVOT}). This is the mechanism that explains why systemic pressure, transmitral inflow, and LV stroke volume all decrease with spontaneous inspiration. The opposite occurs with spontaneous expiration. With positive pressure ventilation, the opposite respiratory pattern exists because intrathoracic pressure increases with inspiration and decreases with expiration. Inferior vena cava plethora simply refers to the dilated inferior vena cava (> 20 mm) with less than 50% inspiratory reduction in diameter seen secondarily to elevated right atrial pressures in patients with pericardial tamponade.

Reference: Otto C. *Textbook of Clinical Echocardiography, Third Edition.* Philadelphia: Elsevier 2004:262.

84. **Answer = E, All impact the hemodynamic severity of a pericardial effusion.** The size of a pericardial effusion is important, but even a small pericardial effusion that develops rapidly can be problematic. Large slowly accumulating effusions sometimes are not as detrimental as small rapidly developing effusions. The location of the effusion also impacts the patient's hemodynamic response. For example, an anterior loculated effusion can increase compression of the thin-walled right heart.

Reference: Otto C. *Textbook of Clinical Echocardiography, Third Edition.* Philadelphia: Elsevier 2004:262.

85. **Answer = A, Isovolumic (isovolumetric) relaxation time (IVRT) would be expected to increase with spontaneous inspiration in a patient with constrictive pericarditis.** The IVRT increases as left ventricular filling decreases. With spontaneous inspiration the negative intrathoracic pressure dilates the thin-walled right ventricle and favors RV filling at the expense of LV filling and LV stroke volume (a reciprocal respiratory filling pattern).

Reference: Otto C. *Textbook of Clinical Echocardiography, Third Edition.* Philadelphia: Elsevier 2004:270–272.

86. **Answer = C, The ratio of neck diameter to aneurysm diameter < 0.5 is seen in a pseudoaneurysm but not a true aneurysm.** Other findings seen in a pseudoaneurysm include the following: abrupt transition from normal myocardium to pseudoaneurysm, and acute angle between the normal myocardium and the pseudoaneurysm. Thrombus and regional wall motion abnormalities are common in both true aneurysms and pseudoaneurysms.

Reference: Otto C. *Textbook of Clinical Echocardiography, Third Edition.* Philadelphia: Elsevier 2004:276.

87. **Answer = B, Myxoma, the most common primary cardiac tumor, accounts for 20 to 30% of intracardiac tumors and is most frequently located in the left atrium attached to the interatrial septum.** This benign tumor can cause mechanical obstruction of left ventricular filling, embolic events, arrhythmias, and left ventricular outflow tract obstruction. It is recommended that these masses be removed if possible to prevent the complications listed.

Reference: Oh JK, Seward JB, Tajik AJ (eds). *The Echo Manual, Second Edition.* Philadelphia: Lippincott Williams & Wilkins 1999:205.

88. **Answer = D, Myxoma, the most common primary cardiac tumor, accounts for 20 to 30% of intracardiac tumors and is most frequently located in the left atrium attached to the interatrial septum.** This **benign tumor** can cause mechanical obstruction of left ventricular filling, embolic events, arrhythmias, and left ventricular outflow tract obstruction. It is recommended that these masses be removed if possible to prevent the complications listed.

Reference: Oh JK, Seward JB, Tajik AJ (eds). *The Echo Manual, Second Edition.* Philadelphia: Lippincott Williams & Wilkins 1999:205.

89. **Answer = A, Angiosarcoma is the most common primary malignant cardiac tumor.**

Reference: Oh JK, Seward JB, Tajik AJ (eds). *The Echo Manual, Second Edition.* Philadelphia: Lippincott Williams & Wilkins 1999:205.

90. **Answer = E, All are possible complications of intraoperative TEE.**

Reference: Savage RM, Aronson S, Thomas JD, Shanewise JS, Shernan SK. *Comprehensive Textbook of Intraoperative Transesophageal Echocardiography.* Philadelphia: Lippincott Williams & Wilkins 2004:106.

91. **Answer = B, 50 microamperes is the maximum leakage current recommended for an electrically safe TEE probe.**

Reference: Savage RM, Aronson S, Thomas JD, Shanewise JS, Shernan SK. *Comprehensive Textbook of Intraoperative Transesophageal Echocardiography.* Philadelphia: Lippincott Williams & Wilkins 2004:106.

92. **Answer = A, Esophageal strictures, webs, or rings are absolute contraindications to TEE.** Other absolute contraindications to TEE include the following: patient refusal, esophageal perforation, obstructing esophageal neoplasms, and cervical spin instability.

Reference: Savage RM, Aronson S, Thomas JD, Shanewise JS, Shernan SK. *Comprehensive Textbook of Intraoperative Transesophageal Echocardiography.* Philadelphia: Lippincott Williams & Wilkins 2004:108.

93. **Answer = D, All of the above.** Comet tail artifact is present. This type of reverberation artifact is also known as ring-down artifact and it occurs when two or more closely spaced strong reflectors reside in a medium with very high propagation speed. The ultrasound beam sound ricochets

back and forth between the two strong reflectors before returning to the transducer.

References: Savage RM, Aronson S, Thomas JD, Shanewise JS, Shernan SK. *Comprehensive Textbook of Intraoperative Transesophageal Echocardiography.* Philadelphia: Lippincott Williams & Wilkins 2004:40; Edelman SK. *Understanding Ultrasound Physics.* Woodlands, TX: ESP, Inc. 1994:56.

94. Answer = B, Segment 8, the mid anterior wall segment, is indicated by arrow 2.

Reference: SCA/ASE Annual Comprehensive Review and Update of Perioperative Hemodynamics Workshop. 17 Feb. 2005, San Diego, CA; discussion lead by Stanton Shernon, et al.

95. Answer = B, The anterior wall is supplied by the left anterior descending coronary artery.

Reference: SCA/ASE Annual Comprehensive Review and Update of Perioperative Hemodynamics Workshop. 17 Feb. 2005, San Diego, CA; discussion lead by Stanton Shernon, et al.

96. Answer = E, Segment 11, the mid inferior wall segment, is indicated by arrow 3.

Reference: SCA/ASE Annual Comprehensive Review and Update of Perioperative Hemodynamics Workshop. 17 Feb. 2005, San Diego, CA; discussion lead by Stanton Shernon, et al.

97. Answer = A, The right coronary artery supplies the mid inferior wall.

Reference: SCA/ASE Annual Comprehensive Review and Update of Perioperative Hemodynamics Workshop. 17 Feb. 2005, San Diego, CA; discussion lead by Stanton Shernon, et al.

98. Answer = D, Enhancement artifact is responsible for the bright appearance of the anterior wall. This results because the blood present in the left ventricle has lower acoustic impedance than the surrounding soft tissue. Enhancement occurs when ultrasound travels through a medium with a lower rate of attenuation than the surrounding soft tissue. Distal to the weakly attenuating medium, objects appear brighter than normal because the ultrasound beam is stronger than expected and the resulting echoes are more intense. Echoes below the weakly attenuating medium are enhanced.

Reference: Savage RM, Aronson S, Thomas JD, Shanewise JS, Shernan SK. *Comprehensive Textbook of Intraoperative Transesophageal Echocardiography.* Philadelphia: Lippincott Williams & Wilkins 2004:40.

99. Answer = B, Lambls' excrescences are mobile connective tissue densities that protrude out linearly from the coaptation point of the aortic valve.

Reference: Savage RM, Aronson S, Thomas JD, Shanewise JS, Shernan SK. *Comprehensive Textbook of Intraoperative Transesophageal Echocardiography.* Philadelphia: Lippincott Williams & Wilkins 2004:45.

100. **Answer = C, Nodules of Arantius are best described as normal leaflet thickenings seen at the central portion of the aortic valve leaflets.**

Reference: Savage RM, Aronson S, Thomas JD, Shanewise JS, Shernan SK. *Comprehensive Textbook of Intraoperative Transesophageal Echocardiography.* Philadelphia: Lippincott Williams & Wilkins 2004:45.

101. **Answer = E, Papillary fibroelastomas are associated with thromboembolic events.** Embolic events are a complication frequently associated with papillary fibroelastomas, and removal is recommended even in asymptomatic patients. Papillary fibroelastomas usually originate from the cardiac valves or adjacent endocardium. These benign tumors tend to originate on the atrial side of the atrioventricular valves and the ventricular surface of the semilunar valves. The aortic valve is most frequently affected and the appearance is similar to that of Lambls' excrescences, but Lambls' excrescences are thinner and broader based.

Reference: Savage RM, Aronson S, Thomas JD, Shanewise JS, Shernan SK. *Comprehensive Textbook of Intraoperative Transesophageal Echocardiography.* Philadelphia: Lippincott Williams & Wilkins 2004:45.

102. **Answer = A, As sound propagates through a physical medium the medium vibrates, resulting in compression and rarefaction of particles in the medium.**

Reference: Savage RM, Aronson S, Thomas JD, Shanewise JS, Shernan SK. *Comprehensive Textbook of Intraoperative Transesophageal Echocardiography.* Philadelphia: Lippincott Williams & Wilkins 2004:49.

103. **Answer = D, Ultrasound (> 20 KHz) is sound that is greater than the audible range.**

Reference: Savage RM, Aronson S, Thomas JD, Shanewise JS, Shernan SK. *Comprehensive Textbook of Intraoperative Transesophageal Echocardiography.* Philadelphia: Lippincott Williams & Wilkins 2004:51.

104. **Answer = A, Decreasing the emitted frequency of the transducer will decrease aliasing artifact.** Decreasing the imaging depth will also decrease aliasing by decreasing the time required to listen for returning echoes and thereby increasing the pulse repetition frequency and the Nyquist limit (NL = 1/2 PRF).

Reference: Edelman SK. *Understanding Ultrasound Physics.* Woodlands, TX: ESP, Inc. 1994:131–137.

105. **Answer = E, Both two-dimensional imaging and pulsed-wave Doppler analysis will be improved when the depth is decreased.** Imaging is best with an incident angle of 90 degrees, whereas Doppler is best with an incident angle of 0 degrees. Imaging is best with high-frequency transducers because spatial resolution is improved. Doppler is best with low-frequency transducers, which decrease aliasing artifact.

Reference: Edelman SK. *Understanding Ultrasound Physics.* Woodlands, TX: ESP, Inc. 1994:131–137.

106. **Answer = C, 3,000 Hz is the Nyquist limit (NL, the highest Doppler shift that can be measured).** The calculation is as follows.

NL = 1/2 PRF

NL = 1/2 (6,000 Hz)

NL = 3,000 Hz

- PRF = pulse repetition frequency

Reference: Edelman SK. *Understanding Ultrasound Physics.* Woodlands, TX: ESP, Inc. 1994:131–137.

107. **Answer = A, The pulmonary artery systolic pressure can be estimated from the tricuspid valve regurgitant jet seen in the midesophageal right ventricular inflow/outflow view.**

Reference: Konstadt SN, Shernon S, Oka Y (eds). *Clinical Transesophageal Echocardiography: A Problem-Oriented Approach, Second Edition.* Philadelphia: Lippincott Williams & Wilkins 2003:427.

108. **Answer = C, 107.2 ml/sec is the mitral valve regurgitant flow rate.** The calculation is as follows.

$Q_{ROA} = Q_{PISA}$

$A_{ROA} * V_{MRpeak} = A_{PISA} * V_{alias} = (2\pi r^2 * \alpha/180) * V_{alias}$

$Q_{ROA} = 2 (3.14) (0.8\ cm)^2 * 160/180 * (30\ cm/sec)$

$Q_{ROA} = 107.2\ ml/sec$

- Q_{ROA} = mitral valve regurgitant flow rate
- Q_{PISA} = proximal isovelocity surface area flow
- A_{ROA} = regurgitant orifice area
- V_{MRpeak} = mitral valve peak regurgitant velocity
- A_{PISA} = PISA area
- PISA = proximal isovelocity surface area
- V_{alias} = aliasing velocity
- α = angle correction factor

Reference: SCA/ASE Annual Comprehensive Review and Update of Perioperative Hemodynamics Workshop. 17 Feb. 2005, San Diego, CA; discussion lead by Stanton Shernon, et al.

109. **Answer = B, 0.214 cm² is the mitral valve regurgitant orifice area.** The calculation is as follows.

$Q_{ROA} = Q_{PISA}$

$A_{ROA} * V_{MRpeak} = A_{PISA} * V_{alias} = (2\pi r^2 * \alpha/180) * V_{alias}$

$A_{ROA} = A_{PISA} * V_{alias} / V_{MRpeak}$

$A_{ROA} = (2\pi r^2 * \alpha/180) * V_{alias} / V_{MRpeak}$

$A_{ROA} = [2(3.14) * (0.8\ cm)^2 * 160/180 * 30\ cm/sec] / 500\ cm/sec$

$A_{ROA} = 0.214\ cm^2$

- Q_{ROA} = mitral valve regurgitant flow rate
- Q_{PISA} = proximal isovelocity surface area flow
- A_{ROA} = regurgitant orifice area
- V_{MRpeak} = mitral valve peak regurgitant velocity
- A_{PISA} = PISA area
- PISA = proximal isovelocity surface area
- V_{alias} = aliasing velocity
- α = angle correction factor

Reference: SCA/ASE Annual Comprehensive Review and Update of Perioperative Hemodynamics Workshop. 17 Feb. 2005, San Diego, CA; discussion lead by Stanton Shernon, et al.

110. **Answer = A, 38.6 ml is the mitral valve regurgitant volume. The calculation is as follows.**

Mitral valve Rvol = ROA $* TVI_{MRjet}$

Mitral valve Rvol = 0.214 cm^2 * 180 cm = 38.6 cm^3

$Q_{ROA} = Q_{PISA}$

$A_{ROA} * V_{MRpeak} = A_{PISA} * V_{alias} = (2\pi r^2 * \alpha/180) * V_{alias}$

$A_{ROA} = A_{PISA} * V_{alias} / V_{MRpeak}$

$A_{ROA} = (2\pi r^2 * \alpha/180) * V_{alias} / V_{MRpeak}$

$A_{ROA} = [2(3.14) * (0.8 \text{ cm})^2 * 160/180 * 30 \text{ cm/sec}] / 500 \text{ cm/sec}$

$A_{ROA} = 0.214$ cm^2

- Q_{ROA} = mitral valve regurgitant flow rate
- Q_{PISA} = proximal isovelocity surface area flow
- A_{ROA} = regurgitant orifice area
- V_{MRpeak} = mitral valve peak regurgitant velocity
- A_{PISA} = PISA area
- PISA = proximal isovelocity surface area
- V_{alias} = aliasing velocity
- α = angle correction factor
- R_{vol} = regurgitant volume
- TVI_{MRjet} = time velocity integral of the mitral regurgitant jet

References: SCA/ASE Annual Comprehensive Review and Update of Perioperative Hemodynamics Workshop. 17 Feb. 2005, San Diego, CA; discussion lead by Stanton Shernon, et al.

111. **Answer = C, Moderate mitral regurgitation is present, given the regurgitant orifice area of 0.214 cm^2 = 21.4 mm^2 (1 cm^2 = 100 mm^2).**

Severity of MR	Mild	Moderate	Severe
MV ROA	< 10 mm^2	10-25 mm^2	25-35 mm^2

References: Perrino AC, Reeves S. *A Practical Approach to TEE.* Philadelphia: Lippincott Williams & Wilkins 2003:137; SCA/ASE Annual Comprehensive Review and Update of Perioperative Hemodynamics Workshop. 17 Feb. 2005, San Diego, CA; discussion lead by Stanton Shernon, et al.

112. **Answer = B, AL/PL = 0.8. The C-sept distance is the distance from the coaptation point to the septum.** A C-sept distance of ≥ 3.0 cm indicates decreased risk for post-repair SAM with LVOT obstruction. A C-sept distance of < 2.5 indicates increased risk for SAM with LVOT obstruction. The ratio of the anterior mitral valve leaflet to the posterior mitral valve leaflet (AL/PL ratio) is also predictive of the post mitral repair SAM with LVOT obstruction. An AL/PL ratio < 1.0 indicates an increased risk; AL/PL > 3.0 indicates decreased risk.

   - AL/PL ratio = ratio of the anterior leaflet to the posterior leaflet
   - C-sept = distance from the coaptation point to the septum
   - LA = left atrial
   - LVOT = left ventricular outflow tract
   - LAP = left atrial pressure
   - SAM = systolic anterior motion of the anterior mitral valve leaflet

Reference: Perrino AC, Reeves S. *A Practical Approach to TEE.* Philadelphia: Lippincott Williams & Wilkins 2003:166.

113. **Answer = C, A left atrial diameter of 52 mm is severely dilated and consistent with dilated cardiomyopathy.** A dp/dt of 1,600 indicates normal systolic function, which would not be consistent with dilated cardiomyopathy. A mitral regurgitant color flow Doppler jet area of 1.2 cm^2 is consistent with trace regurgitation. With this disease at least moderate mitral regurgitation would be expected. A left ventricular end diastolic dimension of 50 mm is at the high end of normal. A right ventricular end diastolic diameter of 30 mm is normal.

Reference: Otto C. *Textbook of Clinical Echocardiography, Third Edition.* Philadelphia: Elsevier 2004:228.

114. **Answer = B, A dagger-shaped continuous-wave Doppler left ventricular outflow pattern with the peak velocity occurring in late systole is indicative of hypertrophic obstructive cardiomyopathy.**

Reference: Otto C. *Textbook of Clinical Echocardiography, Third Edition.* Philadelphia: Elsevier 2004:230–232.

115. **Answer = B, Dynamic LVOT obstruction can occur in hypertrophic cardiomyopathy.** It is divided into four types based on the location of the LV hypertrophy. It is caused by a defect in the beta-myosin heavy chain gene. Hypertrophic cardiomyopathy is inherited and the genetics are best described as autosomal dominant with variable penetrance.

Reference: Otto C. *Textbook of Clinical Echocardiography, Third Edition.* Philadelphia: Elsevier 2004:230–232.

116. **Answer = E, Dynamically occlusive septal hypertrophy is *not* a synonym of hypertrophic cardiomyopathy.** The other choices are all synonyms and can be expected to show up on the test.

Reference: Otto C. *Textbook of Clinical Echocardiography, Third Edition.* Philadelphia: Elsevier 2004:230–232.

117. **Answer = A, The hemodynamic parameters for patient A are the least likely to result in dynamic left ventricular outflow tract obstruction in a patient with hypertrophic cardiomyopathy.** Hemodynamic goals toward decreasing this dynamic obstruction are listed in Table 4.2N. Essentially anything that keeps the heart full will help prevent SAM and decrease LVOT obstruction.

Table 4.2N.

HD parameter:	Preload	Afterload	Contractility	Heart rate
	Increase	Increase	Decrease	Decrease

Reference: Otto C. *Textbook of Clinical Echocardiography, Third Edition.* Philadelphia: Elsevier 2004:230–232.

118. **Answer = C, A lateral mitral annular tissue Doppler E_M < 8 cm/sec would be expected in chronic hypertension.** Impaired relaxation would be expected in this patient, and this form of diastolic dysfunction is characterized by the following findings.

   • Low transmitral peak E-wave velocity
   • Transmitral E/A < 1
   • Color M-mode propagation velocity (VP) < 50 cm/sec
   • Prolonged transmitral E-wave deceleration time (DT)

Reference: Otto C. *Textbook of Clinical Echocardiography, Third Edition.* Philadelphia: Elsevier 2004:245.

119. **Answer = B, Left atrial dilation (left atrial diameter = 52 mm) is consistent with chronic hypertension.** Left ventricular dilation is uncommon and is a sign of heart failure. Other findings seen in chronic hypertension include the following: concentric left ventricular hypertrophy, mitral annular calcification, aortic valve sclerosis, aortic root dilation, left atrial enlargement, and impaired relaxation. Atrial fibrillation may also occur if left atrial pressure is severely elevated.

Reference: Otto C. *Textbook of Clinical Echocardiography, Third Edition.* Philadelphia: Elsevier 2004:245.

120. **Answer = C, Decreasing left ventricular free wall thickness will increase left ventricular wall stress. The other choices will decrease wall stress.** The left ventricle hypertrophies to compensate for increases in wall tension, which result from increased left ventricular end diastolic pressure and left ventricular dilation. Diseases such as aortic stenosis and chronic hypertension are known to increase wall tension and the heart compensates with left ventricular hypertrophy. Wall stress is determined by the law of LaPlace, as follows. Wall stress = P * R / 2T.

   (P = left ventricular end diastolic pressure, R = left ventricular internal radius, T = free wall thickness)

Reference: Otto C. *Textbook of Clinical Echocardiography, Third Edition.* Philadelphia: Elsevier 2004:133.

121. **Answer = C, LVEDP = 11.** The calculation is as follows.

$$\Delta P = 4V^2$$

$$(DBP - LVEDP) = 4(V_{Allate})^2$$

$$LVEDP = DBP - 4\,(3.5)^2$$

$$LVEDP = 60 - 49$$

$$LVEDP = 11\ mmHg$$

- V_{Allate} = late peak aortic regurgitant velocity
- LVEDP = left ventricular end diastolic pressure
- DBP = diastolic blood pressure

Reference: Sidebotham D, Merry A, Legget M (eds.). *Practical Perioperative Transoesophageal Echocardiography.* Burlington, MA: Butterworth Heinemann 2003:241.

122. **Answer = B, 286 mmHg (mm = the wall tension). The calculation is as follows.**

$$Wall\ tension = (P * R)$$

$$Wall\ tension = 11\ mmHg * 26\ mm$$

$$Wall\ tension = 286\ mmHg\ mm$$

$$\Delta P = 4V^2$$

$$(DBP - LVEDP) = 4(V_{Allate})^2$$

$$LVEDP = DBP - 4\,(3.5)^2$$

$$LVEDP = 60 - 49$$

$$LVEDP = 11\ mmHg$$

- V_{Allate} = late peak aortic regurgitant velocity
- P = LVEDP = left ventricular end diastolic pressure
- DBP = diastolic blood pressure
- R = left ventricular end diastolic radius

Reference: Otto C. *Textbook of Clinical Echocardiography, Third Edition.* Philadelphia: Elsevier 2004:133.

123. **Answer = C, 11.9 mmHg = left ventricular wall stress.** Wall stress is determined by the law of LaPlace, which in this case is calculated as follows (P = left ventricular end diastolic pressure, R = left ventricular internal radius, T = free wall thickness). Note that wall tension = P * R and is a component of wall stress.

$$Wall\ stress = wall\ tension\ /\ 2(wall\ thickness)$$

$$Wall\ stress = P * R\ /\ 2T$$

$$Wall\ stress = (11\ mmHg * 26\ mm)\ /\ 2(12\ mm)$$

$$Wall\ stress = 11.9\ mmHg$$

Reference: Otto C. *Textbook of Clinical Echocardiography, Third Edition.* Philadelphia: Elsevier 2004:133.

124. **Answer = A, The numerical value for lateral resolution is decreased as the number of pulses per scan line is increased.** The more pulses per scan line the lower the numerical value for the lateral resolution and the better the lateral resolution. This is how multifocus systems provide better lateral resolution. More pulses per scan line results in a narrower beam width and better lateral resolution. Line density is the number of scan lines per image (not the number of pulses per scan line). As the number of pulses per scan line increases temporal resolution and frame rate decrease.

Reference: Edelman SK. *Understanding Ultrasound Physics.* Woodlands, TX: ESP, Inc. 1994:122.

125. **Answer = E, All are associated with multiple pulses per scan line.** Multifocus systems require multiple pulses, with each pulse having a different focus. Phased-array transducers utilize multiple pulses per scan line to improve lateral resolution. The more pulses per scan line the worse the temporal resolution.

Reference: Edelman SK. *Understanding Ultrasound Physics.* Woodlands, TX: ESP, Inc. 1994:122.

126. **Answer = E, All are possible side effects of dobutamine infusion.** Interestingly, a paradoxical bradycardia occurs in about 8% of patients. This complication usually occurs in patients with coronary artery disease, but it can be related to a vasodepressor effect mediated by the Bezold-Jarisch reflex. It is effectively treated with atropine.

Reference: Oh JK, Seward JB, Tajik AJ (eds). *The Echo Manual, Second Edition.* Philadelphia: Lippincott Williams & Wilkins 1999:96.

127. **Answer = E, The circumflex coronary artery is supplying hibernating myocardium, as indicated by the wall motion seen in the posterior wall.** The posterior wall is akinetic at rest, and then improves in response to low-dose dobutamine (becoming mildly hypokinetic). The posterior wall then reverts to akinesis in response to high-dose dobutamine. This indicates hibernating myocardium, which is supplied by a nonfixed lesion in the circumflex coronary artery. Similarly, the inferior wall also has a DSE pattern indicative of hibernating myocardium. The anterior wall becomes hypokinetic in response to dobutamine, indicating an occult area of reversible ischemia. The anterior wall is not hibernating because it appears normal at rest.

Reference: Oh JK, Seward JB, Tajik AJ (eds). *The Echo Manual, Second Edition.* Philadelphia: Lippincott Williams & Wilkins 1999:96.

128. **Answer = E, The RCA, circumflex, and left anterior descending coronary artery all supply myocardium exhibiting reversible myocardial ischemia.**

Reference: Oh JK, Seward JB, Tajik AJ (eds). *The Echo Manual, Second Edition.* Philadelphia: Lippincott Williams & Wilkins 1999:96.

129. **Answer = B, Right ventricular volume overload causes movement/ displacement/flattening of the septum from the right to the left ventricle during <u>late diastole</u>.** This occurs when the right ventricular volume is highest, which is at end diastole. Note that with right ventricular pressure overload this movement occurs at late systole because this is when right ventricular pressure is highest.

Reference: Sidebotham D, Merry A, Legget M (eds.). *Practical Perioperative Transoesophageal Echocardiography.* Burlington, MA: Butterworth Heinemann 2003:206.

130. **Answer = E, The upper esophageal aortic arch short axis view allows parallel alignment of the ultrasound beam with pulmonic valve flow.** This parallel alignment is essential for determination of the pressure gradient with continuous-wave Doppler ultrasound. The transgastric right ventricular outflow view could also be utilized for determining the pressure gradient across the pulmonic valve.

References: Perrino AC, Reeves S. *A Practical Approach to TEE.* Philadelphia: Lippincott Williams & Wilkins 2003:227.

131. **Answer = C, A cor triatriatum is a congenital abnormal membrane found in the left atrium.** The other choices listed are located on the right side of the heart.

Reference: Sidebotham D, Merry A, Legget M (eds.). *Practical Perioperative Transoesophageal Echocardiography.* Burlington, MA: Butterworth Heinemann 2003:216.

132. **Answer = D, The moderator band is a large muscular band that runs from the septum to the free wall in the right ventricle.**

Reference: Sidebotham D, Merry A, Legget M (eds.). *Practical Perioperative Transoesophageal Echocardiography.* Burlington, MA: Butterworth Heinemann 2003:201.

133. **Answer = C, Increasing the Nyquist limit of the color flow Doppler map will decrease the apparent severity of mitral regurgitation by color flow Doppler examination.** All other changes listed will increase the apparent severity of mitral regurgitation.

References: Perrino AC, Reeves S. *A Practical Approach to TEE.* Philadelphia: Lippincott Williams & Wilkins 2003:138.

134. **Answer = B, In the midesophageal long axis view the A_2 and P_2 scallops are seen.**

Reference: Sidebotham D, Merry A, Legget M (eds.). *Practical Perioperative Transoesophageal Echocardiography.* Burlington, MA: Butterworth Heinemann 2003:137.

135. **Answer = B, Decreased LV compliance can result in an overestimation of MVA by the pressure half time (PHT) method because it causes a shortening of the pressure half time.** Severe aortic insufficiency (AI) will also cause a shortening of the pressure half time and an overestimation of the mitral valve area. Severe mitral

regurgitation (MR) results in elevated left atrial pressures, which cause a shortening of the pressure half time and an overestimation of the mitral valve area. Delayed relaxation of the left ventricle causes an increase in the pressure half time and an underestimation of the mitral valve area.

References: Perrino AC, Reeves S. *A Practical Approach to TEE.* Philadelphia: Lippincott Williams & Wilkins 2003:152.

136. Answer = D, MVA = 220/PHT = 220/110 = 2 cm².

- MVA = mitral valve area
- PHT = pressure half time

Reference: Otto C. *Textbook of Clinical Echocardiography, Third Edition.* Philadelphia: Elsevier 2004:299.

TEST V PART 1

Video Test Booklet

This product is designed to prepare people for the PTEeXAM. This booklet is to be used with the CD-ROM to practice for the video portion of the PTEeXAM.

Preface

As stated previously, this part of this product is designed to prepare people for the video component of the PTEeXAM. Please do not open this test booklet until you have read the instructions. During the PTEeXAM, instructions similar to these will be written on the back of the test booklet. You will be asked to read these instructions by a proctor at the exam. After you have read these instructions you will be asked to break the seal on the test booklet and to remove an answer sheet, similar to the one included with this practice test.

After you have filled out your name, test number, and other identifying information on the answer sheet you will be instructed to open the test booklet and begin. This test will involve video images shown on a computer monitor. You will share this monitor with three other examinees. This portion of the PTEeXAM has about 50 questions. It consists of about 17 cases, with 2 to 5 questions for each case. It is timed. Good luck!

Instructions

This test will consist of several cases, accompanied by 3 to 5 questions per case. Each case will show one or more images. For each case, you are to utilize the information written in this booklet and the information shown in the images to answer questions concerning each case. An audible chime or tone will assist in timing the exam. This tone alerts you when the test advances to the next step.

The order of the exam is as follows.

Tone/chime

1. Read the questions for case 1.

Tone/chime

2. View the images for case 1.

Tone/chime

3. Answer the questions for case 1.

Tone/chime

4. View the images for case 1 again.

Tone/chime

5. Check your answers to the questions for case 1.

Tone/chime

6. Read the questions for case 2.

Tone/chime

The process continues in this manner. In summary: tone, read, tone, view, tone, answer, tone, view, tone, check answers, tone.

Cases

Case 1

1. What is most likely true concerning the color flow Doppler images shown?

   A. A predominantly left-to-right shunt is indicated by the blue color flow.

   B. A predominantly right-to-left shunt is indicated by the blue color flow.

   C. A predominantly left-to-right shunt is indicated by the red color flow.

   D. A predominantly right-to-left shunt is indicated by the red color flow.

2. Q_p/Q_s is most closely approximated by which of the following?

   A. 1:1

   B. 2:1

   C. 3:1

   D. 4:1

Case 2

3. Which of the following statements concerning atrial septal defects is most likely true?

A. Ostium secundum lesions are associated with a cleft mitral valve.

B. Ostium primum lesions are the most common type.

C. Sinus venosus defects are associated with anomalous pulmonary venous return.

D. Ostium primum defects are located in the fossa ovalis.

E. Ostium secundum defects are associated with a persistent left superior vena cava.

Case 3

4. What structure is indicated by the arrow?

A. Eustachian valve

B. Central venous line

C. Christa terminalis

D. Right atrial myxoma

5. In image 2, which letter corresponds most closely to where a wire placed in a femoral vein would first enter the heart?

A. A

B. B

C. C

D. D

6. In image 2, which letter best corresponds to where agitated saline injected into a right-hand intravenous line would first enter the picture?

A. A

B. B

C. C

D. D

7. A patient with a persistent left superior vena cava and a coronary sinus atrial septal defect has a left-hand intravenous line. Where would echo contrast injected into this IV first enter the image?

A. A

B. B

C. C

D. D

Case 4

8. What structure is indicated by arrow 1 in image 2 for case 4?

A. Left coronary cusp

B. Right coronary cusp

C. Noncoronary cusp

D. Posterior coronary cusp

E. Anterior coronary cusp

9. What structure is indicated by arrow 2 in image 3 for case 4?

A. Left coronary cusp

B. Right coronary cusp

C. Noncoronary cusp

D. Posterior coronary cusp

E. Anterior coronary cusp

10. What structure is indicated by arrow 3 in image 4 for case 4?

A. Left coronary cusp

B. Right coronary cusp

C. Noncoronary cusp

D. Posterior coronary cusp

E. Anterior coronary cusp

Case 5

11. Which of the following best describes the degree of aortic insufficiency as determined by the ratio of the AI jet d to LVOT d?

A. Trace (0 to 1+).

B. Mild (1 to 2+).

C. Moderate (2 to 3+).

D. Severe (3 to 4+).

E. There is insufficient information given to answer this question.

(AI jet d = aortic insufficiency jet diameter, LVOT d = left ventricular outflow tract diameter)

12. Which of the following would be indicative of severe aortic regurgitation?

A. Diastolic flow reversal in the descending thoracic aorta

B. Ratio of the AI jet d to LOVT d of 45%

C. AI jet vena contracta of 5 mm

D. Slope of the AI jet by continuous-wave Doppler = 1.8 m/sec

E. Pressure half time = 500 msec by continuous-wave Doppler of the AI jet

(AI jet d = aortic insufficiency jet diameter, LVOT d = left ventricular outflow tract diameter, AI = aortic insufficiency)

Case 6

13. Which of the following best describes the degree of aortic insufficiency as determined by the pressure half time (PHT) method?

A. Trace (0 to 1+).

B. Mild (1 to 2+).

C. Moderate (2 to 3+).

D. Severe (3 to 4+).

E. There is insufficient information given to answer this question.

14. Which of the following best describes the degree of aortic insufficiency as determined by the slope of the AI regurgitant jet?

A. Trace (0 to 1+).

B. Mild (1 to 2+).

C. Moderate (2 to 3+).

D. Severe (3 to 4+).

E. There is insufficient information given to answer this question.

Case 7

15. Which of the following is indicated by arrow 1 in image 2 for case 7?

A. Sinotubular ridge

B. Annulus

C. Sinus of valsalva

D. Bulb of the aortic root

E. Origin of the circumflex coronary ostia

16. What structural measurement is indicated by arrow 2 in image 3 for case 7?

A. Sinotubular ridge diameter

B. Aortic valve annulus diameter

C. Sinus of valsalva diameter

D. Aortic valve diameter

E. Intercusp length

17. Which of the following is indicated by arrow 3 in image 4 for case 7?

A. Aortic valve annulus

B. Sinotubular ridge

C. Sinus of valsavla

D. Apex of the aortic root

E. Origin of the circumflex coronary ostia

Case 8

18. In patients with Marfan's syndrome, an Ao ratio of what value indicates a decreased risk of aortic dissection?

   A. < 2.0

   B. < 1.5

   C. < 1.3

   D. < 1.0

   E. < 0.8

19. Assume a patient of the following statistics: height = 165 cm (65 in), weight = 63 kg, body surface area (BSA) = 1.68m². Which of the following describes the degree of dilation of the sinus of valsalva in case 8?

   A. Normal.

   B. Slightly dilated.

   C. Moderately dilated.

   D. Severely dilated.

   E. It cannot be determined from the given information.

20. Assuming the patient in case 8 is a 54-year-old with Marfan's syndrome, a BSA of 2 m², and a predicted sinus dimension of 3.13 cm, what is the Ao ratio for this patient?

   A. 1.13

   B. 1.23

   C. 1.33

   D. 1.43

   E. 1.53

Case 9

21. What is indicated by the arrow in image 1 for case 9?

    A. Right atrium

    B. Left atrium

    C. Superior vena cava

    D. Inferior vena cava

    E. Coronary sinus

22. Arrow 1 in image 2 for case 9, indicates which of the following?

    A. Pulmonary artery catheter

    B. Coronary sinus catheter

    C. Cardiopulmonary bypass venous cannula

    D. Antegrade cardioplegia catheter

    E. Left atrial catheter

Case 10

23. What view is shown in case 10?

    A. Upper esophageal aortic arch short axis view

    B. Midesophageal ascending aortic short axis view

    C. Midesophageal aortic short axis view

    D. Midesophageal ascending aortic long axis view

    E. Upper esophageal aortic arch long axis view

24. Arrow 1 in images 3 and 4 for case 10 indicates which of the following?

    A. Left pulmonary artery

    B. Right pulmonary artery

    C. Inferior vena cava

    D. Superior vena cava

    E. Aorta

25. Arrow 2 in images 3 and 4 for case 10 indicates which of the following?

    A. Left pulmonary artery

    B. Right pulmonary artery

    C. Inferior vena cava

    D. Superior vena cava

    E. Aorta

26. Arrow 3 in images 3 and 4 for case 10 indicates which of the following?

    A. Left pulmonary artery

    B. Right pulmonary artery

    C. Inferior vena cava

    D. Superior vena cava

    E. Aorta

27. Arrow 1 in images 3 and 4 for case 10 indicates an area that is sometimes difficult to image. Why is this area sometimes difficult to image?

    A. It is obstructed by the trachea and the left main bronchus.

    B. It is obstructed by the trachea and the right main bronchus.

    C. It is located very high in the esophagus.

    D. It is obstructed by the right lung.

    E. It is obstructed by the brachiocephalic trunk.

Case 11

28. Which of the following is indicated by the arrow in image 1 for case 11?

    A. Right upper pulmonary vein

    B. Left upper pulmonary vein

    C. Right lower pulmonary vein

    D. Left lower pulmonary vein

    E. Left atrial appendage

29. Which of the following is indicated by the arrow in image 2 for case 11?

   A. Coumadin ridge

   B. Left atrial thrombus

   C. Left atrial myxoma

   D. Left atrial polyp

   E. Left atrial catheter

30. Which of the following correctly describes the segmental wall motion seen in image 2 for case 11?

   A. Anterior wall hypokinesis

   B. Posterior wall dyskinesis

   C. Lateral wall dyskinesis

   D. Inferior wall hypokinesis

   E. Anteroseptal dyskinesis

31. Systolic flow reversal in the area identified by the arrow in image 3 for case 11 indicates which of the following valvular abnormalities?

   A. Pulmonic stenosis

   B. Pulmonic regurgitation

   C. Tricuspid stenosis

   D. Tricuspid regurgitation

   E. Mitral regurgitation

Case 12

32. What is the diagnosis?

   A. Stanford type B dissection

   B. Reverberation artifact

   C. Stanford type A dissection

   D. Side lobe artifact

   E. Mirror image artifact

33. What is indicated by the arrow in image 3 for case 12?

   A. Dissection flap

   B. Retrograde cardioplegia coronary sinus catheter

   C. Left atrial catheter

   D. Pulmonary artery catheter

   E. Coronary sinus catheter

Case 13

34. Given a central venous pressure of 11 mmHg, what is the right ventricular systolic pressure (RVSP)?

   A. 101 mmHg

   B. 121 mmHg

   C. 141 mmHg

   D. 161 mmHg

   E. 171 mmHg

35. What is the pulmonary artery systolic pressure?

   A. 25 mmHg

   B. 62 mmHg

   C. 97 mmHg

   D. 101 mmHg

   E. 171 mmHg

36. What is the diagnosis?

   A. Tetralogy of fallot

   B. Epstein's anomaly

   C. Pulmonic stenosis

   D. Tricuspid stenosis

   E. Kartagener's syndrome

37. What view is shown in image 3 for case 13?

    A. Midesophageal right ventricular inflow/outflow view

    B. Midesophageal pulmonic outflow view

    C. Transgastric right ventricular outflow view

    D. Transgastric deep long axis view

    E. Transgastric long axis view

38. What is the pressure gradient across the valve interrogated in images 3 and 4 for case 13?

    A. 79 mmHg

    B. 89 mmHg

    C. 99 mmHg

    D. 109 mmHg

    E. 119 mmHg

Case 14

39. Which of the following best describes left ventricular wall thickness in the images shown for case 14 (LVH = left ventricular hypertrophy)?

    A. Normal.

    B. Mild concentric LVH.

    C. Moderate concentric LVH.

    D. Severe LVH.

    E. It cannot be determined from the images shown.

40. Arrow 1 indicates which of the following?

    A. Anterior wall

    B. Anteroseptal wall

    C. Lateral wall

    D. Septal wall

    E. Posterior wall

41. Arrow 2 indicates which of the following?

A. Anterior wall

B. Anteroseptal wall

C. Lateral wall

D. Septal wall

E. Posterior wall

42. Arrow 3 indicates which of the following?

A. Anterior wall

B. Anteroseptal wall

C. Inferior wall

D. Septal wall

E. Posterior wall

43. Arrow 4 indicates which of the following?

A. Anterior wall

B. Anteroseptal wall

C. Lateral wall

D. Septal wall

E. Posterior wall

Case 15

44. Which of the following best describes the degree of tricuspid regurgitation seen in case 15?

A. Trace.

B. Mild.

C. Moderate.

D. Severe.

E. It cannot be determined from the data given.

45. Which of the following findings would be expected in this patient?

   A. Reversal of the pulsed-wave Doppler hepatic vein S wave

   B. Reversal of the pulsed-wave Doppler pulmonary vein S wave

   C. Reversal of the transtricuspid pulsed-wave Doppler E wave

   D. Reversal of the transtricuspid pulsed-wave Doppler A wave

   E. Reversal of the pulsed-wave Doppler hepatic vein D wave

46. Which of the following patients is at increased risk for developing tricuspid regurgitation postoperatively?

   A. Heart transplant

   B. Aortic valve replacement for a bicuspid aortic valve

   C. Mitral valve replacement for endocarditis

   D. Aortic valve replacement for aortic stenosis

   E. CABG patient with decreased systolic function

Case 16

47. Which of the following best describes the degree of tricuspid regurgitation shown?

   A. Trace.

   B. Mild.

   C. Moderate.

   D. Severe.

   E. It cannot be determined from the images shown.

48. A continuous-wave Doppler interrogation of the lesion shown can be used to estimate which of the following?

   A. Right ventricular end diastolic pressure

   B. Pulmonary artery systolic pressure

   C. Pulmonary artery diastolic pressure

   D. Pulmonary artery mean pressure

   E. Pulmonary vascular resistance

49. What is measured in image 3 for case 16?

A. Right coronary artery

B. Left coronary artery

C. Left main coronary artery

D. Coronary sinus

E. Left pulmonary artery

50. The measurement shown could be consistent with which of the following?

A. Persistent left superior vena cava

B. Sinus venosus atrial septal defect

C. Ostium primum atrial septal defect

D. Ostium secundum atrial septal defect

E. None of the above (measurement is within normal limits)

Case 17

51. What is the diagnosis (ASD = atrial septal defect, VSD = ventricular septal defect, AV = atrioventricular)?

A. Ostium secundum ASD and inlet VSD

B. Sinus venosus atrial ASD and muscular VSD

C. Tetralogy of fallot with an ostium primum ASD

D. Complete AV canal defect

E. Tetralogy of fallot with an ostium secundum ASD

52. If mitral regurgitation is present it is most likely due to which of the following?

A. Cleft posterior mitral valve leaflet

B. Cleft anterior mitral valve leaflet

C. Mitral valve prolapse

D. Myxomatous mitral valve disease

E. Restricted mitral valve leaflet motion

53. What type of atrial septal defect is seen?

    A. Ostium primum

    B. Ostium secundum

    C. Sinus venosus

    D. Coronary sinus

    E. Perimembranous

54. What type of ventricular septal defect is shown?

    A. Perimembranous

    B. Aortic outflow

    C. Subarterial

    D. Trabecular (muscular)

    E. Inlet

55. This defect is associated with which of the following?

    A. Kartagener's syndrome

    B. Trisomy 21

    C. Epstein's anomaly

    D. Eulenberg syndrome

    E. Turner's syndrome

Case 18

56. Which of the following is indicated by the arrow in image 1 for case 18?

    A. Posteromedial commissure

    B. Posterolateral commissure

    C. Anteromedial commissure

    D. Anterolateral commissure

    E. Inferior commissure

57. According to the American Society of Echocardiography 16-segment model, what numerical segment of the left ventricle is described by arrow 1 in image 2?

   A. 1

   B. 2

   C. 3

   D. 4

   E. 5

58. According to the American Society of Echocardiography 16-segment model, what numerical segment of the left ventricle is described by arrow 2 in image 2?

   A. 3

   B. 4

   C. 5

   D. 6

   E. 7

59. According to the American Society of Echocardiography 16-segment model, what numerical segment of the left ventricle is described by arrow 3 in image 2?

   A. 1

   B. 2

   C. 3

   D. 4

   E. 5

60. According to the American Society of Echocardiography 16-segment model, what numerical segment of the left ventricle is described by arrow 4 in image 2?

   A. 1

   B. 2

   C. 3

   D. 4

   E. 5

61. According to the American Society of Echocardiography 16-segment model, what numerical segment of the left ventricle is described by arrow 5 in image 2?

   A. 1

   B. 2

   C. 3

   D. 4

   E. 5

62. According to the American Society of Echocardiography 16-segment model, what numerical segment of the left ventricle is described by arrow 6 in image 2?

   A. 1

   B. 2

   C. 3

   D. 4

   E. 5

Case 19

63. Arrow 1 indicates which of the following?

    A. Moderator band

    B. Left ventricular band

    C. Chiari network

    D. Eustachian valve

    E. Ventricular septation

64. Arrow 2 indicates which of the following?

    A. Posteromedial papillary muscle

    B. Anterolateral papillary muscle

    C. Posterolateral papillary muscle

    D. Anteromedial papillary muscle

    E. None of the above

65. Arrow 3 indicates which of the following?

    A. Right atrium

    B. Left atrium

    C. Right ventricle

    D. Left ventricle

    E. Pulmonary artery

Case 20

66. Arrow 1 indicates which of the following?

    A. Right upper pulmonary vein

    B. Right lower pulmonary vein

    C. Left upper pulmonary vein

    D. Left lower pulmonary vein

    E. Coronary sinus

67. Arrow 2 indicates which of the following?

   A. Right upper pulmonary vein

   B. Right lower pulmonary vein

   C. Left upper pulmonary vein

   D. Left lower pulmonary vein

   E. Coronary sinus

Case 21

68. Arrow 2 indicates which of the following?

   A. Christa terminalis

   B. Moderator band

   C. Eustachian valve

   D. Chairi network

   E. Cor triatriatum

69. Arrow 1 indicates which of the following?

   A. Right upper pulmonary vein

   B. Right lower pulmonary vein

   C. Left upper pulmonary vein

   D. Left lower pulmonary vein

   E. Coronary sinus

70. Arrow 3 indicates which of the following?

   A. Right upper pulmonary vein

   B. Right lower pulmonary vein

   C. Left upper pulmonary vein

   D. Left lower pulmonary vein

   E. Coronary sinus

Answers:

1. A	25. D	49. D
2. C	26. E	50. A
3. C	27. A	51. D
4. A	28. B	52. B
5. C	29. A	53. A
6. B	30. C	54. E
7. A	31. D	55. B
8. B	32. D	56. A
9. A	33. D	57. E
10. C	34. E	58. D
11. B	35. B	59. A
12. A	36. C	60. B
13. C	37. C	61. C
14. D	38. D	62. D
15. C	39. D	63. B
16. B	40. D	64. B
17. B	41. B	65. B
18. C	42. A	66. A
19. D	43. C	67. B
20. D	44. D	68. D
21. B	45. A	69. A
22. A	46. A	70. A
23. B	47. D	
24. A	48. B	

Explanations

Case 1

1. **Answer = A, The image shows an ostium secundum ASD with a prominent left-to-right shunt (as indicated by the blue color flow Doppler).** This is the most common type of ASD, accounting for greater than 70% of all atrial septal defects.

References: Perrino AC, Reeves S. *A Practical Approach to TEE.* Philadelphia: Lippincott Williams & Wilkins 2003:287; Otto C. *Textbook of Clinical Echocardiography, Third Edition.* Philadelphia: Elsevier 2004:466.

2. **Answer = C, Q_p/Q_s = 9.74/3.12 = 3:1.** Q_p/Q_s = pulmonary flow / systemic flow. The images shown illustrate that pulmonic flow is greater than systemic flow. This is what would be expected for the left-to-right shunt indicated by the color flow Doppler images. Flow through the LVOT and the pulmonary artery was calculated using the TEE machine's software package. For the LVOT: $CO = HR * SV = HR * (A_{lvot} * TVI_{lvot})$. For the PA: $CO = HR * SV = HR * (A_{PA} * TVI_{PA})$. The CO is given in the images, and thus these calculations are not necessary in solving this problem (however, this knowledge is essential for passing the PTEeXAM).

Reference: Perrino AC, Reeves S. *A Practical Approach to TEE.* Philadelphia: Lippincott Williams & Wilkins 2003:94–106.

Case 2

3. **Answer = C, Sinus venosus defects are associated with anomalous pulmonary venous return.** Mnemonic: Sinus venosus defects → anomalous pulmonary venous return. Ostium primum ASDs are associated with a cleft mitral valve. Ostium primum ASDs + inlet VSD = endocardial cushion defect = AV canal defect. Secundum ASDs are the most common type of ASD, comprising greater than 70% of all ASDs. Coronary sinus ASDs are very rare, and they are associated with a persistent left superior vena cava.

Reference: Perrino AC, Reeves S. *A Practical Approach to TEE.* Philadelphia: Lippincott Williams & Wilkins 2003:287.

Case 3

4. **Answer = A, A eustachian valve is shown.** This is a benign embryologic remnant. Its purpose in the fetus is to divert well-oxygenated blood across the foramen ovale into the left atrium so that this blood can travel to vital areas such as the brain and the coronary circulation.

Reference: Savage RM, Aronson S, Thomas JD, Shanewise JS, Shernan SK. *Comprehensive Textbook of Intraoperative Transesophageal Echocardiography.* Philadelphia: Lippincott Williams & Wilkins 2004:43.

5. **Answer = C, A wire placed in the femoral vein will travel up the inferior vena cava (IVC) and enter the right atrium at the point indicated by letter C.** The structures indicated are as follows: A = LA, B = SVC, C = IVC, D = RA.

   - LA = left atrium
   - SVC = superior vena cava
   - IVC = inferior vena cava
   - RA = right atrium

Reference: Otto C. *Textbook of Clinical Echocardiography, Third Edition.* Philadelphia: Elsevier 2004:80.

6. **Answer = B, A bubble injected into a right-hand IV will first enter the heart through the superior vena cava (SVC), indicated by the letter B in image 2.** The structures indicated are as follows: A = LA, B = SVC, C = IVC, D = RA.

   - LA = left atrium
   - SVC = superior vena cava
   - IVC = inferior vena cava
   - RA = right atrium

Reference: Perrino AC, Reeves S. *A Practical Approach to TEE.* Philadelphia: Lippincott Williams & Wilkins 2003:30.

7. **Answer = A, A persistent left superior vena cava will drain into the coronary sinus.** If a coronary sinus defect is present and echo contrast is injected into the left-hand IV, the left atrium will fill with contrast before the right atrium. This is one method of testing for this anomaly when a patient has a dilated coronary sinus. A coronary sinus greater than 10 mm is suspicious. It is important to evaluate the size of the coronary sinus prior to cardiopulmonary bypass if retrograde cardioplegia is to be utilized, because in the presence of a persistent left SVC retrograde cardioplegia will not be effective.

References: Perrino AC, Reeves S. *A Practical Approach to TEE.* Philadelphia: Lippincott Williams & Wilkins 2003:287; Otto C. *Textbook of Clinical Echocardiography, Third Edition.* Philadelphia: Elsevier 2004:80.

Case 4

8. **Answer = B, The right coronary cusp is indicated by arrow 1.**
   The midesophageal aortic valve short axis view is shown.

Reference: Savage RM, Aronson S, Thomas JD, Shanewise JS, Shernan SK. *Comprehensive Textbook of Intraoperative Transesophageal Echocardiography.* Philadelphia: Lippincott Williams & Wilkins 2004:224.

9. **Answer = A, The left coronary cusp is indicated by arrow 2.**
   The midesophageal aortic valve short axis view is shown.

Reference: Savage RM, Aronson S, Thomas JD, Shanewise JS, Shernan SK. *Comprehensive Textbook of Intraoperative Transesophageal Echocardiography.* Philadelphia: Lippincott Williams & Wilkins 2004:224.

10. **Answer = C, the noncoronary cusp is indicated by arrow 3.** The midesophageal aortic valve short axis view is shown.

Reference: S Savage RM, Aronson S, Thomas JD, Shanewise JS, Shernan SK. *Comprehensive Textbook of Intraoperative Transesophageal Echocardiography.* Philadelphia: Lippincott Williams & Wilkins 2004:224.

Case 5

11. **Answer = B, Mild aortic insufficiency is present according to the ratio of the AI jet d to LVOT d = 0.35 to 0.44, which is consistent with mild aortic insufficiency.** Note that this is at the very high end of mild according to this method, and therefore may be more accurately described as mild to moderate (2+). However, when given the choice between mild or moderate mild is the best answer.

AI jet d = Aortic insufficiency jet diameter.

LVOT d = left ventricular outflow tract diameter.

Degree of AI:	Trace (0-1+)	Mild (1-2+)	Moderate (2-3+)	Severe (3-4+)
AIJetd/LVoTd	1–24%	25–46%	47–64%	> 65%

Reference: Perrino AC, Reeves S. *A Practical Approach to TEE.* Philadelphia: Lippincott Williams & Wilkins 2003:180.

12. **Answer = A, Diastolic flow reversal in the descending thoracic aorta is indicative of severe AI.** The other parameters listed are less than severe AI.

Reference: Perrino AC, Reeves S. *A Practical Approach to TEE.* Philadelphia: Lippincott Williams & Wilkins 2003:180.

Case 6

13. **Answer = C, A pressure half time (PHT) of 339 msec is consistent with moderate aortic insufficiency (AI).** The pressure half time is the time it takes for the pressure gradient between two chambers/vessels to decrease from the maximum to half the maximum. The smaller the PHT the less time it takes for the pressure to equilibrate between two chambers, and therefore the larger the hole between the two chambers. A big hole leads to fast equilibration of pressures and a shorter PHT. A small hole leads to slower equilibration of pressures and a longer PHT.

Big hole→fast equilibration of pressures→short PHT.

Small hole→slower equilibration of pressures→longer PHT

Obviously, the bigger the hole in the aortic valve the worse the degree of regurgitation.

Some books consider < 300 ms (not < 200 ms) to indicate severe AI

Degree of AI: PHT	Trace (0-1+)	Mild (1-2+) > 500 ms	Moderate (2-3+) 200–500 ms	Severe (3-4+) < 200 (300?) ms

Reference: Perrino AC, Reeves S. *A Practical Approach to TEE.* Philadelphia: Lippincott Williams & Wilkins 2003:180.

14. **Answer = D, A slope of 335 cm/sec or 3.35 m/s is indicative of severe AI.**

Degree of AI: Stope	Trace (0-1+)	Mild (1-2+)	Moderate (2-3+) 200–500 cm/sec	Severe (3-4+) ≥ 300 cm/sec

Reference: Perrino AC, Reeves S. *A Practical Approach to TEE.* Philadelphia: Lippincott Williams & Wilkins 2003:180.

Case 7

15. **Answer = C, The diameter of the sinus of valsalva is indicated by arrow 1 in image 2 for case 7.**

Reference: Gott VL, Greene PS, Alejo DE, Cameron DE, Naftel DC, et al. Replacement of the aortic root in patients with Marfan's syndrome. *N Engl J Med* 1999;340:1307–1316.

16. **Answer = B, The diameter of the aortic valve annulus is indicated by arrow 2 in image 3 for case 7.**

Reference: Gott VL, Greene PS, Alejo DE, Cameron DE, Naftel DC, et al. Replacement of the aortic root in patients with Marfan's syndrome. *N Engl J Med* 1999;340:1307–1316.

17. **Answer = B, The sinotubular ridge (ST ridge) is indicated by arrow 1 in image 2 for case 7.**

Reference: Gott VL, Greene PS, Alejo DE, Cameron DE, Naftel DC, et al. Replacement of the aortic root in patients with Marfan's syndrome. *N Engl J Med* 1999;340:1307–1316.

Case 8

18. **Answer = C, An Ao ratio < 1.3 indicates a low-risk group for aortic dissection in patients with Marfan's syndrome.** Ao ratio is the sinus of valsalva diameter divided by the predicted sinus diameter for a given age and BSA. An Ao ratio < 1.3 or an annual rate of change < 5% indicates a low-risk group for aortic dissection in patients with Marfan's syndrome. For adults (> 40 years): predicted sinus dimension (cm) = 1.92 + [0.74 * BSA (m^2)].

Reference: Legget M, Unger TA, O'Sullivan CK, Zwink TR, Bennett RL, Byers PH, Otto CM. Aortic root complications in Marfan's syndrome: Identification of a lower risk group. *British Heart Journal* 1996;74(4):389–395.

19. **Answer = D, The sinus of valsalva is severely dilated.** The upper limit of normal for a sinus of valsalva is about 3.1 cm in adults. This patient is relatively small (height = 165 cm (65 in), weight = 63 kg, and BSA = 1.68 m^2. For a small patient this is a severely dilated sinus of valsalva.

Reference: Legget M, Unger TA, O'Sullivan CK, Zwink TR, Bennett RL, Byers PH, Otto CM. Aortic root complications in Marfan's syndrome: Identification of a lower risk group. *British Heart Journal* 1996;74(4):389–395.

20. **Answer = D, 1.43 = the Ao ratio.** Ao ratio is the sinus of valsalva diameter divided by the predicted sinus diameter for a given age and BSA. For adults (> 40 years): predicted sinus dimension (cm) = 1.92 + [0.74 * BSA (m^2)] = 1.92 + (0.74 * 2) = 3.13 cm → Ao ratio = 4.5/3.13 = 1.43. An Ao ratio < 1.3 or an annual rate of change < 5% indicates a low-risk group in patients with Marfan's syndrome.

Reference: Legget M, Unger TA, O'Sullivan CK, Zwink TR, Bennett RL, Byers PH, Otto CM. Aortic root complications in Marfan's syndrome: Identification of a lower risk group. *British Heart Journal* 1996;74(4):389–395.

Case 9

21. **Answer = B, The arrow indicates the left atrium.**

22. **Answer = A, Arrow 1 indicates a pulmonary artery catheter.**

Case 10

23. **Answer = B, The midesophageal ascending aortic short axis view is shown.**

Reference: Perrino AC, Reeves S. *A Practical Approach to TEE.* Philadelphia: Lippincott Williams & Wilkins 2003:334.

24. **Answer = A, The left pulmonary artery is shown by arrow 1.**

25. **Answer = D, Arrow 2 indicates the superior vena cava.**

26. **Answer = E, Arrow 3 points to the aorta.**

27. **Answer = A, Arrow 1 indicates the left pulmonary artery, which is sometimes difficult to visualize because the air-filled trachea and left main bronchus can lie between the esophagus and this structure and occlude its view.**

Case 11

28. **Answer = B, The left upper pulmonary vein is shown.**

29. **Answer = A, The Coumadin ridge is shown.**

30. **Answer = C, The lateral wall is dyskinetic.**

31. **Answer = D, Tricuspid regurgitation will result in systolic flow reversal in the hepatic veins and inferior vena cava.**

Reference: Perrino AC, Reeves S. *A Practical Approach to TEE.* Philadelphia: Lippincott Williams & Wilkins 2003:225.

Case 12

32. **Answer = D, A side lobe artifact is shown.** A pulmonary artery catheter (PAC) appears in the wrong location on the image. Significant acoustic energy can be emitted by the transducer outside the main axis of the ultrasound beam. These side lobes are normally too weak to generate recognizable echoes. However, when a very strong (bright) reflector such as a PAC lies in the path of a side lobe a reflection may be generated on the image. The machine incorrectly assumes that this reflection was produced by structures lying along the main axis of the ultrasound beam and places the structure in the wrong location on the image. Reflections received by the TEE probe from these off-axis side lobe pulses appear on the image as if they reside in the main axis of the ultrasound beam. A dissection must be confirmed by imaging the region of interest from multiple views. If you see the same finding in multiple views from different angles, it is likely not an artifact. When in doubt pull the PA catheter out!

References: Edelman SK. *Understanding Ultrasound Physics.* Woodlands, TX: ESP, Inc. 1994:205; Perrino AC, Reeves S. *A Practical Approach to TEE.* Philadelphia: Lippincott Williams & Wilkins 2003:311.

33. **Answer = D, A pulmonary artery catheter is shown.**

Case 13

34. **Answer = E, The right ventricular systolic pressure (RVSP) = 171 mmHg.** The calculation is as follows.

$$\Delta P = 4V_2$$

$$(RVSP - RAP) = 4V_{TR}^2$$

$$(RVSP - CVP) = 4V^2$$

$$RVSP = 4V^2 + CVP$$

$$RVSP = 4(6.41 \text{ m/s})^2 + 11$$

$$RVSP = 171 \text{ mmHg}$$

- RVSP = right ventricular systolic pressure
- RAP = right atrial pressure
- CVP = central venous pressure

Reference: Otto C. *Textbook of Clinical Echocardiography, Third Edition.* Philadelphia: Elsevier 2004:463.

35. **Answer = B, The pulmonary artery systolic pressure (PASP) = 62 mmHg.** The calculation is as follows.

$$PASP = (RVSP - \Delta P_{ps})$$

$$PASP = [RVSP - 4(V_{ps})^2]$$

$$PASP = [171 - 109] = 62 \text{ mmHg}$$

$$\Delta P = 4V^2$$

$$(RVSP - RAP) = 4V_{TR}^2$$

$$(RVSP - CVP) = 4V^2$$

$$RVSP = 4V^2 + CVP$$

$$RVSP = 4(6.41 \text{ m/s})^2 + 7$$

$$RVSP = 171 \text{ mmHg}$$

- RVSP = right ventricular systolic pressure
- RAP = right atrial pressure
- CVP = central venous pressure
- PASP = pulmonary artery systolic pressure
- V_{ps} = pulmonic stenosis peak flow velocity by Doppler = velocity of systolic flow across the pulmonic valve
- V_{TR} = peak velocity of the tricuspid valve regurgitant jet

Reference: Otto C. *Textbook of Clinical Echocardiography, Third Edition.* Philadelphia: Elsevier 2004:463.

36. **Answer = C, Pulmonic stenosis is shown.**

37. **Answer = C, The transgastric right ventricular outflow view is shown.** This is sometimes called the transgastric right ventricular inflow/outflow view.

38. **Answer = D, 109 mmHg is the peak instantaneous systolic pressure gradient across the pulmonic valve (ΔP_{PV}), which is interrogated in case 13.** The calculation is as follows.

$$\Delta P = 4V^2$$

$$\Delta P_{PV} = 4 (V_{PVsystolic\ peak})^2$$

$$\Delta P_{PV} = 4 (5.22 \text{ m/s})^2$$

$$\Delta P_{PV} = 109 \text{ mmHg}$$

- $V_{PVsystolic\ peak}$ = peak velocity of systolic flow across the pulmonic valve
- ΔP_{PV} = the peak instantaneous systolic pressure gradient across the pulmonic valve

Reference: Otto C. *Textbook of Clinical Echocardiography, Third Edition.* Philadelphia: Elsevier 2004:463.

Case 14

39. **Answer = D, Severe concentric left ventricular hypertrophy is present.**

40. **Answer = D, Arrow 1 indicates the septal wall.**

41. **Answer = B, Arrow 2 indicates the anteroseptal wall.**

42. **Answer = A, Arrow 3 indicates the anterior wall.**

43. **Answer = C, Arrow 4 indicates the lateral wall.**

Case 15

44. **Answer = D, Severe tricuspid regurgitation is present.**

45. **Answer = A, Reversal of the pulsed-wave Doppler hepatic venous S wave would be expected in this patient with severe tricuspid regurgitation.**

Reference: Perrino AC, Reeves S. *A Practical Approach to TEE.* Philadelphia: Lippincott Williams & Wilkins 2003:225.

46. **Answer = A, A heart transplant patient is at increased risk for the development of tricuspid regurgitation.** This develops following right heart catheterization and right ventricular tissue biopsy, which can damage the tricuspid subvalvular apparatus.

Case 16

47. **Answer = D, Severe tricuspid regurgitation is shown.** The color flow Doppler TR jet fills more than half of the right atrium, which is consistent with severe tricuspid regurgitation (TR).

Reference: Perrino AC, Reeves S. *A Practical Approach to TEE.* Philadelphia: Lippincott Williams & Wilkins 2003:224.

48. **Answer = B, The pulmonary artery systolic pressure can be estimated by a continuous-wave Doppler of the tricuspid regurgitant jet if no pulmonic stenosis is present.** The formula is as follows.

$$\Delta P = 4V^2$$

$$(RVSP - RAP) = 4V_{TR}^2$$

$$(RVSP - CVP) = 4V^2$$

$$RVSP = 4V^2 + CVP$$

$$PASP = RVSP$$

- PASP = pulmonary artery systolic pressure
- RVSP = right ventricular systolic pressure

- RAP = right atrial pressure
- CVP = central venous pressure
- V_{TR} = peak velocity of the tricuspid valve regurgitant jet

Reference: Otto C. *Textbook of Clinical Echocardiography, Third Edition.* Philadelphia: Elsevier 2004:463.

49. **Answer = D, A dilated coronary sinus is shown.**

50. **Answer = A, A persistent left superior vena cava is associated with a dilated coronary sinus.** The dilated coronary sinus shown likely resulted from increased right atrial pressure due to severe tricuspid regurgitation. Normally, the coronary sinus is less than 10 mm in diameter.

Case 17

51. **Answer = D, A complete AV canal defect is shown.** This is composed of an ostium primum atrial septal defect and an inlet ventricular septal defect. It is associated with mitral regurgitation due to a cleft anterior mitral valve leaflet and trisomy 21 (Down's syndrome).

Reference: Otto C. *Textbook of Clinical Echocardiography, Third Edition.* Philadelphia: Elsevier 2004:466.

52. **Answer = B, Mitral regurgitation in this patient would likely be due to a cleft anterior mitral valve leaflet, which is associated with the complete AV canal defect shown.**

Reference: Otto C. *Textbook of Clinical Echocardiography, Third Edition.* Philadelphia: Elsevier 2004:466.

53. **Answer = A, An ostium primum atrial septal defect is present.**

Reference: Otto C. *Textbook of Clinical Echocardiography, Third Edition.* Philadelphia: Elsevier 2004:466.

54. **Answer = E, An inlet ventricular septal defect is shown.**

Reference: Otto C. *Textbook of Clinical Echocardiography, Third Edition.* Philadelphia: Elsevier 2004:466.

55. **Answer = B, Trisomy 21 (Down's syndrome) is associated with this defect.**

Reference: Otto C. *Textbook of Clinical Echocardiography, Third Edition.* Philadelphia: Elsevier 2004:466.

Case 18

56. **Answer = A, The posteromedial commissure is indicated by the arrow in image 1.**

57. **Answer = E, Segment 5, the basal inferior wall segment, is indicated by arrow 1.**

Reference: ASE/SCA Guidelines for Performing a Comprehensive Intraoperative Multiplane Transesophageal Echocardiography Examination. *J Am Soc Echocardiog* 1999;12:884–900.

58. **Answer = D, Segment 6, the basal septal wall segment, is indicated by arrow 2.**

Reference: ASE/SCA Guidelines for Performing a Comprehensive Intraoperative Multiplane Transesophageal Echocardiography Examination. *J Am Soc Echocardiog* 1999;12:884–900.

59. **Answer = A, Segment 1, the basal anteroseptal segment, is indicated by arrow 3.**

Reference: ASE/SCA Guidelines for Performing a Comprehensive Intraoperative Multiplane Transesophageal Echocardiography Examination. *J Am Soc Echocardiog* 1999;12:884–900.

60. **Answer = B, Segment 2, the basal anterior wall segment, is indicated by arrow 4.**

Reference: ASE/SCA Guidelines for Performing a Comprehensive Intraoperative Multiplane Transesophageal Echocardiography Examination. *J Am Soc Echocardiog* 1999;12:884–900.

61. **Answer = C, Segment 3, the basal lateral wall segment, is indicated by arrow 5.**

Reference: ASE/SCA Guidelines for Performing a Comprehensive Intraoperative Multiplane Transesophageal Echocardiography Examination. *J Am Soc Echocardiog* 1999;12:884–900.

62. **Answer = D, Segment 4, the basal posterior wall segment, is indicated by arrow 6.**

Reference: ASE/SCA Guidelines for Performing a Comprehensive Intraoperative Multiplane Transesophageal Echocardiography Examination. *J Am Soc Echocardiog* 1999;12:884–900.

Case 19

63. **Answer = B, A left ventricular band is shown.**

64. **Answer = B, The anterolateral papillary muscle is shown.**

65. **Answer = B, The left atrium is shown.**

Case 20

66. **Answer = A, The right upper pulmonary vein is shown.**

67. **Answer = B, The right lower pulmonary vein is shown.**

Case 21

68. **Answer = D, A chiari network is shown.**

69. **Answer = A, The right upper pulmonary vein is shown.**

70. **Answer = A, The right upper pulmonary vein is shown.**

TEST V PART 2

Written Test Booklet

NOTE: Use Table 5.2A to answer the next six (6) questions.

Table 5.2A.

LVEDd = 55 mm	LVEDVol = 130 ml	PHT_{MV} = 62 msec
LVESd = 32 mm	LVESVol = 42 ml	$TVI_{MVinflow}$ = 24.7 cm
LVEDA = 23.8 cm^2	$\Delta t_{MR100-300}$ = 0.02 sec	HR = 100 beats/min
LVESA = 8.1 cm^2	BSA = 2 M^2	BP = 130/80 mmHg

Abbreviations: LVEDd = left ventricular end diastolic dimension, LVESd = left ventricular end systolic dimension, LVEDA = left ventricular end diastolic diameter, LVESA = left ventricular end systolic area, LVEDVol = left ventricular end diastolic volume, LVESVol = left ventricular end systolic volume, $\Delta t_{MR100-300}$ = delta t = dt = the time required for a mitral regurgitant jet to accelerate from a velocity of 100 cm/sec to a velocity of 300 cm/sec during isovolumic left ventricular contraction, BSA = body surface area, PHT_{MV} = mitral valve inflow pressure half time, BP = blood pressure, $TVI_{MVinflow}$ = time velocity integral of diastolic mitral inflow, HR = heart rate.

1. What is the fractional shortening?

   A. 12%

   B. 22%

   C. 32%

   D. 42%

   E. 52%

2. What is the fractional area change?

   A. 35%

   B. 45%

   C. 55%

   D. 65%

   E. 75%

3. What is the ejection fraction?

   A. 38%

   B. 48%

   C. 58%

   D. 68%

   E. 78%

4. What is the change in pressure with respect to time during isovolumic left ventricular contraction (dp/dt)?

   A. 800 mmHg/sec

   B. 1,000 mmHg/sec

   C. 1,200 mmHg/sec

   D. 1,400 mmHg/sec

   E. 1,600 mmHg/sec

5. What is the cardiac index?

   A. 1.2 L/min/m^2

   B. 2.2 L/min/m^2

   C. 4.4 L/min/m^2

   D. 4.8 L/min/m^2

   E. 5.2 L/min/m^2

6. Which of the following best describes this patient's systolic function?

   A. Normal.

   B. Mildly decreased.

   C. Moderately decreased.

   D. Severely decreased.

   E. It cannot be determined from the given information.

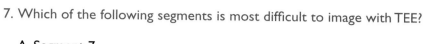

7. Which of the following segments is most difficult to image with TEE?

    A. Segment 7

    B. Segment 8

    C. Segment 11

    D. Segment 12

    E. Segment 13

8. Which of the following is a distinction between true septal dyskinesis (DK) and paradoxical septal motion (PSM = paradoxical septal motion, DK = dyskinesis, RV = right ventricular)?

    A. Septal DK occurs with RV epicardial pacing; PSM does not.

    B. Systolic septal wall thickening occurs with PSM but not with septal DK.

    C. A left bundle branch block can cause septal DK, but not PSM.

    D. Septal DK occurs with right ventricular pressure overload; PSM does not.

    E. There is no difference between PSM and septal DK.

9. Which of the following views allows visualization of myocardial segments supplied by all three coronary arteries, as well as calculation of fractional shortening and fractional area change?

    A. Transgastric two-chamber view

    B. Transgastric long axis view

    C. Midesophageal four-chamber view

    D. Transgastric mid papillary short axis view

    E. Midesophageal two-chamber view

10. Which of the following views allows assessment of end diastolic area (volume status), fractional area change, and fractional shortening?

    A. Transgastric two-chamber view

    B. Transgastric long axis view

    C. Midesophageal four-chamber view

    D. Transgastric mid papillary short axis view

    E. Midesophageal two-chamber view

11. Which of the following best indicates mitral valve annular dilatation?

   A. End systolic anterior posterior midesophageal long axis annulus measurement > 3.6 cm.

   B. End diastolic anterior posterior midesophageal long axis annulus measurement > 3.6 cm.

   C. End systolic intercommissural measurement > 36 mm.

   D. End diastolic intercommissural measurement > 36 mm.

   E. End systolic four-chamber view measurement > 36 mm.

12. Which of the following views is best for accurately measuring the mitral regurgitation vena contracta?

   A. Midesophageal four-chamber view

   B. Midesophageal mitral valve commissural view

   C. Midesophageal two-chamber view

   D. Midesophageal long axis view

   E. Transgastric basal short axis view

13. Which of the following indicates severe acute mitral regurgitation?

   A. Vena contracta width = 4 mm

   B. Color flow Doppler mitral regurgitant jet area = 4 cm^2

   C. Systolic suppression of the pulmonary venous pulsed-wave Doppler flow profile

   D. V-wave cut-off sign on the continuous-wave Doppler mitral regurgitant flow profile

   E. Color flow Doppler jet area = 33% of the left atrial area

NOTE: Use Table 5.2B to answer the next eight (8) questions.

Table 5.2B.

LVOT diameter = 20 mm	V_{TRpeak} = 200 cm/sec	CVP = 10 mmHg
PA diameter = 24 mm	$TVI_{TV\ inflow}$ = 20 cm	BP = 110/70 mmHg
TVI_{AV} = 8.85 cm	TVI_{MV} = 30 cm	HR = 100 beats/min
TVI_{PA} = 13.26 cm	PHT_{MV} = 110 msec	BSA = 2 m^2

Abbreviations: LVOT = left ventricular outflow tract, V_{TRpeak} = peak velocity of the tricuspid regurgitant jet, CVP = central venous pressure, PA = pulmonary artery, TVI_{AV} = time velocity integral of blood flow through the aortic valve, LA = left atrial, $TVI_{TV\ inflow}$ = time velocity integral of diastolic transtricuspid inflow, TVI_{MV} = time velocity integral of diastolic mitral inflow, PHT_{MV} = mitral valve inflow pressure half time, HR = heart rate, BSA = body surface area.

14. Which of the following is the best estimate of the right ventricular systolic pressure?

    A. 16 mmHg

    B. 18 mmHg

    C. 26 mmHg

    D. 28 mmHg

    E. 30 mmHg

15. Which of the following is the best estimate of the mitral valve area?

    A. 0.5 cm^2

    B. 1.0 cm^2

    C. 1.3 cm^2

    D. 2.0 cm^2

    E. 2.2 cm^2

16. Which of the following is the best estimate of the mitral valve stroke volume?

    A. 20 ml

    B. 30 ml

    C. 40 ml

    D. 50 ml

    E. 60 ml

17. Which of the following is the best estimate of the mitral valve cardiac output?

   A. 2 L/min

   B. 3 L/min

   C. 4 L/min

   D. 5 L/min

   E. 6 L/min

18. Which of the following is the best estimate of the mitral valve cardiac index?

   A. 1 L/min/m^2

   B. 2 L/min/m^2

   C. 3 L/min/m^2

   D. 4 L/min/m^2

   E. 6 L/min/m^2

19. Which of the following is the best estimate of the tricuspid valve area?

   A. 2 cm^2

   B. 3 cm^2

   C. 4 cm^2

   D. 5 cm^2

   E. Cannot be detemined from the given information

20. Which of the following is the best estimate of the pulmonary artery stroke volume?

   A. 20 ml

   B. 30 ml

   C. 40 ml

   D. 50 ml

   E. 60 ml

21. This patient has no pulmonary insufficiency. How would you describe the degree of mitral regurgitation present?

   A. No mitral regurgitation is present.

   B. Mild mitral regurgitation.

   C. Moderate mitral regurgitation.

   D. Severe mitral regurgitation.

   E. It cannot be determined from the given data.

NOTE: Use Figure 5.2A to answer the next five (5) questions.

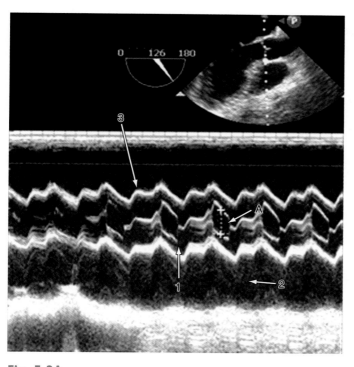

Fig. 5-2A

22. Arrow 1 indicates which of the following?

   A. Left coronary cusp

   B. Right coronary cusp

   C. Non coronary cusp

   D. Anterior leaflet

   E. Posterior leaflet

23. Arrow 2 indicates which of the following?

    A. Right atrium

    B. Left atrium

    C. Right ventricle

    D. Left ventricle

    E. Pericardial effusion

24. A narrowing of the area (labeled A) between the caliper marks is indicative of which of the following?

    A. Hypertrophic obstructive cardiomyopathy

    B. Dilated cardiomyopathy

    C. Restrictive cardiomyopathy

    D. Aortic stenosis

    E. Mitral stenosis

25. Midsystolic closure (area labeled A) followed by coarse fluttering of the leaflets is indicative of which of the following?

    A. Hypertrophic obstructive cardiomyopathy

    B. Dilated cardiomyopathy

    C. Aortic regurgitation

    D. Aortic stenosis

    E. Mitral regurgitation

26. Which of the following is indicated by arrow 3?

    A. Right atrium

    B. Left atrium

    C. Right ventricle

    D. Pericardial effusion

    E. Left ventricular outflow tract

27. Which of the following are directly proportional?

   A. Spatial pulse length and lateral resolution

   B. Beam width and lateral resolution

   C. Wavelength and pulse duration

   D. Pulse repetition frequency and image depth

   E. Pulse repetition frequency and pulse repetition period

28. Which of the following is true concerning intensity?

   A. The units of intensity are Watts/cm^3.

   B. It is proportional to the amplitude squared.

   C. It is initially determined by both the ultrasound system and the medium through which the beam travels.

   D. It is attenuated more with low-frequency transducers than with high-frequency transducers.

   E. It varies with duty factor.

29. Which of the following types of intensities correlates most readily with the heating of tissues and is therefore the most relevant with regard to the bioeffects of ultrasound?

   A. SPTP

   B. SATP

   C. SPTA

   D. SATA

   E. SAPA

   (SP = spatial peak, SA = spatial average, TP = temporal peak, TA = temporal average, PA = pulsed average)

30. Which of the following is true regarding continuous-wave ultrasound?

   A. It can be used to produce two-dimensional images.

   B. It is subject to aliasing.

   C. SPTP intensity = SPTA intensity for continuous-wave ultrasound.

   D. Duty factor = 0.5.

   E. All of the above are correct.

   (SP = spatial peak, SA = spatial average, TP = temporal peak, TA = temporal average, PA = pulsed average)

31. The output of a TEE probe is increased such that the intensity of the ultrasound system is doubled. This can be represented as (dB = decibels):

   A. +3 dB

   B. +6 dB

   C. +8 dB

   D. +10 dB

   E. +12 dB

32. A TEE probe has an ultrasound frequency of 20 MHz. What is the attenuation coefficient?

   A. 2 dB/cm

   B. 5 dB/cm

   C. 10 dB/cm

   D. 20 dB/cm

   E. None of the above

33. How many decibels (dB) of attenuation occur at 8 cm when a 20-MHz TEE probe is used?

   A. 20 dB

   B. 40 dB

   C. 80 dB

   D. 160 dB

   E. 320 dB

34. Which of the following most closely estimates the *thickness* of tissue required to reduce the *power* of an 18-MHz TEE transducer by *half*?

A. 0.33 cm

B. 0.67 cm

C. 0.90 cm

D. 1.80 cm

E. 2.40 cm

NOTE: Use Table 5.2C to answer question 35.

Table 5.2C.

Medium 1	Medium 2	Medium 3	Medium 4
Density = 1	Density = 3	Density = 1	Density = .05
Velocity = 1.54	Velocity = 1.6	Velocity = 2	Velocity = 1
Elasticity = 1	Elasticity = 0.9	Elasticity = 3	Elasticity = 0.9
Specific heat = 1	Specific heat = 0.9	Specific heat = 1.5	Specific heat = 2

35. A 10-MHz ultrasound beam from a TEE probe travels through the four media outlined in the table. Which of these media most likely has the highest acoustic impedance?

A. Medium 1

B. Medium 2

C. Medium 3

D. Medium 4

36. Which of the following is most likely true concerning the matching layer?

A. It shortens the spatial pulse length.

B. It increases the Q factor.

C. It has acoustic impedance between that of the skin and the active element in the transducer.

D. It decreases the bandwidth.

NOTE: Use Table 5.2D to answer question 37.

Table 5.2D.

Parameter	Crystal A	Crystal B	Crystal C	Crystal D
Wavelength (λ)	1	2	2	1
Crystal diameter (D)	0.5	0.5	1	1
Acoustic impedance (Z)	0.3	0.4	0.4	0.3
Velocity (V)	1.3	0.5	1	1.5

37. Given Table 5.2D, which of the following TEE piezoelectric crystals will have the longest focal length?

A. Crystal A

B. Crystal B

C. Crystal C

D. Crystal D

38. Which of the following is most likely true concerning the frequency of a TEE piezoelectric crystal?

A. As frequency increases spatial pulse length increases.

B. As frequency increases attenuation decreases.

C. As frequency increases propagation velocity increases.

D. As frequency increases focal depth (near-zone length) increases

E. As frequency increases piezoelectric thickness increases.

39. Which of the following will most likely create an ultrasound beam with a shallow focus (short near-zone length)?

A. Increasing the acoustic impedance

B. Decreasing the ultrasound frequency

C. Increasing the piezoelectric crystal diameter

D. Decreasing the crystal thickness

40. An unfocused ultrasound beam has a near-zone length of 6 cm. The diameter of the piezoelectric crystal in the transducer is 6 mm. What is the best estimate of the lateral resolution at a depth of 7 cm?

A. 2.7 mm

B. 3 mm

C. 3.4 mm

D. 6 mm

41. Which of the following is most likely to be true concerning an increase in the spatial pulse length (SPL)?

A. As SPL increases the numerical value for axial resolution increases.

B. As SPL increases lateral resolution increases.

C. As SPL increases depth resolution increases.

D. As SPL increases image quality increases.

E. As SPL increases spatial resolution increases.

42. Which of the following describes most TEE probes?

A. Linear sequential array

B. Linear phased array

C. Curvilinear sequential array

D. Curvilinear phased array

43. Which of the following most correctly describes the X and Y axes of an M-mode (motion mode) tracing?

A. X axis = time, Y axis = velocity

B. Y axis = time, X axis = velocity

C. X axis = time, Y axis = depth

D. X axis = depth, Y axis = time

44. A TEE probe uses multiple sound beams with different focal depths to create a single scan line. Which of the following is true concerning this use of multiple focal zones?

   A. Frame rate is increased.

   B. Lateral resolution is improved.

   C. Line density is increased.

   D. There are fewer pulses per scan line.

45. Which of the following is a major advantage of continuous-wave ultrasound?

   A. It produces superior two-dimensional images.

   B. Range resolution is superior.

   C. It can be used to measure very high velocities.

   D. Azimuthal resolution is superior.

   E. None of the above.

46. Which of the following is true concerning pulsed-wave Doppler?

   A. It can be used to measure very high velocities.

   B. A sample volume or gate provides range resolution.

   C. It is not subject to aliasing.

   D. The Nyquist limit of pulsed-wave Doppler is greater than the Nyquist limit of continuous-wave Doppler.

   E. None of the above.

47. Which of the following angles of incidence will provide the best two-dimensional grayscale TEE image?

   A. 120 degrees

   B. 100 degrees

   C. 90 degrees

   D. 60 degrees

   E. 0 degrees

48. Which of the following is most likely to decrease aliasing of pulsed-wave Doppler?

    A. Increasing the pulse repetition frequency

    B. Increasing the line density

    C. Increasing the depth of the sample volume

    D. Increasing the frequency of the transducer

    E. Increasing the spatial pulse length

49. Which of the following can help decrease aliasing artifact?

    A. Using a continuous-wave Doppler ultrasound beam

    B. Using a higher-frequency transducer

    C. Placing the sample volume at a deeper depth

    D. Decreasing the pulse repetition frequency (PRF)

    E. All of the above

50. Which of the following is associated with continuous-wave Doppler (CWD)?

    A. Range resolution

    B. Aliasing

    C. Sample volume

    D. High-velocity measurements

    E. None of the above

51. Which of the following is associated with pulsed-wave Doppler?

    A. Range ambiguity

    B. High-velocity measurements

    C. Aliasing

    D. Optimal with orthogonal incidence

    E. None of the above

NOTE: Use Table 5.2E to answer the following nine (9) questions.

Table 5.2E.

	HR = 80	TVI LVOT = 15 cm
V_{VSD} = 500 cm/s	CVP = 10 mmHg	TVI PA = 20 cm
$V_{PIearly}$ = 300 cm/s	SBP = 120 mmHg	LVOT diameter = 20 mm
V_{PIlate} = 255 cm/s	DBP = 80 mmHg	PA diameter = 22 mm
V_{MRpeak} = 1,200 cm/s	MAP = 83 mmHg	Sinus of valsalva diameter = 32 mm

Abbreviations: V_{PI} = velocity of the pulmonic insufficiency jet,
V_{VSD} = velocity of the flow across the ventricular septal defect,
V_{MRpeak} = the peak velocity of the mitral regurgitant jet, V_{ASD} = velocity of flow across the atrial septal defect,
HR = heart rate, SBP = systolic blood pressure, DBP = diastolic blood pressure, MAP = mean arterial pressure,
LVOT = left ventricular outflow tract, PA = pulmonary artery (main PA), TVI = time velocity integral.

52. What is the right ventricular systolic pressure?

    A. 5 mmHg

    B. 10 mmHg

    C. 15 mmHg

    D. 20 mmHg

    E. 25 mmHg

53. What is the pulmonary artery mean pressure?

    A. 16 mmHg

    B. 26 mmHg

    C. 36 mmHg

    D. 46 mmHg

    E. 56 mmHg

54. What is the pulmonary artery diastolic pressure?

    A. 16 mmHg

    B. 26 mmHg

    C. 36 mmHg

    D. 46 mmHg

    E. 56 mmHg

55. Which of the following is the best estimate of the pulmonary artery systolic pressure?

   A. 5 mmHg

   B. 10 mmHg

   C. 15 mmHg

   D. 20 mmHg

   E. 25 mmHg

56. What is the right ventricular stroke volume?

   A. 36 cm^3

   B. 46 cm^3

   C. 56 cm^3

   D. 66 cm^3

   E. 76 cm^3

57. What is the right ventricular cardiac output?

   A. 7.1 L/min

   B. 6.1 L/min

   C. 5.1 L/min

   D. 4.1 L/min

   E. 3.1 L/min

58. What is the left ventricular stroke volume?

   A. 37 cm^3

   B. 47 cm^3

   C. 57 cm^3

   D. 67 cm^3

   E. 77 cm^3

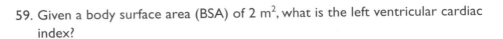
59. Given a body surface area (BSA) of 2 m², what is the left ventricular cardiac index?

   A. 1.89 L/min/m²

   B. 2.51 L/min/m²

   C. 3.64 L/min/m²

   D. 4.13 L/min/m²

   E. 5.14 L/min/m²

60. What is the ratio of pulmonic flow to systemic flow (Q_P/Q_S)?

   A. 1.62

   B. 1.91

   C. 2.20

   D. 2.31

   E. 2.63

NOTE: Use the information in Table 5.2F to answer the next five (5) questions.

Table 5.2F.

$DT_{MVinflow} = 253$ msec	BP = 130/80 mmHg	$V_{AVpeak} = 250$ cm/sec
$TVI_{AV} = 20$ cm	HR = 100 beats/min	$V_{LVOTpeak} = 60$ cm/sec
$TVI_{MVinflow} = 15$ cm	CVP = 10 mmHg	Sinus of valsalva diameter = 32 mm
$TVI_{LVOT} = 18.7$ cm	BSA = 2 m²	Sinotubular ridge diameter = 24 mm

Abbreviations: $DT_{MVinflow}$ = the deceleration time of the diastolic mitral inflow continuous-wave Doppler spectrum, TVI_{AV} = the time velocity integral of systolic flow through the aortic valve, $TVI_{MVinflow}$ = the time velocity integral of flow through the mitral valve into the LV in diastole, TVI_{LVOT} = the time velocity integral of flow through the left ventricular outflow tract, BP = blood pressure, HR = heart rate, CVP = central venous pressure, V_{AVpeak} = the peak systolic flow velocity across the aortic valve, $V_{LVOTpeak}$ = the peak systolic flow velocity in the left ventricular outflow tract.

61. Which of the following is the best estimate of the mitral valve area as calculated from the data in the table?

   A. 1.0 cm²

   B. 2.0 cm²

   C. 2.5 cm²

   D. 3.0 cm²

   E. 3.5 cm²

62. Which of the following is the best estimate of the aortic valve area as calculated from the data in the table?

A. 0.75 cm^2

B. 1.25 cm^2

C. 2.00 cm^2

D. 2.25 cm^2

E. 3.00 cm^2

63. Which of the following is the best estimate of the peak instantaneous pressure gradient across the aortic valve?

A. 9 mmHg

B. 12 mmHg

C. 17 mmHg

D. 25 mmHg

E. 36 mmHg

64. Which of the following is the best estimate of this patient's cardiac output?

A. 4.0 L/min

B. 4.5 L/min

C. 5.0 L/min

D. 5.5 L/min

E. 6.0 L/min

65. Which of the following is the best estimate of this patient's cardiac index?

A. 2.00 L/min/m^2

B. 2.25 L/min/m^2

C. 2.50 L/min/m^2

D. 2.75 L/min/m^2

E. 3.00 L/min/m^2

NOTE: Use Table 5.2G to answer the next seven (7) questions concerning a patient with a pulmonary artery catheter (PAC) in place and scheduled to undergo cardiac surgery.

Table 5.2G.

$TVI_{MVinflow} = 60$ cm	CVP = 10 mmHg	Thermodilution CI from PAC = 1.5 L/min/m^2
$PHT_{MVinflow} = 169$ msec	HR = 100 beats/min	LVOT diameter = 20 mm
$TVI_{MR} = 100$ cm	BP = 110/70 mmHg	Pulmonary artery diameter = 24 mm
$TVI_{AV} = 22$ cm	BSA = 2.2 m^2	Sinus of valsalva diameter = 32 mm

Abbreviations: $TVI_{MVinflow}$ = time velocity integral of diastolic mitral inflow, CVP = central venous pressure, CI = cardiac index, $PHT_{MVinflow}$ = pressure half time of diastolic mitral inflow, HR = heart rate, BP = systemic blood pressure, TVI_{MR} = time velocity integral of diastolic mitral inflow, TVI_{AV} = time velocity integral of aortic systolic flow, BSA = body surface area, PAC = pulmonary artery catheter, LVOT = left ventricular outflow tract.

66. Which of the following is the best estimate of the mitral valve area?

    A. 0.8 cm^2

    B. 1.3 cm^2

    C. 2.2 cm^2

    D. 2.5 cm^2

    E. 3.0 cm^2

67. Which of the following is the best estimate of the mitral valve stroke volume?

    A. 38 cm^3

    B. 48 cm^3

    C. 58 cm^3

    D. 68 cm^3

    E. 78 cm^3

68. Which of the following is the best estimate of the mitral valve regurgitant volume?

    A. 45 cm^3

    B. 40 cm^3

    C. 35 cm^3

    D. 30 cm^3

    E. 25 cm^3

69. Which of the following is the best estimate of mitral valve regurgitant orifice area as calculated from the data in the table?

    A. 0.25 cm^2

    B. 0.35 cm^2

    C. 0.45 cm^2

    D. 0.55 cm^2

    E. 0.65 cm^2

70. Which of the following is the best estimate of the mitral valve regurgitant fraction?

    A. 28%

    B. 38%

    C. 48%

    D. 58%

    E. 68%

71. Which of the following best describes the degree of mitral regurgitation?

    A. Trace.

    B. Mild.

    C. Moderate.

    D. Severe.

    E. It cannot be determined from the given data.

72. Which of the following best describes the degree of mitral stenosis?

    A. Normal (no stenosis).

    B. Mild.

    C. Moderate.

    D. Severe.

    E. It cannot be determined from the given data.

73. In which of the following aortic lesions is deep hypothermic circulatory arrest most likely to be required to facilitate surgical repair?

    A. DeBakey type I dissection

    B. Crawford type III aneurysm

    C. Crawford type IV aneurysm

    D. Crawford type V aneurysm

    E. DeBakey type IIIb dissection starting 2 cm distal to the left subclavian artery

NOTE: Use Figure 5.2B1–3 to answer the next four (4) questions.

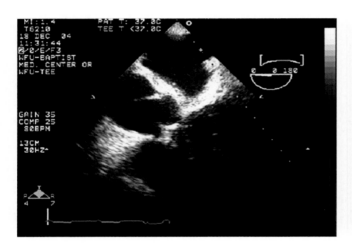

Fig. 5-2B1

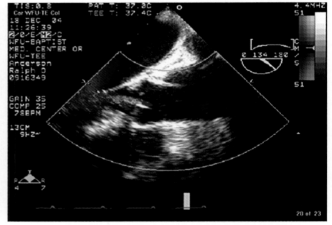

Fig. 5-2B2

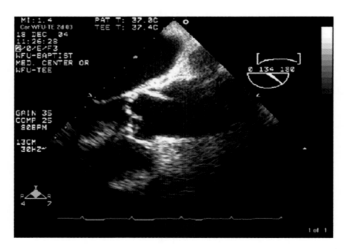

Fig. 5-2B3

74. Which of the following statements is true concerning the disorder illustrated?

    A. The mortality rate is 72% with surgical management.

    B. The mortality rate is 32% with medical management.

    C. Beta blockers are beneficial because they decrease the ejection velocity.

    D. The incidence of coronary artery involvement is 30%.

    E. None of the above is correct.

75. Which of the following is the most likely diagnosis of the patient shown?

    A. Aortic tear at the ligamentum arteriosum

    B. Aortic dissection, DeBakey type IIIa

    C. Aortic dissection, Stanford class B

    D. Aortic dissection, Stanford class A

    E. Aortic dissection, DeBakey type IIIb

76. Which of the following is true concerning the disorder illustrated (Ao ratio = the ratio of the patient's measured sinus of valsalva diameter to the predicted sinus of valsalva diameter for the same age and body surface area. CABG = coronary artery bypass graft surgery)?

    A. Patients with Marfan's syndrome with an Ao ratio < 1.3 are at decreased risk of developing this complication.

    B. Patients with an aortic root diameter of 50 mm undergoing CABG are at increased risk of developing this disorder.

    C. Patients with this disorder may present with hoarseness secondary to compression of the recurrent laryngeal nerve.

    D. Patients with this disorder may have asymmetry of pulses.

    E. All of the above are true.

77. Which of the following is true concerning the disorder illustrated?

   A. Atherosclerosis is an independent risk factor for this disorder.

   B. This disorder may occur during cannulation for cardiopulmonary bypass.

   C. An intimal tear just distal to the left subclavian artery at the level of the ligamentum arteriosum is the most common cause of this disorder.

   D. All of the above.

   E. None of the above.

78. Which of the following is true concerning the systolic component of the pulsed-wave Doppler venous flow profile?

   A. It has three components: PVS_1, PVS_2, and PVS_3.

   B. PVS_2 depends on left atrial relaxation and the subsequent decrease in left atrial pressure.

   C. PVS_1 is influenced by right ventricular stroke volume.

   D. Pulmonary systolic flow reversal is indicative of severe MR.

   E. Diastolic flow reversal is indicative of severe pulmonary insufficiency.

79. Which of the following is most likely true concerning the pulsed-wave Doppler pulmonary vein A wave (PV_{AR} wave)?

   A. In restrictive diastolic dysfunction the PV_{AR} wave may be elevated secondarily to decreased left ventricular compliance.

   B. In restrictive diastolic dysfunction the PV_{AR} wave may be decreased due to left atrial mechanical failure.

   C. In delayed relaxation (impaired relaxation) PV_{AR} < A-wave velocity.

   D. PV_{AR} may be increased in patients with mitral stenosis.

   E. All of the above are correct.

80. Which of the following valvular abnormalities would most likely result in a large increase in the PV$_{AR}$ wave?

    A. Mitral stenosis (MS)

    B. Aortic stenosis (AS)

    C. Mitral regurgitation (MR)

    D. Pulmonic stenosis (PS)

    E. Tricuspid regurgitation (TR)

81. Which of the following is true of constrictive pericarditis but **not** true of restrictive cardiomyopathy due to amyloidosis?

    A. Lateral mitral annular tissue Doppler E$_M$ > 8 cm/sec.

    B. Transmitral color M-mode Doppler flow propagation velocity (V$_P$) < 50 cm/sec.

    C. Transmitral pulsed-wave Doppler peak flow velocities showing E >> A.

    D. Transmitral E-wave deceleration time (DT) is shortened.

    E. Isovolumic relaxation time (IVRT) is shortened.

82. Which of the following disorders is most likely to produce a restrictive transmitral pulsed-wave Doppler flow velocity profile with a normal lateral mitral annular tissue Doppler E$_M$?

    A. Myocardial ischemia

    B. Constrictive pericarditis

    C. Severe concentric left ventricular hypertrophy

    D. Hypertrophic cardiomyopathy

    E. Amyloidosis

NOTE: Use Figure 5.2C to answer the next question.

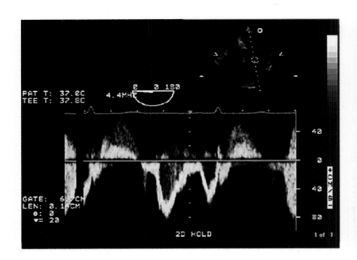

Fig. 5-2C1

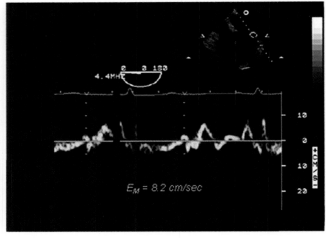

Fig. 5-2C2

83. Given the transmitral pulsed-wave Doppler flow velocities and the lateral mitral annular tissue Doppler E_M velocity shown, which of the following best describes this patient's diastolic function?

A. Normal

B. Pseudonormal

C. Impaired relaxation

D. Constrictive

E. Restrictive

NOTE: Use the pulmonary vein flow velocities shown in Figure 5.2D to answer the next three (3) questions.

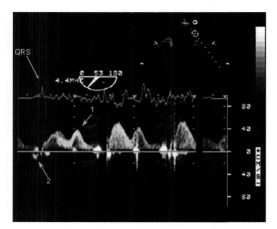

Fig. 5-2D

84. Which of the following patients would most likely have a pulmonary vein Doppler flow velocity profile similar to that shown?

   A. A healthy 42-year-old

   B. A patient with end-stage infiltrative amyloidosis

   C. A patient with constrictive pericarditis

   D. A patient with a 34-mm pericardial effusion with RV diastolic collapse

   E. None of the above

85. Which of the following best describes the wave labeled 1?

   A. PV_{AR} wave

   B. S wave

   C. D wave

   D. V wave

   E. A wave

86. Which of the following best describes the wave labeled 2?

   A. PV_{AR} wave

   B. S wave

   C. D wave

   D. V wave

   E. A wave

NOTE: Use the pulmonary vein pulsed-wave Doppler flow velocity profile shown in Figure 5.2E to answer the next three (3) questions.

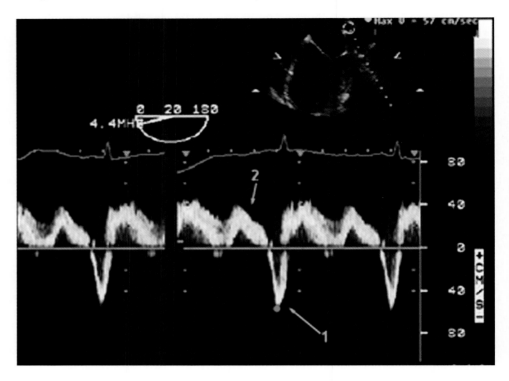

Fig. 5-2E

87. Which of the following disease states would be expected to increase the size of the pulmonary venous wave labeled 1?

    A. Impaired relaxation

    B. Complete heart block

    C. Severe mitral regurgitation

    D. Severe aortic stenosis

    E. Severe aortic regurgitation

88. Which of the following best describes the wave labeled 1?

    A. PV_{AR} wave

    B. S wave

    C. D wave

    D. E wave

    E. A wave

89. Which of the following best describes the wave labeled 2?

   A. PV$_{AR}$ wave

   B. S wave

   C. D wave

   D. E wave

   E. A wave

NOTE: Use the hepatic venous pulsed-wave Doppler flow velocity profile shown in Figure 5.2F to answer the next three (3) questions.

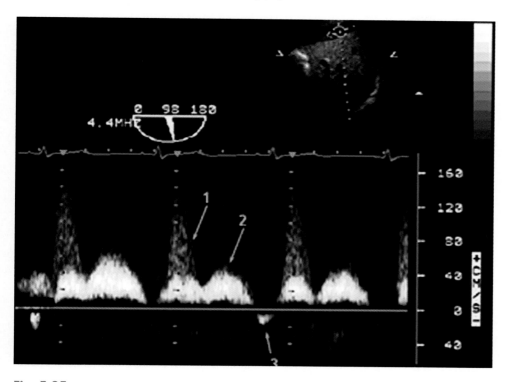

Fig. 5-2F

90. Which of the following best describes the hepatic venous wave labeled 1?

   A. V wave

   B. S wave

   C. E wave

   D. D wave

   E. A wave

91. Which of the following best describes the hepatic venous wave labeled 2?

A. V wave

B. S wave

C. E wave

D. D wave

E. A wave

92. Which of the following best describes the hepatic venous wave labeled 3?

A. V wave

B. S wave

C. E wave

D. D wave

E. A wave

93. Which of the following is a typical finding in pericardial tamponade?

A. Moderate to severe pericardial effusion

B. Right ventricular systolic collapse

C. Right atrial diastolic collapse

D. Increase in LV filling (transmitral inflow) with spontaneous inspiration

E. Decrease in RV filling (transtricuspid) with spontaneous expiration

NOTE: Use Table 5.2H to answer the next four (4) questions.

Table 5.2H.

HD Scenario	VTI$_{PA}$	Transtricuspid E	Transmitral E	VTI$_{LVOT}$	SBP
A	Increase	Increase	Decrease	Decrease	Decrease
B	Decrease	Decrease	Increase	Increase	Increase
C	Increase	Increase	Increase	Increase	Increase
D	Decrease	Decrease	Decrease	Decrease	Decrease
E	Increase	Decrease	Increase	Decrease	Decrease

Abbreviations: HD = hemodynamic, VTI$_{PA}$ = time velocity integral of flow through the pulmonary artery, Transtricuspid E = peak early transtricuspid flow velocity, SBP = systolic blood pressure, VTI$_{LVOT}$ = time velocity integral of flow through the left ventricular outflow tract, Transmitral E = transmitral peak early-filling velocity by pulsed wave Doppler.

94. Which of the hemodynamic scenarios would be expected with spontaneous inspiration in a patient with a hemodynamically significant pericardial effusion?

    A. Scenario A

    B. Scenario B

    C. Scenario C

    D. Scenario D

    E. Scenario E

95. Which of the hemodynamic scenarios would be expected in an intubated patient with a hemodynamically significant pericardial effusion undergoing positive pressure inspiration?

    A. Scenario A

    B. Scenario B

    C. Scenario C

    D. Scenario D

    E. Scenario E

96. Which of the hemodynamic scenarios would be expected with spontaneous expiration in a patient with a hemodynamically significant pericardial effusion?

    A. Scenario A

    B. Scenario B

    C. Scenario C

    D. Scenario D

    E. Scenario E

97. Which of the hemodynamic scenarios would be expected during expiration in an intubated patient with a hemodynamically significant pericardial effusion undergoing positive pressure ventilation?

    A. Scenario A

    B. Scenario B

    C. Scenario C

    D. Scenario D

    E. Scenario E

98. Cardiac rhabdomyoma is associated with which of the following?

    A. Down's syndrome

    B. Tuberous sclerosis

    C. Kartagener's syndrome

    D. Noonan's syndrome

    E. Ebstein's anomaly

99. Which of the following is the most likely location of a rhabdomyoma?

    A. Right ventricle

    B. Left ventricle

    C. Left atrium

    D. Right atrium

    E. Aortic root

100. Which of the following tumors usually originates from the cardiac valves or adjacent endocardium?

    A. Papillary fibroelastomas

    B. Myxoma

    C. Angiosarcoma

    D. Fibroma

    E. Rhabdomyoma

101. Which of the following is an absolute contraindication to perioperative TEE?

    A. Obstructing esophageal neoplasms

    B. Esophageal diverticulum

    C. Deformities of the oral pharynx

    D. Large hiatal hernia

    E. Recent esophageal surgery

102. Which of the following is *not* a relative contraindication to TEE probe placement?

    A. Esophageal diverticulum.

    B. Large hiatal hernia.

    C. Recent esophageal or gastric surgery.

    D. Esophageal varices.

    E. All of the above are relative contraindications.

NOTE: Use Table 5.21 to answer the next four (4) questions concerning a patient with left-to-right flow across a patent foramen ovale.

Table 3.21.

CVP = 10 mmHg	V_{AVPeak} = 300 cm/sec	$V_{PFOPeak}$ = 100 cm/sec
TVI_{LVOT} = 9 cm	HR = 100 beats/min	PADP = 12 mmHg
TVI_{AV} = 27 cm	LVOT diameter = 2 cm	BP = 120/80 mmHg

Abbreviations: CVP = central venous pressure, TVI = time velocity integral, BP = systemic blood pressure, LVOT = left ventricular outflow tract, TVI_{LVOT} = time velocity integral in the left ventricular outflow tract, $V_{LVOTPeak}$ = peak velocity in the left ventricular outflow tract, TVI_{AV} = time velocity integral of flow through the aortic valve, HR = heart rate, $V_{PFOPeak}$ = peak left to right flow across a patent foramen ovale, PADP = pulmonary artery diastolic pressure.

103. Given the information in the table, what is the left atrial pressure?

    A. 6 mmHg

    B. 8 mmHg

    C. 10 mmHg

    D. 12 mmHg

    E. 14 mmHg

104. What is the left ventricular stroke volume?

    A. 18 ml

    B. 28 ml

    C. 38 ml

    D. 48 ml

    E. 58 ml

105. What is the left ventricular cardiac output?

    A. 1,800 ml/min

    B. 2,800 ml/min

    C. 3,800 ml/min

    D. 4,800 ml/min

    E. 5,800 ml/min

106. What is the aortic valve area?

    A. 0.8 cm^2

    B. 1.2 cm^2

    C. 2.1 cm^2

    D. 3.4 cm^2

    E. 4.0 cm^2

107. An ultrasound probe interrogates a blood vessel with an incident angle of 0 degrees. The probe emits a frequency of 10 MHz and the returning echoes have a frequency of 10.5 MHz. What is the velocity of blood flow in the vessel?

    A. 8.5 m/s

    B. 18.5 m/s

    C. 28.5 m/s

    D. 38.5 m/s

    E. 48.5 m/s

108. Which of the following views can be used to estimate the right ventricular stroke volume?

    A. Midesophageal ascending aortic short axis view

    B. Upper esophageal aortic arch long axis view

    C. Midesophageal right ventricular inflow/outflow view

    D. Transgastric right ventricular inflow view

    E. Midesophageal bicaval view

109. Which of the following is generally an advantage of the transthoracic echocardiography over TEE?

    A. Superior aortic valve evaluation

    B. Superior mitral valve evaluation

    C. Superior interatrial septum evaluation

    D. Superior sinus of valsalva evaluation

    E. Superior left ventricular apex evaluation

110. Which of the following views is useful for detecting thrombus in the main pulmonary artery?

    A. Midesophageal ascending aortic short axis view

    B. Midesophageal bicaval view

    C. Transgastric right ventricular inflow/outflow view

    D. Midesophageal ascending aortic long axis view

    E. Upper esophageal aortic arch long axis view

111. Which of the following causes of left atrial dilation is least likely to be associated with a left atrial appendage thrombus?

    A. Severe mitral stenosis

    B. Severe mitral regurgitation

    C. Severe left ventricular failure secondary to a dilated cardiomyopathy

    D. Protein C deficiency and ischemic cardiomyopathy

    E. Postpartum cardiomyopathy

112. Which of the following is most likely to present with a holosystolic hepatic venous flow reversal pattern and a normal pulmonary venous flow pattern?

    A. Rheumatic heart disease

    B. History of intravenous drug abuse

    C. Noonan's syndrome

    D. Down's syndrome

    E. Marfan's syndrome

113. Which of the following is the most likely location for bacterial vegetation?

    A. Left ventricular side of the mitral valve.

    B. Left ventricular outflow tract side of the aortic valve.

    C. Right ventricular outflow tract side of the pulmonic valve.

    D. Right ventricular side of the tricuspid valve.

    E. None of the above is a likely location for vegetation.

114. Which of the following is the most common malignant tumor seen extending into the inferior vena cava and the right atrium?

    A. Rhabdomyoma

    B. Melanoma

    C. Colon carcinoma

    D. Renal cell carcinoma

    E. Breast carcinoma

115. Which of the following is true concerning rhabdomyomas?

    A. They are primary intracardiac malignancies.

    B. They are the most common primary cardiac tumors in children.

    C. They are usually found in the left atrium.

    D. They are frequently attached to the aortic valve.

    E. They are more common in patients with Down's syndrome.

116. Which of the following is a benign primary cardiac tumor?

   A. Angiosarcoma

   B. Rhabdomyosarcoma

   C. Mesothelioma

   D. Myxoma

   E. Lymphoma

117. Which of the following would be expected in a patient with dilated cardiomyopathy?

   A. V_{TRpeak} = 100 cm/sec and RAP = 10

   B. Fractional shortening (FS) = 34%

   C. Fractional area change (FAC) = 34%

   D. Mitral valve color flow Doppler regurgitant jet area of 1.6 cm^2

   E. Cardiac index of 4.1 L/min/m^2

118. Which of the following left ventricular wall thickness measurements is consistent with normal left ventricular wall thickness in an adult?

   A. 4 mm

   B. 11 mm

   C. 15 mm

   D. 17 mm

   E. 19 mm

119. A continuous-wave Doppler ultrasound beam is positioned parallel to the left ventricular outflow tract and aortic valve outflow. The patient has a normal Doppler profile at rest. Amyl nitrate is administered and a late-peaking high-velocity systolic jet is observed. Which of the following is the most likely diagnosis?

   A. Hypertrophic cardiomyopathy

   B. Aortic stenosis due to a bicuspid aortic valve

   C. Obstruction due to a subaortic membrane

   D. Aortic stenosis due to rheumatic heart disease

   E. Aortic stenosis due to senile degenerative calcification

120. Which of the following can cause a restrictive cardiomyopathy?

   A. Amyloidosis

   B. Hemochromatosis

   C. Glycogen storage diseases

   D. Sarcoidosis

   E. All of the above

121. A patient has restrictive diastolic dysfunction, normal systolic function, and an apical left ventricular thrombus. The disease also affects the brain, bone marrow, and lungs. Which of the following is the most likely diagnosis?

   A. Hypertrophic cardiomyopathy

   B. Amyloidosis

   C. Hypereosinophilic syndrome

   D. Sarcoidosis

   E. Hemochromatosis

122. Which of the following cannot be measured or estimated reliably by echocardiography in patients with dilated cardiomyopathy?

   A. Pulmonary artery systolic pressure (PASP)

   B. Pulmonary artery mean pressure (PAMP)

   C. Right ventricular systolic pressure (RVSP)

   D. Pulmonary vascular resistance (PVR)

   E. Pulmonary artery diastolic pressure (PADP)

123. Which of the following statements concerning Doppler ultrasound is most likely true?

   A. Continuous-wave ultrasound produces images with better two-dimensional temporal resolution than pulsed-wave ultrasound.

   B. In the best views for obtaining blood flow velocities with Doppler ultrasound the blood flow is perpendicular to the direction of the ultrasound beam.

   C. In the best views for two-dimensional imaging the object of interest is parallel to the path of the ultrasound beam.

   D. None of the above.

NOTE: Use Table 5.2J to answer the next five (5) questions.

Table 5.2J.

LVOT diameter = 2 cm	Heart rate = 100 beats/min
TVI_{AV} = 20 cm	BSA = 2.0 M^2
$V_{peak\ AV}$ = 200 cm/s	MAP = 73 mmHg
$V_{peak\ LVOT}$ = 100 cm/s	$V_{peak\ MV}$ = 76 cm/s

124. Given that the angle between the direction of blood flow through both the aortic valve and the left ventricular outflow tract and the TEE transducer beam is 60 degrees, which of the following is the best estimate of the aortic valve area?

   A. 3.14 cm^2

   B. 1.57 cm^2

   C. 6.28 cm^2

   D. 3.89 cm^2

   E. Cannot be accurately determined because of the 60-degree angle between the ultrasound beam and blood flow

125. If the data in the table were obtained without correcting for the 60-degree angle, what is the best estimate of the pressure gradient across the aortic valve?

   A. 16 mmHg

   B. 32 mmHg

   C. 36 mmHg

   D. 77 mmHg

   E. 144 mmHg

126. What is the best estimate of the stroke volume?

   A. 31.4 cm^3

   B. 62.3 cm^3

   C. 89 cm^3

   D. 100 cm^3

   E. 112 cm^3

127. Which of the following is the best estimate of the cardiac output?

    A. 3,140 ml/min

    B. 6,230 ml/min

    C. 8,900 ml/min

    D. 10,000 ml/min

    E. 11,200 ml/min

128. Which of the following is the best estimate of the cardiac index?

    A. 1.57 L/min/m^2

    B. 3.12 L/min/m^2

    C. 4.45 L/min/m^2

    D. 5.0 L/min/m^2

    E. 5.6 L/min/m^2

129. Which of the following structures is located in the right atrium?

    A. Crista supraventricualris

    B. Cor triatriatum

    C. Coumadin ridge

    D. Chiari network

    E. Moderator band

NOTE: Use Figure 5.2G to answer question 130.

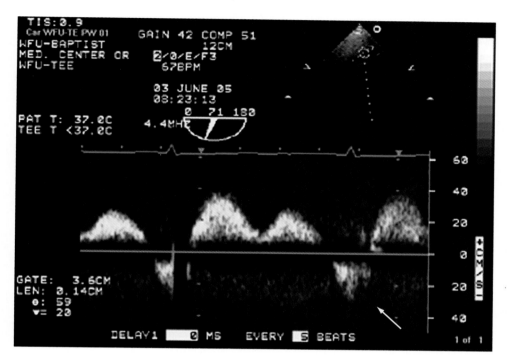

Fig. 5-2G

130. What valvular disorder would most likely be consistent with an abnormal enlargement of the hepatic venous flow wave indicated by the arrow?

    A. Tricuspid regurgitation

    B. Mitral regurgitation

    C. Tricuspid stenosis

    D. Pulmonic stenosis

    E. Mitral stenosis

131. Which of the following views allows assessment of the tricuspid annulus systolic excursion?

    A. Transgastric right ventricular outflow view

    B. Midesophageal right ventricular inflow/outflow view

    C. Transgastric right ventricular inflow view

    D. Transgastric mid papillary short axis view

    E. Midesophageal four-chamber view

132. The deceleration time for the transmitral inflow velocity spectrum by continuous-wave Doppler is 759 ms. What is the mitral valve area?

    A. 1.0 cm^2

    B. 1.5 cm^2

    C. 1.75 cm^2

    D. 2 cm^2

    E. 2.5 cm^2

NOTE: Table 5.2K outlines data from patients who underwent mitral valve repair with a ring annuloplasty and a posterior leaflet resection. Use this information to answer the next question (C-sept distance = distance from the coaptation point to the septum, AL/PL ratio = anterior leaflet length versus post leaflet length TG LVEDd = transgastric left ventricular end diastolic dimension).

Table 5.2K.

Parameter	A	B	C	D	E
C-sept distance (cm)	2.6 cm	1.9 cm	2.2 cm	3.4 cm	3.1 cm
TG LVEDd (mm)	29 mm	27 mm	27 mm	48 mm	51 mm
AL/PL ratio	3.4	0.8	2.7	2.8	0.9
Ring size (mm)	29 mm	27 mm	27 mm	31 mm	31 mm

133. Which of the patients is at highest risk of left ventricular outflow tract obstruction after mitral valve repair?

    A. Patient A

    B. Patient B

    C. Patient C

    D. Patient D

    E. Patient E

134. What percentage of patients develops systolic anterior motion of the anterior mitral valve leaflet with left ventricular outflow tract obstruction after mitral valve repair?

    A. < 1%

    B. 2 to 16%

    C. 16 to 18%

    D. 18 to 20%

    E. > 20%

135. What valve is most commonly affected by rheumatic valvular disease?

    A. Aortic valve.

    B. Mitral valve.

    C. Tricuspid valve.

    D. Pulmonic valve.

    E. The aortic and mitral valves are affected with equal frequency.

Answers:

1. D	23. C	45. C
2. D	24. D	46. B
3. D	25. A	47. C
4. E	26. B	48. A
5. C	27. C	49. A
6. A	28. B	50. D
7. E	29. C	51. C
8. B	30. C	52. D
9. D	31. A	53. D
10. D	32. C	54. C
11. A	33. C	55. D
12. D	34. A	56. E
13. D	35. B	57. B
14. C	36. C	58. B
15. D	37. D	59. A
16. E	38. D	60. A
17. E	39. B	61. D
18. C	40. C	62. D
19. E	41. A	63. D
20. E	42. B	64. B
21. A	43. C	65. B
22. B	44. B	66. B

Answers:—continued

67. E	90. B	113. B
68. A	91. D	114. D
69. C	92. E	115. B
70. D	93. A	116. D
71. D	94. A	117. C
72. C	95. B	118. B
73. A	96. B	119. A
74. C	97. A	120. E
75. D	98. B	121. C
76. E	99. A	122. D
77. B	100. A	123. D
78. D	101. A	124. B
79. E	102. E	125. B
80. A	103. E	126. A
81. A	104. B	127. A
82. B	105. B	128. A
83. A	106. C	129. D
84. A	107. D	130. C
85. C	108. A	131. E
86. A	109. E	132. A
87. B	110. A	133. B
88. A	111. B	134. B
89. C	112. B	135. B

Explanations

1. **Answer = D, 42% is the fractional shortening.** The calculation is as follows.

FS = (LVEDd − LVESd) / LVEDd = (55 mm − 32 mm) / 55 mm = <u>42%</u>.

- FS = fractional shortening
- LVEDd = left ventricular end diastolic dimension
- LVESd = left ventricular end systolic dimension

Reference: Perrino AC, Reeves S. *A Practical Approach to TEE.* Philadelphia: Lippincott Williams & Wilkins 2003:37.

2. **Answer = D, 65% is the fractional area change.** The calculation is as follows.

FAC = (LVEDA − LVESA) / LVEDA = (23.8 cm^2 − 8.1 cm^2) / 23.8 cm^2 = <u>65%</u>.

- FAC = fractional area change
- LVEDA = left ventricular end diastolic area
- LVESA = left ventricular end systolic area

Reference: Sidebotham D, Merry A, Legget M (eds.). *Practical Perioperative Transoesophageal Echocardiography.* Burlington, MA: Butterworth Heinemann 2003:103.

3. **Answer = D, The left ventricular ejection fraction (LVEF) is 68%.** The calculation is as follows.

LVEF = (LVEDVol − LVESVol) / LVEDVol = (130 ml − 42 ml) / 130 ml = <u>68%</u>.

- LVEF = left ventricular ejection fraction
- LVEDVol = left ventricular end diastolic volume
- LVESVol = left ventricular end systolic volume

Reference: Sidebotham D, Merry A, Legget M (eds.). *Practical Perioperative Transoesophageal Echocardiography.* Burlington, MA: Butterworth Heinemann 2003:105.

4. **Answer = E, 1,600 mmHg/sec is the change in pressure with respect to time during isovolumic left ventricular contraction (Dp/dt).** The calculation is as follows.

dp/dt = 32 mmHg / $\Delta t_{MR100-300}$ = 32 mmHg / 0.02 sec = <u>1,600 mmHg/sec</u>.

$\Delta t_{MR100-300}$ = delta t = dt = the time required for a mitral regurgitant jet to accelerate from a velocity of 100 cm/sec to a velocity of 300 cm/sec during isovolumic left ventricular contraction

References: Perrino AC, Reeves S. *A Practical Approach to TEE.* Philadelphia: Lippincott Williams & Wilkins 2003:45; Sidebotham D, Merry A, Legget M (eds.). *Practical Perioperative Transoesophageal Echocardiography.* Burlington, MA: Butterworth Heinemann 2003:107.

5. **Answer = C, 4.4 L/min/m² is the cardiac index.** The calculation is as follows.

$$CI = CO/BSA = 8.8 \text{ L/min} / 2 \text{ m}^2 = 4.4 \text{ L/min/m}^2$$

$$CO = HR * SV = HR * [\text{ TVI}_{MVinflow} * AMV]$$

$$CO = HR * [\text{TVI}_{MVinflow} * 220/PHT_{MV}]$$

$$CO = 100 \text{ beats/min} * [24.7 \text{ cm} * 220/62]$$

$$CO = 8.8 \text{ L/min}$$

Alternative method: SV = [LVEDVol - LVESVol] = 88 ml.

Reference: Sidebotham D, Merry A, Legget M (eds.). *Practical Perioperative Transoesophageal Echocardiography.* Burlington, MA: Butterworth Heinemann 2003:232.

6. **Answer = A, This patient has normal systolic function. All of the parameters calculated in the previous questions are normal.**

Reference: Sidebotham D, Merry A, Legget M (eds.). *Practical Perioperative Transoesophageal Echocardiography.* Burlington, MA: Butterworth Heinemann 2003:102.

7. **Answer = E, Segment 13, the apical anterior wall, is often difficult to image with TEE.** Transthoracic echocardiography usually provides better images of the left ventricular apex, and this is one of the limitations of TEE.

Reference: Sidebotham D, Merry A, Legget M (eds.). *Practical Perioperative Transoesophageal Echocardiography.* Burlington, MA: Butterworth Heinemann 2003:110.

8. **Answer = B, Systolic septal wall thickening occurs with paradoxical septal motion but not with septal dyskinesis.** Paradoxical septal motion occurs with conduction abnormalities and with right ventricular pressure overload. This can be distinguished from true septal dyskinesis, which occurs as a result of septal infarction. In both true septal dyskinesis and paradoxical septal motion the movement of the septum during systole is toward the right ventricle, but with true septal dyskinesis the septum does *not* thicken.

Reference: Sidebotham D, Merry A, Legget M (eds.). *Practical Perioperative Transoesophageal Echocardiography.* Burlington, MA: Butterworth Heinemann 2003:111–112.

9. **Answer = D, The transgastric mid papillary short axis view allows visualization of myocardial segments supplied by all three coronary arteries as wall as calculation of fractional shortening and fractional area change.**

Reference: Sidebotham D, Merry A, Legget M (eds.). *Practical Perioperative Transoesophageal Echocardiography.* Burlington, MA: Butterworth Heinemann 2003:114.

10. **Answer = D, The transgastric mid papillary short axis view allows assessment of volume status (EDA), as well as calculation of fractional shortening and fractional area change.**

Reference: Sidebotham D, Merry A, Legget M (eds.). *Practical Perioperative Transoesophageal Echocardiography.* Burlington, MA: Butterworth Heinemann 2003:114.

11. **Answer = A, An end systolic anterior posterior mid esophageal long axis measurement of greater that 3.6 cm is the best definition of mitral valve annular dilatation.** An end systolic intercommissural measurement of > 4.6 cm is also consistent with mitral valve annular dilatation.

Reference: Sidebotham D, Merry A, Legget M (eds.). *Practical Perioperative Transoesophageal Echocardiography.* Burlington, MA: Butterworth Heinemann 2003:133, 250.

12. **Answer = D, The mid esophageal long axis view is the best view for accurately measuring the mitral regurgitation vena contracta.**

Reference: Sidebotham D, Merry A, Legget M (eds.). *Practical Perioperative Transoesophageal Echocardiography.* Burlington, MA: Butterworth Heinemann 2003:138.

13. **Answer = D, The V-wave cut-off sign on the continuous-wave Doppler profile of the mitral regurgitant jet indicates severe acute mitral regurgitation.** The shape of the mitral regurgitant profile can be diagnostic of the type of mitral regurgitation. Acute regurgitation of a large volume of blood into the left atrium causes a late systolic reduction in the transmitral gradient due to a sharp rise in the left atrial pressure. This causes a late systolic reduction in the mitral regurgitant jet velocity, which gives the Doppler profile an asymmetrical shape known as the V-wave cut-off sign. The large increase in left atrial pressure is seen as a V-wave on a left atrial catheter tracing and hence the name V-wave cut-off sign.

Reference: Sidebotham D, Merry A, Legget M (eds.). *Practical Perioperative Transoesophageal Echocardiography.* Burlington, MA: Butterworth Heinemann 2003:146 (Figure 9.14).

14. **Answer = C, 26 mmHg is the right ventricular systolic pressure (RVSP).** The calculation is as follows.

$$\Delta P = 4V^2$$

$$(RVSP - RAP) = 4V_{TR}^2$$

$$(RVSP - CVP) = 4V^2$$

$$RVSP = 4V^2 + CVP$$

$$RVSP = 4(2 \text{ m/s})^2 + 10$$

$$RVSP = 26 \text{ mmHg}$$

$$PASP = RVSP = 26 \text{ mmHg}$$

- PASP = pulmonary artery systolic pressure
- RVSP = right ventricular systolic pressure
- RAP = right atrial pressure
- CVP = central venous pressure
- V_{TR} = peak velocity of the tricuspid valve regurgitant jet

Reference: Otto C. *Textbook of Clinical Echocardiography, Third Edition.* Philadelphia: Elsevier 2004:463.

15. **Answer = D, 2.0 cm^2 is the mitral valve area.** The calculation is as follows.

MVA = 220/PHT

MVA = 220/110

MVA = 2.0 cm^2

- $PHT_{MVinflow}$ = pressure half time of diastolic mitral inflow
- MVA = mitral valve area

Reference: Perrino AC, Reeves S. *A Practical Approach to TEE.* Philadelphia: Lippincott Williams & Wilkins 2003:105.

16. **Answer = E, 60 ml is the mitral valve stroke volume.** The calculation is as follows.

SV_{MV} = A_{MV} * $TVI_{MVinflow}$

SV_{MV} = 2.0 cm^2 * 30 cm

SV_{MV} = 60 cm^3

MVA = 220/PHT

MVA = 220/110

MVA = 2.0 cm^2

- $PHT_{MVinflow}$ = pressure half time of diastolic mitral inflow
- MVA = mitral valve area
- SV_{MV} = mitral valve stroke volume
- A_{MV} = mitral valve area
- $TVI_{MVinflow}$ = time velocity integral of mitral valve inflow

Reference: Sidebotham D, Merry A, Legget M (eds.). *Practical Perioperative Transoesophageal Echocardiography.* Burlington, MA: Butterworth Heinemann 2003:231.

17. **Answer = E, 6 L/min is the mitral valve cardiac output.** The calculation is as follows.

$$\text{CO} = \text{HR} * \text{SV} = (100 \text{ beats/min}) * (60 \text{ ml/beat}) = 6 \text{ L/min}$$

$$\text{SV}_{MV} = \text{A}_{MV} * \text{TVI}_{MVinflow}$$

$$\text{SV}_{MV} = 2.0 \text{ cm}^2 * 30 \text{ cm}$$

$$\text{SV}_{MV} = 60 \text{ cm}^3$$

$$\text{MVA} = 220/\text{PHT}$$

$$\text{MVA} = 220/110$$

$$\text{MVA} = 2.0 \text{ cm}^2$$

- $\text{PHTM}_{Vinflow}$ = pressure half time of diastolic mitral inflow
- MVA = mitral valve area = A_{MV}
- SV_{MV} = mitral valve stroke volume
- A_{MV} = mitral valve area
- HR = heart rate
- $\text{TVI}_{MVinflow}$ = time velocity integral of mitral valve inflow
- CO = cardiac output

Reference: Sidebotham D, Merry A, Legget M (eds.). *Practical Perioperative Transoesophageal Echocardiography.* Burlington, MA: Butterworth Heinemann 2003:231.

18. **Answer = C, 3 L/min/m² is the cardiac index.** The calculation is as follows.

$$\text{CI} = \text{CO}/\text{BSA} = (6 \text{ L/min}) / (2 \text{ m}^2) = 3 \text{ L/min/m}^2$$

- CI = cardiac index
- BSA = body surface area

Reference: Sidebotham D, Merry A, Legget M (eds.). *Practical Perioperative Transoesophageal Echocardiography.* Burlington, MA: Butterworth Heinemann 2003:231.

19. **Answer = E, It cannot be determined from the given data.** The continuity principle cannot be utilized in this case because tricuspid regurgitation is present. You are given the velocity of the tricuspid regurgitant jet (V_{TRpeak}), and this is the hint that alerts you to the presence of tricuspid regurgitation.

Reference: Sidebotham D, Merry A, Legget M (eds.). *Practical Perioperative Transoesophageal Echocardiography.* Burlington, MA: Butterworth Heinemann 2003:233.

20. **Answer = E, 60 cm³ is the stroke volume of blood flow through the pulmonary artery (SV$_{PA}$).** The calculation is as follows.

$SV_{PA} = A_{PA} * TVI_{PA}$

$SV_{PA} = \pi r^2 * TVI_{PA}$

$SV_{PA} = \pi (1.2)^2 * (13.26)$

$SV_{PA} = 60 \text{ cm}^3$

Reference: Sidebotham D, Merry A, Legget M (eds.). *Practical Perioperative Transoesophageal Echocardiography.* Burlington, MA: Butterworth Heinemann 2003:231.

21. **Answer = A, No mitral regurgitation is present.** The continuity principle works for the mitral valve (SV$_{PA}$ = SV$_{MV}$). Thus, no MR is present.

Reference: Sidebotham D, Merry A, Legget M (eds.). *Practical Perioperative Transoesophageal Echocardiography.* Burlington, MA: Butterworth Heinemann 2003:233.

22. **Answer = B, The right coronary cusp of the aortic valve is indicated by arrow 1.**

23. **Answer = C, The right ventricle is shown by arrow 2.**

24. **Answer = D, Aortic stenosis is indicated by a narrowing of the aortic valve leaflets.**

25. **Answer = A, Hypertrophic obstructive cardiomyopathy is indicated by midsystolic closure of the aortic valve followed by a coarse fluttering of the aortic valve leaflets.**

Reference: Otto C. *Textbook of Clinical Echocardiography, Third Edition.* Philadelphia: Elsevier 2004:237.

26. **Answer = B, Arrow 3 indicates the left atrium.**

27. **Answer = C, Wavelength (λ) and pulse duration are directly related.** As wavelength increases pulse duration increases. Spatial pulse length and lateral resolution are not related, as lateral resolution is determined by beam width. Pulse repetition frequency (PRF) and imaging depth are inversely related. PRF and pulse repetition period (PRP) are reciprocals.

Reference: Kremkau FW. *Diagnostic Ultrasound: Principles Instruments and Exercises, Third Edition.* Philadelphia: Saunders 1989:22.

28. **Answer = B, Intensity is proportional to the amplitude squared.** The units of intensity are watts/cm², as intensity = power divided by the cross sectional area of the ultrasound beam. Both intensity and power are proportional to the amplitude squared. Intensity is initially determined by the ultrasound system only, not the medium. The intensity of an ultrasound beam is attenuated more by high-frequency transducers than by low-frequency transducers.

Reference: Kremkau FW. *Diagnostic Ultrasound: Principles Instruments and Exercises, Third Edition.* Philadelphia: Saunders 1989:27–30.

29. **Answer = C, Spatial peak temporal average intensity (SPTA) correlates most readily with the heating of tissues and this makes it the most relevant with regard to the bioeffects of ultrasound.**

Reference: Edelman SK. *Understanding Ultrasound Physics.* Woodlands, TX: ESP, Inc. 1994:45.

30. **Answer = C, SPTP intensity for CW ultrasound is the same as SPTA because the beam is continuous over time.** Continuous-wave (CW) ultrasound cannot produce two-dimensional images, is not subject to aliasing, and has a duty factor of 1.0. The duty factor is 1.0 (100%) because with continuous-wave ultrasound the beam is always "on."

Reference: Edelman SK. *Understanding Ultrasound Physics.* Woodlands, TX: ESP, Inc. 1994.

31. **Answer = A, A doubling of the intensity can be represented as +3 dB.** For intensity, dB = 10 Log I_2/I_1, where I_2 is the new intensity and I_1 is the initial or reference intensity. In this case, 10 Log I_2/I_1 = ?. If the intensity is doubled, I_2/I_1 is equal to 2 and this substitution yields 10 Log2 = X, → X = 3.

Reference: http://www.phys.unsw.edu.au/~jw/dB.html.

32. **Answer = C, 10 dB/cm.** In soft tissue, the attenuation coefficient can be estimated as half the frequency. Attenuation coefficient = 1/2 frequency (dB = decibels).

Reference: Edelman SK. *Understanding Ultrasound Physics.* Woodlands, TX: ESP, Inc. 1994:54.

33. **Answer = C, 80 decibels (dB) of attenuation.** For soft tissue, the attenuation coefficient (AC) = 1/2 frequency. The amount of attenuation is equal to the attenuation coefficient times the path length. Therefore, the total amount of attenuation is 10 dB/cm * 8 cm = 80 dB.

Reference: Edelman SK. *Understanding Ultrasound Physics.* Woodlands, TX: ESP, Inc. 1994:54.

34. **Answer = A, 0.33 cm = the thickness of tissue required to reduce the power of an 18-MHz transducer by half.** For ultrasound in soft tissue:

Half *power distance* = 3 dB/AC = 3 dB/9 db/cm = 0.33 cm.
  • AC = attenuation coefficient = 1/2 frequency

Reference: Edelman SK. *Understanding Ultrasound Physics.* Woodlands, TX: ESP, Inc. 1994:56.

35. **Answer = B, Medium 2. Impedance = density * velocity.**

Reference: Kremkau FW. *Diagnostic Ultrasound: Principles Instruments and Exercises, Third Edition.* Philadelphia: Saunders 1989:293.

36. **Answer = C, The matching layer has an acoustic impedance between that of the piezoelectric crystal (PZT) and the skin.** The matching layer serves to decrease the amount of reflection that occurs at the interface of the crystal and the skin. This will maximize the amount of transmission through the skin. Spatial pulse length, Q factor, and bandwidth are all altered by the damping material (backing material), not the matching layer.

(Acoustic impedance: PZT > matching layer > gel > skin.)

Reference: Edelman SK. *Understanding Ultrasound Physics.* Woodlands, TX: ESP, Inc. 1994:74.

37. **Answer = D, Crystal D has the longest focal length.** For ultrasound: focal length = length of the near field = $L_n = r^2/\lambda$, where r = radius of the piezoelectric crystal and λ = wavelength.

Reference: Perrino AC, Reeves S. *A Practical Approach to TEE.* Philadelphia: Lippincott Williams & Wilkins 2003:10.

38. **Answer = D, As frequency increases focal depth (near-zone length) increases.** This seems somewhat counterintuitive, given that higher-frequency transducers are more subject to attenuation and therefore penetrate soft tissues less readily. Crystal manufacturers use small-diameter crystals to decrease the focal depth of high-frequency transducers to allow high resolution of shallow structures. Choice A is incorrect because frequency does not increase as spatial pulse length increases. Choice B is incorrect because as frequency increases attenuation increases. Choice C is wrong because velocity is determined by the medium through which sound travels, not the frequency. Choice E is wrong because as piezoelectric crystal thickness increases frequency increases.

Reference: Edelman SK. *Understanding Ultrasound Physics.* Woodlands, TX: ESP, Inc. 1994:81–82.

39. **Answer = B, *Decreasing the ultrasound frequency* will most likely create an ultrasound beam with a *shallow focus* (short near-zone length).** Acoustic impedance has nothing to do with the length of the focal zone (near-zone length)(focal depth). Increasing the piezoelectric crystal diameter will increase the near-zone length (focal depth). Decreasing the crystal thickness will increase the frequency of the ultrasound beam, and thereby increase the focal depth (near-zone length). Focal length = length of the near field = $L_n = r^2/\lambda$, r = radius of the piezoelectric crystal, λ = wavelength.

Reference: Edelman SK. *Understanding Ultrasound Physics.* Woodlands, TX: ESP, Inc. 1994:81–82.

40. **Answer = C, 3.4 mm = the best estimate of the lateral resolution at a depth of 7 cm.** If the near-zone length is 6 cm, the focus lies at 6 cm. For an unfocused ultrasound beam, the beam diameter at the focus is 1/2 the crystal diameter (in this case, 3 mm). Therefore, at 7 cm (just distal to the focus) the beam diameter should be a little greater than 1/2 the crystal diameter (about 3.4 mm). Because lateral resolution is equal to the beam diameter the lateral resolution is equal to 3.4 mm.

Reference: Edelman SK. *Understanding Ultrasound Physics.* Woodlands, TX: ESP, Inc. 1994:83, 92.

41. **Answer = A, As spatial pulse length (SPL) increases the numerical value of axial resolution increases.** Axial resolution = 1/2 SPL. The lower the numerical value the better the image quality and thus the higher the spatial resolution. *Depth resolution* is a synonym of *axial resolution*. Therefore, it is decreased (numerical value increased) by increasing SPL. Lateral resolution is determined by beam width. It is not related to SPL. Note that *spatial resolution* is a term that includes both lateral and axial (depth) resolution. It refers to the ability to accurately image two small closely located structures and display them in their correct anatomic location.

Reference: Edelman SK. *Understanding Ultrasound Physics.* Woodlands, TX: ESP, Inc. 1994:89, 90.

42. **Answer = B, Most TEE probes are linear phased-array transducers.**

Reference: Perrino AC, Reeves S. *A Practical Approach to TEE.* Philadelphia: Lippincott Williams & Wilkins 2003:10.

43. **Answer = C, X axis = time, Y axis = depth.**

44. **Answer = B, Lateral resolution is improved.** When multiple focal zones are used, the beam width along each scan line is decreased and lateral resolution is improved. Multiple focal zones means multiple narrow focal points exist along the scan line and the overall beam width is narrower. This requires more pulses per scan line and thereby it takes more time to produce each scan line. Because it takes more time to produce each scan line, it takes more time to create each image/frame and the frame rate (frames/sec) is decreased. Line density (the number of lines per image/frame) is not affected.

Reference: Edelman SK. *Understanding Ultrasound Physics.* Woodlands, TX: ESP, Inc. 1994:124.

45. **Answer = C, Measurement of very high velocities is a major advantage of continuous-wave ultrasound.** Continuous-wave Doppler cannot produce images. Only pulsed ultrasound can produce images. There are two definitions for range resolution: (1) range resolution = depth or axial resolution and (2) range resolution = the ability to determine the location/origin of a returning echo. In neither case is range resolution a property of continuous-wave ultrasound. Axial resolution refers to image quality and continuous-wave ultrasound cannot create images. In addition, continuous-wave ultrasound cannot determine the origin of echoes (range ambiguity). Similarly, azimuthal (lateral) resolution is a property of pulsed ultrasound, as only pulsed ultrasound is capable of image production.

Reference: Edelman SK. *Understanding Ultrasound Physics.* Woodlands, TX: ESP, Inc. 1994:134–137.

46. **Answer = B, A sample gate or sample volume provides range resolution with pulsed-wave Doppler (PWD).** High velocities cannot be measured with pulsed-wave Doppler, and this is the major disadvantage of PWD. High velocities are best measured with continuous-wave Doppler.

The Nyquist limit (Nyquist frequency) is a property of pulsed ultrasound. It is the Doppler frequency shift above which aliasing occurs. Continuous-wave Doppler (CWD) is not subject to aliasing and therefore does not have a Nyquist frequency.

Reference: Edelman SK. *Understanding Ultrasound Physics.* Woodlands, TX: ESP, Inc. 1994:137.

47. **Answer = C, 90 degrees = the angle of incidence that will provide the best two-dimensional TEE images.**

Reference: Edelman SK. *Understanding Ultrasound Physics.* Woodlands, TX: ESP, Inc. 1994:137.

48. **Answer = A, Increasing the pulse repetition frequency (PRF) will decrease the aliasing of pulsed-wave Doppler.** Aliasing occurs when $\Delta F \geq$ the Nyquist limit = 1/2 PRF. Therefore, if PRF increases aliasing will decrease. Line density is unrelated to aliasing. Increasing the depth of the sample volume will increase aliasing because PRF decreases as depth increases. Increasing the transmitted frequency (Ft) will increase aliasing by increasing ΔF because $\Delta F = V \cos \theta\, 2\, (F_t)\, /\, C$.

Reference: Edelman SK. *Understanding Ultrasound Physics.* Woodlands, TX: ESP, Inc. 1994:134–137.

49. **Answer = A, Using a continuous-wave Doppler ultrasound transducer will eliminate aliasing artifact and allow high flow velocities to be measured.** Using a higher frequency, placing the sample volume at a deeper depth, and decreasing the pulse repetition frequency will all increase aliasing artifact.

Reference: Edelman SK. *Understanding Ultrasound Physics.* Woodlands, TX: ESP, Inc. 1994:133–137.

50. **Answer = D, The ability to measure high velocities is a property of continuous-wave Doppler (CWD).** Range resolution, aliasing artifact, and sample volume are associated with pulsed-wave Doppler (PWD). There are two definitions for range resolution: (1) range resolution = depth or axial resolution and (2) range resolution = the ability to determine the location/origin of a returning echo. In neither case is range resolution a property of continuous-wave ultrasound. Aliasing artifact occurs when $\Delta F \geq$ 1/2 PRF = Nyquist frequency, with pulsed-wave Doppler. For continuous-wave Doppler the pulse repetition frequency is essentially infinite, and a Doppler shift of 1/2 infinity is impossible. Thus, continuous-wave Doppler is not subject to aliasing. The sample volume or sample gate is the region of interest where blood flow velocities are interrogated with pulsed-wave Doppler.

Reference: Edelman SK. *Understanding Ultrasound Physics.* Woodlands, TX: ESP, Inc. 1994:137.

51. **Answer = C, Aliasing artifact is associated with pulsed-wave Doppler.** Aliasing artifact occurs when $\Delta F \geq$ 1/2 PRF = Nyquist frequency, with pulsed-wave Doppler. When this occurs, velocity measurements are

inaccurate, ambiguous, and indeterminate. Range ambiguity refers to the inability of continuous-wave Doppler measurements to determine the location/position of a given velocity measurement. Pulsed-wave Doppler cannot measure high velocities because of aliasing artifact. Doppler detection of blood flow velocities cannot occur with orthogonal or perpendicular incidence.

Reference: Edelman SK. *Understanding Ultrasound Physics.* Woodlands, TX: ESP, Inc. 1994:137.

52. **Answer = D, 20 mmHg is the right ventricular systolic pressure (RVSP).** This is calculated as follows.

$\Delta P = 4V^2$

$\Delta P = 4 (V_{VSD})^2$

$(LVSP - RVSP) = 4 (V_{VSD})^2$

$(SBP - RVSP) = 4 (V_{VSD})^2$

$-RVSP = 4 (V_{VSD})^2 - SBP$

$RVSP = SBP - 4 (V_{VSD})^2$

$RVSP = 120 - 4(5 \text{ m/s})^2$

$RVSP = 20 \text{ mmHg}$

- LVSP = left ventricular systolic pressure
- SBP = systolic blood pressure
- RVSP = right ventricular systolic pressure
- V_{VSD} = velocity of flow across the ventricular septal defect

Reference: Perrino AC, Reeves S. *A Practical Approach to TEE.* Philadelphia: Lippincott Williams & Wilkins 2003:291.

53. **Answer = D, 46 mmHg is the pulmonary artery mean pressure.** This is calculated as follows.

$\Delta P = 4V^2$

$(PAMP - RVDP) = 4 (V_{Plearly})^2$

$(PAMP - CVP) = 4 (V_{Plearly})^2$

$PAMP = 4 (V_{Plearly})^2 + CVP$

$PAMP = 4 (V_{Plearly})^2 + CVP$

$PAMP = 4(3 \text{ m/s})^2 + 10$

$PAMP = 46 \text{ mmHg}$

- PAMP = pulmonary artery mean pressure
- CVP = central venous pressure
- RVDP = right ventricular diastolic pressure
- $V_{Plearly}$ = the early peak velocity of the pulmonic insufficiency jet obtained with CWD
- CWD = continuous-wave Doppler
- ΔP = change in pressure (pressure gradient)

Reference: Perrino AC, Reeves S. *A Practical Approach to TEE.* Philadelphia: Lippincott Williams & Wilkins 2003:104.

54. **Answer = C, 36 = the pulmonary artery diastolic pressure.** This is calculated as follows.

$$\Delta P = 4V^2$$

$$(PADP - RVDP) = 4\,(V_{PIlate})^2$$

$$(PADP - CVP) = 4\,(V_{PIlate})^2$$

$$PADP = 4\,(V_{PIlate})^2 + CVP$$

$$PADP = 4\,(V_{PIlate})^2 + CVP$$

$$PADP = 4(2.55\ m/s)^2 + 10$$

$$PADP = 36\ mmHg$$

- PADP = pulmonary artery diastolic pressure
- CVP = central venous pressure
- RVDP = right ventricular diastolic pressure
- V_{PIlate} = the late peak velocity of the pulmonic insufficiency jet obtained with CWD
- CWD = continuous-wave Doppler
- ΔP = change in pressure (pressure gradient)

Reference: Perrino AC, Reeves S. *A Practical Approach to TEE.* Philadelphia: Lippincott Williams & Wilkins 2003:104.

55. **Answer = D, 20 mmHg is the best estimate of the pulmonary artery systolic pressure.** Assuming there is no pulmonary artery stenosis, the right ventricular systolic pressure is equal to the pulmonary artery systolic pressure (PASP). This is calculated as follows.

$$\Delta P = 4V^2$$

$$\Delta P = 4\,(V_{VSD})^2$$

$$(LVSP - RVSP) = 4\,(V_{VSD})^2$$

$$(SBP - RVSP) = 4\,(V_{VSD})^2$$

$$-RVSP = 4\,(V_{VSD})^2 - SBP$$

$$RVSP = SBP - 4\,(V_{VSD})^2$$

$$RVSP = 120 - 4(5\ m/s)^2$$

$$RVSP = 20\ mmHg = PASP$$

- LVSP = left ventricular systolic pressure
- SBP = systolic blood pressure
- RVSP = right ventricular systolic pressure
- V_{VSD} = velocity of flow across the ventricular septal defect

Reference: Perrino AC, Reeves S. *A Practical Approach to TEE.* Philadelphia: Lippincott Williams & Wilkins 2003:291.

56. Answer = E, 76 cm³ = the right ventricular stroke volume (SV_RV).

The calculation is as follows.

$$SV_{RV} = TVI_{PA} * \pi r^2$$

$$SV_{RV} = (20 \text{ cm}) * \pi (1.1)^2$$

$$SV_{RV} = 76 \text{ cm}^3$$

- SV_{RV} = right ventricular stroke volume
- TVI_{PA} = main pulmonary artery time velocity integral
- r = radius of the main pulmonary artery

Reference: Sidebotham D, Merry A, Legget M (eds.). *Practical Perioperative Transoesophageal Echocardiography.* Burlington, MA: Butterworth Heinemann 2003:231.

57. Answer = B, 6.1 L = the right ventricular cardiac output. The

calculation is as follows.

$$CO_{RV} = SV_{PA} * HR$$

$$CO_{RV} = TVI_{PA} * \pi r^2 * HR$$

$$CO_{RV} = (20 \text{ cm}) * \pi (1.1)^2 * 80 \text{ beats/min}$$

$$CO_{RV} = 76 \text{ cm}^3 * 80 \text{ beats/min}$$

$$CO_{RV} = 6.1 \text{ L/min}$$

- CO_{RV} = right ventricular cardiac output
- SV_{PA} = stroke volume in the main pulmonary artery
- HR = heart rate
- TVI_{PA} = time velocity integral of flow in the main pulmonary artery

Reference: Sidebotham D, Merry A, Legget M (eds.). *Practical Perioperative Transoesophageal Echocardiography.* Burlington, MA: Butterworth Heinemann 2003:231.

58. Answer = B, 47 cm³ = the left ventricular stroke volume. The

calculation is as follows.

$$SV_{LVOT} = A_{LVOT} * TVI_{LVOT}$$

$$SV_{LVOT} = \pi r^2 * TVI_{LVOT}$$

$$SV_{LVOT} = \pi (1)^2 * (15)$$

$$SV_{LVOT} = 47 \text{ cm}^3$$

- SV_{LVOT} = stroke volume in the left ventricular outflow tract
- TVI_{LVOT} = time velocity integral of flow through the left ventricle outflow tract
- A = area of the left ventricular outflow tract
- r = radius of the left ventricular outflow tract

Reference: Sidebotham D, Merry A, Legget M (eds.). *Practical Perioperative Transoesophageal Echocardiography.* Burlington, MA: Butterworth Heinemann 2003:231.

59. **Answer = A, 1.89 L/min/m² = the left ventricular cardiac index (CI).**
The calculation is as follows.

$$SV_{LVOT} = A_{LVOT} * TVI_{LVOT}$$

$$SV_{LVOT} = \pi r^2 * TVI_{LVOT}$$

$$SV_{LVOT} = \pi (1)^2 * (15)$$

$$SV_{LVOT} = 47 \text{ cm}^3$$

$$CI_{LVOT} = CO_{LVOT} / BSA$$

$$CI_{LVOT} = SV * HR / BSA$$

$$CI_{LVOT} = (47 \text{ cm}^3) * (80 \text{ beats/min}) / 2 \text{ m}^2$$

$$CI_{LVOT} = 1.89 \text{ L/min/m}^2$$

- SV_{LVOT} = stroke volume in the left ventricular outflow tract
- TVI_{LVOT} = time velocity integral of flow through the left ventricle outflow tract
- A = area of the left ventricular outflow tract
- r = radius of the left ventricular outflow tract

Reference: Sidebotham D, Merry A, Legget M (eds.). *Practical Perioperative Transoesophageal Echocardiography.* Burlington, MA: Butterworth Heinemann 2003:231.

60. **Answer = A, 1.62 = the ratio of pulmonic flow to systemic flow (Q_P/Q_S).** The calculation is as follows.

$$Q_P/Q_S = CO_{RV}/CO_{LV} = SV_{RV}/SV_{LVOT} = 76/47 = 1.62$$

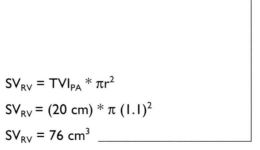

$$SV_{LVOT} = A_{LVOT} * TVI_{LVOT}$$

$$SV_{LVOT} = \pi r^2 * TVI_{LVOT}$$

$$SV_{LVOT} = \pi (1)^2 * (15)$$

$$SV_{LVOT} = 47 \text{ cm}^3$$

$$SV_{RV} = TVI_{PA} * \pi r^2$$

$$SV_{RV} = (20 \text{ cm}) * \pi (1.1)^2$$

$$SV_{RV} = 76 \text{ cm}^3$$

- SV_{RV} = right ventricular stroke volume
- TVI_{PA} = main pulmonary artery time velocity integral
- r = radius of the main pulmonary artery
- CO_{RV} = right ventricular cardiac output
- CO_{LV} = left ventricular cardiac output
- Q_P/Q_S = the ratio of pulmonic to systemic (LV) flow

Reference: Sidebotham D, Merry A, Legget M (eds.). *Practical Perioperative Transoesophageal Echocardiography.* Burlington, MA: Butterworth Heinemann 2003:231.

61. **Answer = D, 3.0 cm² is the mitral valve area.** This is calculated using the deceleration time (DT) of the diastolic mitral inflow continuous-wave Doppler spectrum. The calculation is as follows.

MVA = 759/DT

MVA = 759/253

MVA = 3.0 cm^2

Reference: Perrino AC, Reeves S. *A Practical Approach to TEE.* Philadelphia: Lippincott Williams & Wilkins 2003:152.

62. **Answer = D, 2.25 cm² is the aortic valve area (AVA) (A_{AV}).** The calculation involves the continuity principle.

$Q_{AV} = Q_{MV}$

$SV_{AV} = SV_{MV}$

$A_{AV} * TVI_{AV} = A_{MV} * TVI_{MV}$

$A_{AV} = A_{MV} * TVI_{MV} / TVI_{AV}$

$A_{AV} = 3.0 \text{ cm}^2 * 15 \text{ cm} / 20 \text{ cm}$

$A_{AV} = 2.25 \text{ cm}^2$

Reference: Otto C. *Textbook of Clinical Echocardiography, Third Edition.* Philadelphia: Elsevier 2004:287.

63. **Answer = D, 25 mmHg is the peak instantaneous systolic pressure gradient across the aortic valve.** The calculation is as follows.

$\Delta P = 4V^2$

$\Delta P_{AV} = 4(V_{AV})^2$

$\Delta P_{AV} = 4(2.5 \text{ m/s})^2$

$\Delta P_{AV} = 25 \text{ mmHg}$

Reference: Savage RM, Aronson S, Thomas JD, Shanewise JS, Shernan SK. *Comprehensive Textbook of Intraoperative Transesophageal Echocardiography.* Philadelphia: Lippincott Williams & Wilkins 2004:15.

64. **Answer = B, 4.5 L/min is the cardiac output.** The calculation is as follows.

CO = HR * SV

CO = HR * SV_{MV}

CO = HR * A_{MV} * TVI_{MV}

CO = 100 beats/min * 3.0 cm^2 * 15 cm

- CO = 4.5 L/min
- CO = cardiac output
- HR = heart rate
- SV = stroke volume
- MV = mitral valve

- A_{MV} = mitral valve area
- TVI_{MV} = time velocity integral of diastolic mitral inflow
- SV_{MV} = stroke volume through the mitral valve

Reference: Sidebotham D, Merry A, Legget M (eds.). *Practical Perioperative Transoesophageal Echocardiography.* Burlington, MA: Butterworth Heinemann 2003:232.

65. **Answer = B, 2.25 L/min/m^2 is the cardiac index.** The calculation is as follows.

$$CI = CO/BSA = 4.5/2 = 2.25 \text{ L/min/m}^2$$

$CO = HR * SV$

$CO = HR * SV_{MV}$

$CO = HR * A_{MV} * TVI_{MV}$

$CO = 100 \text{ beats/min} * 3.0 \text{ cm}^2 * 15 \text{ cm}$

$CO = 4.5 \text{ L/min}$

Reference: Sidebotham D, Merry A, Legget M (eds.). *Practical Perioperative Transoesophageal Echocardiography.* Burlington, MA: Butterworth Heinemann 2003:232.

66. **Answer = B, 1 valve area by the pressure half time method.** The calculation is as follows.

$MVA = 220/PHT$

$MVA = 220/169$

$MVA = 1.3 \text{ cm}^2$

- $PHT_{MVinflow}$ = pressure half time of diastolic mitral inflow
- MVA = mitral valve area

Reference: Perrino AC, Reeves S. *A Practical Approach to TEE.* Philadelphia: Lippincott Williams & Wilkins 2003:105.

67. **Answer = E, 78 cm^3 is the mitral valve stroke volume.** The calculation is as follows.

$SV_{MV} = A_{MV} * TVI_{MVinflow}$

$SV_{MV} = 1.3 \text{ cm}^2 * 60 \text{ cm}$

$SV_{MV} = 78 \text{ cm}^3$

$MVA = 220/PHT$

$MVA = 220/169$

$MVA = 1.3 \text{ cm}^2$

Reference: Sidebotham D, Merry A, Legget M (eds.). *Practical Perioperative Transoesophageal Echocardiography.* Burlington, MA: Butterworth Heinemann 2003:231.

68. **Answer = A, 45 cm³ is the mitral valve regurgitant volume (MVRVol).** The calculation is as follows.

$$MVRVol = SV_{MV} - SV_{PA}$$

$$MVRVol = 78\ cm^3 - 33\ cm^3$$

$$MVRVol = 45\ cm^3$$

$$SV_{PA} = CI_{PA} * BSA\ /\ HR$$

$$SV_{PA} = 1.5\ L/min/m^2 * 2.2\ m^2\ /\ 100\ beats/min$$

$$SV_{PA} = 33\ cm^3$$

$$SV_{MV} = A_{MV} * TVI_{MVinflow}$$

$$SV_{MV} = 1.3\ cm^2 * 60\ cm$$

$$SV_{MV} = 78\ cm^3$$

$$MVA = 220/PHT$$

$$MVA = 220/169$$

$$MVA = 1.3\ cm^2$$

- MVA = A_{MV} = mitral valve area
- SV = stroke volume
- CI = cardiac index
- PA = pulmonary artery
- BSA = body surface area
- HR = heart rate
- TVI = time velocity integral
- MV = mitral valve

Reference: SCA/ASE Annual Comprehensive Review and Update of Perioperative Hemodynamics Workshop. 17 Feb. 2005, San Diego, CA; discussion lead by Stanton Shernon, et al.

69. **Answer = C 0.45 cm² is the mitral valve regurgitant orifice area (MVROA).** The calculation is as follows.

$$MVROA = RVol\ /\ TVI_{MR}$$

$$MVROA = 45\ cm^3\ /\ 100\ cm$$

$$MVROA = 0.45\ cm^2$$

- RVol = mitral valve regurgitant volume
- TVI_{MR} = time velocity integral of the mitral valve regurgitant jet

Reference: SCA/ASE Annual Comprehensive Review and Update of Perioperative Hemodynamics Workshop. 17 Feb. 2005, San Diego, CA; discussion lead by Stanton Shernon, et al.

70. **Answer = D, 58% is the mitral valve regurgitant fraction (MVRegFx).** The calculation is as follows.

MVRegFx = RVol / SV_{MV}

MVRegFx = 45 cm^3 / 78 cm^3

MVRegFx = 58%

- RVol = mitral valve regurgitant volume
- SV_{MV} = stroke volume of diastolic mitral inflow

Reference: SCA/ASE Annual Comprehensive Review and Update of Perioperative Hemodynamics Workshop. 17 Feb. 2005, San Diego, CA; discussion lead by Stanton Shernon, et al.

71. **Answer = D, Severe mitral regurgitation is present.** A mitral valve regurgitant fraction (MVRegFx) of 58% and a mitral valve regurgitant orifice area (MVROA) of 0.45 cm^2 are consistent with severe mitral regurgitation. (See Table 5.2L.)

Reference: Perrino AC, Reeves S. *A Practical Approach to TEE.* Philadelphia: Lippincott Williams & Wilkins 2003:137.

Table 5.2L.   GRADING OF MR

Method	Mild	Moderate	Severe
MVROA	< 0.1 cm^2	0.10–0.25 cm^2	> 0.25 cm^2
MVRegFx	< 30%	30–50%	> 50%

72. **Answer = C, Moderate mitral stenosis is present.** A mitral valve area of 1.3 cm^2 is consistent with moderate mitral stenosis. (See Table 5.2M.)

Reference: Perrino AC, Reeves S. *A Practical Approach to TEE.* Philadelphia: Lippincott Williams & Wilkins 2003:150.

Table 5.2M.   GRADING OF MS

Method	Mild	Moderate	Severe
MVA	1.6–2.0 cm^2	1.0–1.5 cm^2	< 1.0 cm^2

73. **Answer = A, a DeBakey type I dissection involves the aortic arch and therefore will most likely require deep hypothermic circulatory arrest to facilitate repair.** (See Tables 5.2N and 5.2O.)

Table 5.2N.   CRAWFORD CLASSIFICATION FOR THORACOABDOMINAL ANEURYSMS

Type	Origin	Extends Distally to:
I	Near left subclavian artery	Above renal arteries
II	Near left subclavian artery	Below renal arteries
III	More distal than types I or II but above the diaphragm	Below renal arteries
IV	Below the diaphragm (abdominal)	Below renal arteries

Table 5.2O. DEBAKEY CLASSIFICATION FOR AORTIC DISSECTIONS

Type	Origin	Extends Distally to:	Stanford Classification
I	Ascending thoracic aorta	Aortic bifurcation	A
II	Ascending thoracic aorta	Brachiocephalic trunk (ends before the arch)	A
IIIa	Near the left subclavian A.	Above the diaphragm	B
IIIb	Near the left subclavian A.	Aortic bifurcation	B

Reference: Perrino AC, Reeves S. *A Practical Approach to TEE.* Philadelphia: Lippincott Williams & Wilkins 2003:252–254.

74. **Answer = C, Beta blockers are beneficial because they decrease the ejection velocity.** A Stanford class A dissection is shown. The mortality rate is 72% with medical management and 32% with surgical management. Therefore, surgery is recommended. The coronary arteries are involved in < 20% of acute aortic dissections.

Reference: Hensley FA, Martin DE, Gravlee GP. *A Practical Approach to Cardiac Anesthesia, Third Edition.* Philadelphia: Lippincott Williams & Wilkins. 2002:621.

75. **Answer = D, A Stanford type A dissection is shown.** The Stanford classification is simple and clinically relevant. Stanford class A includes all dissections involving the ascending aorta regardless of where the intimal tear is located and regardless of how far the dissection propagates. The mortality rate is 72% with medical management and 32% with surgical management. Therefore, surgery is recommended for type A dissections. Stanford type B dissections are those that involve the aorta distal to the origin of the left subclavian artery. Mortality rates for medical and surgical management are similar for type B dissections.

Reference: Hensley FA, Martin DE, Gravlee GP. *A Practical Approach to Cardiac Anesthesia, Third Edition.* Philadelphia: Lippincott Williams & Wilkins. 2002:621.

76. **Answer = E, All are correct.** An Ao ratio < 1.3 indicates a low-risk group in patients with Marfan's syndrome. The Ao ratio is the sinus of valsalva diameter divided by the predicted sinus diameter for a given age and BSA. Ao ratio < 1.3 or annual rate of change < 5% indicates a low-risk group in patients with Marfan's syndrome. For adults (> 40 years): predicted sinus dimension (cm) = 1.92 + [0.74 * BSA (m^2)]. Patients with an aortic root diameter of 50 mm undergoing CABG are at increased risk of aortic dissection. Patients with aortic dissections may present with hoarseness secondary to compression of the recurrent laryngeal nerve. Patients may also present with asymmetry of pulses.

References: Hensley FA, Martin DE, Gravlee GP. *A Practical Approach to Cardiac Anesthesia, Third Edition.* Philadelphia: Lippincott Williams & Wilkins. 2002:621; Legget ME, Unger TA, O'Sullivan CK, Zwink TR, Bennett RL, Byers PH, Otto CM. Aortic root complications in Marfan's syndrome: Identification of a lower risk group. *British Heart Journal* 1996;74(4):389–395.

77. **Answer = B, Stanford type A dissections may occur as a result of aortic cannulation for cardiopulmonary bypass surgery.** An intimal tear just distal to the level of the ligamentum arteriosum is the most common cause of a type B dissection. Atherosclerosis is a risk factor for the development of aortic aneurysms, but surprisingly has not been shown to be a risk factor for the development of aortic dissections.

Reference: Hensley FA, Martin DE, Gravlee GP. *A Practical Approach to Cardiac Anesthesia, Third Edition.* Philadelphia: Lippincott Williams & Wilkins. 2002:621.

78. **Answer = D, Systolic reversal of pulmonic flow is indicative of severe mitral regurgitation (MR).** The systolic component of the pulmonary venous flow profile has two components: PVS_1 and PVS_2. The size of PVS_1 depends on left atrial relaxation and the subsequent decrease in left atrial pressure. The size of PVS_2 is influenced by the right ventricular stroke volume.

Reference: Perrino AC, Reeves S. *A Practical Approach to TEE.* Philadelphia: Lippincott Williams & Wilkins 2003:117.

79. **Answer = E, All are correct concerning the pulmonary vein atrial flow reversal wave (pulmonary vein A-wave = PV_{AR} wave).** In restrictive diastolic dysfunction the PV_{AR} wave may be elevated secondary to decreased LV compliance or it may be decreased due to left atrial mechanical failure. Left atrial failure results from the increased left atrial workload seen in restrictive disease due to decreased LV compliance. In delayed relaxation the PV_{AR} peak velocity is less than the A-wave peak velocity because the forward flow through the mitral valve is greater than backward flow into the pulmonary veins. The PV_{AR} wave is increased in mitral stenosis because the stenotic mitral valve inhibits forward flow and promotes backward flow into the pulmonary veins.

Reference: Perrino AC, Reeves S. *A Practical Approach to TEE.* Philadelphia: Lippincott Williams & Wilkins 2003:117–118.

80. **Answer = A, Mitral stenosis results in a large pulmonary vein atrial reversal wave (PV_{AR} wave = pulmonary vein A wave) because the stenotic mitral valve inhibits forward flow and promotes backward flow into the pulmonary veins.**

Reference: Perrino AC, Reeves S. *A Practical Approach to TEE.* Philadelphia: Lippincott Williams & Wilkins 2003:117–118.

81. **Answer = A, Lateral mitral annular tissue Doppler is normal (E_M > 8 cm/sec) in constrictive pericarditis but not in a restrictive cardiomyopathy due to an infiltrative process such as amyloidosis.** This intuitively makes sense. In constrictive pericarditis the tissue is normal but filling is restricted by the noncompliant pericardium encasing the heart. Because in constrictive pericarditis the tissue is normal, tissue Doppler imaging will be normal. In an infiltrative disease such as amyloidosis, the

cardiac tissue itself is abnormal and noncompliant (resulting in abnormal tissue Doppler imaging).

Reference: Perrino AC, Reeves S. *A Practical Approach to TEE.* Philadelphia: Lippincott Williams & Wilkins 2003:126.

82. **Answer = B, Constrictive pericarditis will produce a restrictive transmitral pulsed-wave Doppler velocity profile and a normal lateral mitral annular tissue Doppler velocity profile.** In constrictive pericarditis the tissue is normal but filling is restricted by the noncompliant pericardium encasing the heart. Because in constrictive pericarditis the tissue is normal, tissue Doppler imaging will be normal. In an infiltrative disease such as amyloidosis, the cardiac tissue itself is abnormal and noncompliant (resulting in abnormal tissue Doppler imaging).

Reference: Oh JK, Seward JB, Tajik AJ (eds). *The Echo Manual, Second Edition.* Philadelphia: Lippincott Williams & Wilkins 1999:52.

83. **Answer = A, Normal diastolic function is present.** A normal-appearing transmitral pulsed-wave Doppler diastolic velocity profile is shown. This normal-appearing E- and A-wave profile could result from normal or pseudonormal diastolic function. A normal lateral mitral annular tissue Doppler E_M peak velocity is also present and this confirms the diagnosis of normal diastolic function. If pseudonormal diastolic function were present the lateral mitral annular tissue Doppler E_M peak velocity would be decreased (< 8 cm/sec).

Reference: Groban L, Dolinski SY. Evaluation of diastolic function. *Chest* 2005;128;3652–3663.

84. **Answer = A, A healthy 42-year-old male would be expected to have a normal pulmonary vein pulsed-wave Doppler flow velocity profile (as is shown).** All other choices listed would be expected to result in restrictive diastolic dysfunction. In restrictive disease the S wave is typically less than the D wave.

Reference: Groban L, Dolinski SY. Evaluation of diastolic function. *Chest* 2005;128;3652–3663.

85. **Answer = C, The pulmonary vein diastolic wave (D wave) is shown.**

Reference: Groban L, Dolinski SY. Evaluation of diastolic function. *Chest* 2005;128;3652–3663.

86. **Answer = A, The pulmonary vein atrial flow reversal wave (PV$_{AR}$ wave) is shown.**

Reference: Groban L, Dolinski SY. Evaluation of diastolic function. *Chest* 2005;128;3652–3663.

87. **Answer = B, Complete heart block can produce an increased PV**$_{AR}$ **wave.** This increased retrograde flow velocity results from a loss of AV synchrony. When the left atrium contracts against a closed mitral valve a large pulmonary venous reversal wave PV$_{AR}$ results. An enlarged PV$_{AR}$ wave can also occur with mitral stenosis and pseudonormal diastolic dysfunction.

Reference: Perrino AC, Reeves S. *A Practical Approach to TEE.* Philadelphia: Lippincott Williams & Wilkins 2003:117–118.

88. **Answer = A, Arrow 1 indicates the pulmonary vein atrial flow reversal wave (PV**$_{AR}$ **wave).**

Reference: Groban L, Dolinski SY. Evaluation of diastolic function. *Chest* 2005;128;3652–3663.

89. **Answer = C, Arrow 2 indicates the pulmonary vein diastolic flow wave (D wave).**

Reference: Groban L, Dolinski SY. Evaluation of diastolic function. *Chest* 2005;128;3652–3663.

90. **Answer = B, Arrow 1 indicates the hepatic venous systolic flow wave (S wave).**

Reference: Groban L, Dolinski SY. Evaluation of diastolic function. *Chest* 2005;128;3652–3663.

91. **Answer = D, Arrow 2 indicates the hepatic venous diastolic flow wave (D wave).**

Reference: Groban L, Dolinski SY. Evaluation of diastolic function. *Chest* 2005;128;3652–3663.

92. **Answer = E, Arrow 3 indicates the hepatic venous A wave.** This retrograde flow wave results from atrial contraction. This wave is enlarged in patients with tricuspid stenosis and decreased right ventricular compliance.

Reference: Groban L, Dolinski SY. Evaluation of diastolic function. *Chest* 2005;128;3652–3663.

93. **Answer = A, A moderate to severe pericardial effusion is typical with pericardial tamponade.** Right ventricular diastolic (*not* systolic) and right atrial systolic (*not* diastolic) collapse are seen with pericardial tamponade. During ventricular systole the ventricular pressure is high, preventing ventricular collapse and favoring collapse of the low-pressure right atria. During diastole the ventricular pressure falls and right ventricular diastolic collapse occurs. Reciprocal respiratory changes can be explained as follows. Fluid is not compressible and with pericardial tamponade the total pericardial volume (heart chambers plus pericardial fluid) is fixed. If right ventricular volume is high, left ventricular volume will be low (and vice versa). During spontaneous inspiration intrathoracic pressure decreases and the thin-walled right ventricle dilates, increasing venous return. This increases right ventricular filling and transmitral flow velocities. As the right ventricle fills, right ventricular pressure exceeds left ventricular pressure and the interventricular septum shifts to the

left (compressing the left ventricle). This LV compression decreases transmitral inflow and left ventricular stroke volume (TVI$_{LVOT}$). This is the mechanism that explains why systemic pressure, transmitral inflow, and LV stroke volume all decrease with spontaneous inspiration. The opposite occurs with spontaneous expiration. With positive-pressure ventilation, the opposite respiratory pattern exists because intrathoracic pressure increases with inspiration and decreases with expiration.

Reference: Otto C. *Textbook of Clinical Echocardiography, Third Edition.* Philadelphia: Elsevier 2004:262.

94. **Answer = A, Scenario A would be expected with spontaneous inspiration.** During spontaneous inspiration intrathoracic pressure decreases and the thin-walled right ventricle dilates (increasing venous return). This increases right ventricular filling and transmitral flow velocities. As the right ventricle fills, right ventricular pressure exceeds left ventricular pressure and the interventricular septum shifts to the left (compressing the left ventricle). This LV compression decreases transmitral inflow and left ventricular stroke volume (TVI$_{LVOT}$). This is the mechanism that explains why systemic pressure, transmitral inflow, and LV stroke volume all decrease with spontaneous inspiration. The opposite occurs with spontaneous expiration. With positive-pressure ventilation, the opposite respiratory pattern exists because intrathoracic pressure increases with inspiration and decreases with expiration.

Reference: Otto C. *Textbook of Clinical Echocardiography, Third Edition.* Philadelphia: Elsevier 2004:262.

95. **Answer = B, Scenario B would be expected with positive pressure inspiration.** With positive-pressure inspiration the thin-walled RV is compressed, favoring LV filling and left ventricular cardiac output at the expense of right ventricular filling and right ventricular output. During spontaneous inspiration, intrathoracic pressure decreases and the thin-walled right ventricle dilates (increasing venous return). This increases right ventricular filling and transmitral flow velocities. As the right ventricle fills, right ventricular pressure exceeds left ventricular pressure and the interventricular septum shifts to the left (compressing the left ventricle). This LV compression decreases transmitral inflow and left ventricular stroke volume (TVI$_{LVOT}$). This is the mechanism that explains why systemic pressure, transmitral inflow, and LV stroke volume all decrease with spontaneous inspiration. The opposite occurs with spontaneous expiration. With positive-pressure ventilation, the opposite respiratory pattern exists because intrathoracic pressure increases with inspiration and decreases with expiration.

Reference: Otto C. *Textbook of Clinical Echocardiography, Third Edition.* Philadelphia: Elsevier 2004:262.

96. **Answer = B, Scenario B would be expected with spontaneous expiration.** With spontaneous expiration the thin-walled RV is compressed, favoring LV filling and left ventricular cardiac output at the expense of right ventricular filling and right ventricular output. During spontaneous inspiration intrathoracic pressure decreases and the thin-walled right ventricle dilates (increasing venous return). This increases right ventricular filling and transmitral flow velocities. As the right ventricle fills, right ventricular pressure exceeds left ventricular pressure and the interventricular septum shifts to the left (compressing the left ventricle). This LV compression decreases transmitral inflow and left ventricular stroke volume (TVI$_{LVOT}$). This is the mechanism that explains why systemic pressure, transmitral inflow, and LV stroke volume all decrease with spontaneous inspiration. The opposite occurs with spontaneous expiration. With positive-pressure ventilation, the opposite respiratory pattern exists because intrathoracic pressure increases with inspiration and decreases with expiration.

Reference: Otto C. *Textbook of Clinical Echocardiography, Third Edition.* Philadelphia: Elsevier 2004:262.

97. **Answer = A, Scenario A would be expected during expiration in an intubated patient with a hemodynamically significant pericardial effusion undergoing positive-pressure ventilation.** During expiration in an intubated patient undergoing positive-pressure ventilation, the intrathoracic pressure decreases and the thin-walled right ventricle dilates (increasing venous return). This increases right ventricular filling and transmitral flow velocities at the expense of left ventricular filling. During spontaneous inspiration intrathoracic pressure decreases and the thin-walled right ventricle dilates, increasing venous return. This increases right ventricular filling and transmitral flow velocities. As the right ventricle fills, right ventricular pressure exceeds left ventricular pressure and the interventricular septum shifts to the left (compressing the left ventricle). This LV compression decreases transmitral inflow and left ventricular stroke volume (TVI$_{LVOT}$). This is the mechanism that explains why systemic pressure, transmitral inflow, and LV stroke volume all decrease with spontaneous inspiration. The opposite occurs with spontaneous expiration. With positive-pressure ventilation, the opposite respiratory pattern exists because intrathoracic pressure increases with inspiration and decreases with expiration.

Reference: Otto C. *Textbook of Clinical Echocardiography, Third Edition.* Philadelphia: Elsevier 2004:262.

98. **Answer = B, Rhabdomyoma is associated with tuberous sclerosis.** This malignant tumor is the most common intracardiac tumor in children and multiple masses are frequently seen in the right ventricle.

Reference: Oh JK, Seward JB, Tajik AJ (eds). *The Echo Manual, Second Edition.* Philadelphia: Lippincott Williams & Wilkins 1999:209.

99. **Answer = A, Rhabdomyoma, the most common cardiac tumor in children, is usually found in the right ventricle.** This malignant tumor is associated with tuberous sclerosis and multiple tumors are frequently present.

Reference: Oh JK, Seward JB, Tajik AJ (eds). *The Echo Manual, Second Edition.* Philadelphia: Lippincott Williams & Wilkins 1999:209.

100. **Answer = A, Papillary fibroelastomas usually originate from the cardiac valves or adjacent endocardium.** These benign tumors tend to originate on the atrial side of the atrioventricular valves and the ventricular surface of the similunar valves. The aortic valve is most frequently affected and the appearance is similar to that of lambl excrescences, but lambl excrescences are thinner and broader based. Embolic events can result from papillary fibroelastomas, and removal is recommended even in asymptomatic patients.

Reference: Oh JK, Seward JB, Tajik AJ (eds). *The Echo Manual, Second Edition.* Philadelphia: Lippincott Williams & Wilkins 1999:209–210.

101. **Answer = A, An obstruction esophageal neoplasm is an absolute contraindication to TEE.** Absolute contraindications to TEE include esophageal strictures, webs or rings, patient refusal, esophageal perforation, obstruction esophageal neoplasms, and cervical spin instability.

Reference: Savage RM, Aronson S, Thomas JD, Shanewise JS, Shernan SK. *Comprehensive Textbook of Intraoperative Transesophageal Echocardiography.* Philadelphia: Lippincott Williams & Wilkins 2004:108.

102. **Answer = E, All of the above are relative contraindication to TEE.** Relative contraindications to TEE include the following: esophageal diverticulum, large hiatal hernia, recent esophageal or gastric surgery, esophageal varices, history of dysphagia or odynophagia, cervical arthritis, history of radiation to the mediastinum, deformities of the oral pharynx, and severe coagulopathy.

Reference: Savage RM, Aronson S, Thomas JD, Shanewise JS, Shernan SK. *Comprehensive Textbook of Intraoperative Transesophageal Echocardiography.* Philadelphia: Lippincott Williams & Wilkins 2004:108.

103. **Answer = E, 14 mmHg is the left atrial pressure.** The calculation is as follows.

$$\Delta P = 4V^2$$

$$\Delta P = 4V^2$$

$$(LAP - RAP) = (4V_{PFOPeak})^2$$

$$LAP = 4(V_{PFO})^2 + RAP$$

$$LAP = 4 + 10$$

$$LAP = 14 \text{ mmHg}$$

- ΔP = change in pressure
- LAP = left atrial pressure
- RAP = right atrial pressure
- V_{PFO} = peak velocity of left to right flow across a patent foramen ovale

Reference: Perrino AC, Reeves S. *A Practical Approach to TEE.* Philadelphia: Lippincott Williams & Wilkins 2003:102.

104. **Answer = B, 28 ml is the left ventricular stroke volume.** The calculation is as follows.

$$SV_{LVOT} = TVI_{LVOT} * A_{LVOT}$$

$$SV_{LVOT} = 9 \text{ cm} * \pi r^2$$

$$SV_{LVOT} = (9 \text{ cm}) * (3.14 \text{ cm}^2)$$

$$SV_{LVOT} = 28 \text{ ml}$$

- SV_{LVOT} = stroke volume of flow through the left ventricular outflow tract
- TVI_{LVOT} = time velocity integral of flow through the left ventricular outflow tract
- A_{LVOT} = area of the left ventricular outflow tract

Reference: Perrino AC, Reeves S. *A Practical Approach to TEE.* Philadelphia: Lippincott Williams & Wilkins 2003:96.

105. **Answer = B, 2,800 ml/min is the left ventricular cardiac output.** The calculation is as follows.

CO = SV * HR = 28 ml/beat * 100 beats/min = 2,800 ml/min

$$SV_{LVOT} = TVI_{LVOT} * A_{LVOT}$$

$$SV_{LVOT} = 9 \text{ cm} * \pi r^2$$

$$SV_{LVOT} = (9 \text{ cm}) * (3.14 \text{ cm}^2)$$

$$SV_{LVOT} = 28 \text{ ml}$$

- SV_{LVOT} = stroke volume of flow through the left ventricular outflow tract
- TVI_{LVOT} = time velocity integral of flow through the left ventricular outflow tract
- A_{LVOT} = area of the left ventricular outflow tract
- HR = heart rate

Reference: Perrino AC, Reeves S. *A Practical Approach to TEE.* Philadelphia: Lippincott Williams & Wilkins 2003:96.

106. **Answer = C, 2.1 cm² is the aortic valve area.** The calculation is as follows.

$$Q_{AV} = Q_{LVOT}$$

$$SV_{AV} = SV_{LVOT}$$

$$TVI_{AV} * A_{AV} = TVI_{LVOT} * A_{LVOT}$$

$$A_{AV} = TVI_{LVOT} * A_{LVOT} / TVI_{AV}$$

$$A_{AV} = 9 \text{ cm} * \pi r^2 / 27 \text{ cm}$$

$$A_{AV} = 2.1 \text{ cm}^2$$

- Q_{AV} = flow through the aortic valve
- Q_{LVOT} = flow through the left ventricular outflow tract
- SV_{AV} = stroke volume in the aortic valve
- SV_{LVOT} = stroke volume through the left ventricular outflow tract
- TVI_{AV} = time velocity integral of flow through the aortic valve
- A_{AV} = area of the aortic valve
- TVI_{LVOT} = time velocity integral of flow through the left ventricular outflow tract
- ALVOT = area of the left ventricular outflow tract

Reference: Perrino AC, Reeves S. *A Practical Approach to TEE.* Philadelphia: Lippincott Williams & Wilkins 2003:100.

107. **Answer = D, 38.5 m/s is the velocity of blood flow in the vessel.** The calculation is as follows.

$V = \Delta F/\cos\theta * C/2F_T$

$V = (0.5\ \text{MHz}) / 1 * 1540\ \text{m/s} / (20\ \text{MHz})$

$V = 38.5\ \text{m/s}$

- V = velocity of blood flow = Doppler shift $(F_T - F_R)$
- F_T = transmitted frequency
- F_R = reflected frequency

Reference: Edelman SK. *Understanding Ultrasound Physics.* Woodlands, TX: ESP, Inc. 1994:131.

108. **Answer = A, The mid esophageal ascending aortic valve short axis view can be used to estimate the right ventricular stroke volume.**

Reference: Konstadt SN, Shernon S, Oka Y (eds). *Clinical Transesophageal Echocardiography: A Problem-Oriented Approach, Second Edition.* Philadelphia: Lippincott Williams & Wilkins 2003:428.

109. **Answer = E, The LV apex is usually better visualized with transthoracic echocardiography.**

Reference: Sidebotham D, Merry A, Legget M (eds.). *Practical Perioperative Transoesophageal Echocardiography.* Burlington, MA: Butterworth Heinemann 2003:82.

110. **Answer = A, The midesophageal ascending aortic short axis view provides images of the main pulmonary artery and is a good view for evaluating thrombus in the main pulmonary artery.**

Reference: Sidebotham D, Merry A, Legget M (eds.). *Practical Perioperative Transoesophageal Echocardiography.* Burlington, MA: Butterworth Heinemann 2003:83.

111. **Answer = B, Severe mitral regurgitation is unlikely to be associated with a left atrial appendage thrombus because flow into the left atrium is increased.**

Reference: Sidebotham D, Merry A, Legget M (eds.). *Practical Perioperative Transoesophageal Echocardiography.* Burlington, MA: Butterworth Heinemann 2003:83.

112. **Answer = B, Intravenous drug use is a common cause of tricuspid valve endocarditis and this can result in severe tricuspid regurgitation (which causes holosystolic hepatic venous flow reversal).**

Reference: Sidebotham D, Merry A, Legget M (eds.). *Practical Perioperative Transoesophageal Echocardiography.* Burlington, MA: Butterworth Heinemann 2003:83.

113. **Answer = B, The LVOT side of the aortic valve is the most common location of a bacterial vegetation listed.** Vegetations typically arise on the upstream or low pressure side of a valve. The least common valve affected by endocarditis is the pulmonic valve, possibly due to the lower flow velocities across the pulmonic valve. Pulmonic valve vegetations would be expected to occur on the right ventricular outflow tract side of the valve, but these are not as common as aortic valve vegetations. Mitral and tricuspid vegetations usually occur on the atrial side of the valve (upstream low-pressure side).

Reference: Sidebotham D, Merry A, Legget M (eds.). *Practical Perioperative Transoesophageal Echocardiography.* Burlington, MA: Butterworth Heinemann 2003:83.

114. **Answer = D, Renal cell carcinoma is the most common malignant tumor seen extending into the right atrium.**

Reference: Sidebotham D, Merry A, Legget M (eds.). *Practical Perioperative Transoesophageal Echocardiography.* Burlington, MA: Butterworth Heinemann 2003:84.

115. **Answer = B, Rhabdomyomas are the most common primary cardiac tumors in children.** They are benign tumors usually found in the right ventricle. They are not associated with Down's syndrome.

Reference: Sidebotham D, Merry A, Legget M (eds.). *Practical Perioperative Transoesophageal Echocardiography.* Burlington, MA: Butterworth Heinemann 2003:84.

116. **Answer = D, Myxomas are benign cardiac tumors.** These are the most common primary intracardiac tumor. They usually occur in the left atrium attached to the interatrial septum. They can cause embolic phenomenon and valvular obstruction. Thus, surgical excision is warranted.

Reference: Sidebotham D, Merry A, Legget M (eds.). *Practical Perioperative Transoesophageal Echocardiography.* Burlington, MA: Butterworth Heinemann 2003:89.

117. **Answer = C, Fractional area change (FAC) of 34% is indicative of decreased systolic function and this is consistent with dilated cardiomyopathy.** V_{TRpeak} = 100 cm/sec and RAP = 10 would indicate a right ventricular systolic pressure of 14 mmHg. This is not consistent with dilated cardiomyopathy. The calculation is as follows.

$$\Delta P = 4V^2$$

$$(RVSP - RAP) = 4V_{TR}^{2}$$

$$(RVSP - CVP) = 4V^2$$

$$RVSP = 4V^2 + CVP$$

$$RVSP = 4(1 \ m/s)^2 + 10$$

$$RVSP = 14 \ mmHg$$

A fractional shortening (FS) of 34% indicates normal systolic function (normal FS = 25 to 40%). A mitral valve color flow Doppler regurgitant jet area of 1.6 cm^2 is consistent with trace regurgitation. With dilated cardiomyopathy, moderate to severe mitral regurgitation would be expected.

Reference: Otto C. *Textbook of Clinical Echocardiography, Third Edition.* Philadelphia: Elsevier 2004:228.

118. **Answer = B, 11 mm is consistent with normal left ventricular wall thickness.** (See Table 5.2P.)

Table 5.2P.

Degree of LVH	LV Free Wall Thickness
Normal	6–11 mm
Mild LVH	12–14 mm
Moderate LVH	15–19 mm
Severe LVH	≥ 20 mm

Abbreviations: LV = left ventricle, LVH = left ventricle hypertrophy.

119. **Answer = A, Development of a late-peaking high-velocity systolic jet on continuous-wave Doppler after amyl nitrate administration is indicative of dynamic left ventricular outflow tract due to hypertrophic cardiomyopathy.**

Reference: Otto C. *Textbook of Clinical Echocardiography, Third Edition.* Philadelphia: Elsevier 2004:238.

120. **Answer = E, All are causes of restrictive cardiomyopathy.**

Reference: Otto C. *Textbook of Clinical Echocardiography, Third Edition.* Philadelphia: Elsevier 2004:241.

121. **Answer = C, Hypereosinophilic syndrome is a systemic disease characterized by hypereosinophilia with involvement of the lungs, bone marrow, brain, and heart.** The heart findings are unique. Restrictive diastolic dysfunction and left ventricular thrombus are common. Thrombus formation occurs despite normal left ventricular wall motion. Thrombus formation usually occurs in the apex, gradually filling it in (apical obliteration). Thrombus may also form under the posterior mitral valve leaflet, causing it to adhere to the endocardium (which results in mitral regurgitation).

Reference: Otto C. *Textbook of Clinical Echocardiography, Third Edition.* Philadelphia: Elsevier 2004:241.

122. **Answer = D, The pulmonary vascular resistance cannot be measured or estimated reliably by echocardiography in patients with dilated cardiomyopathy.** This must be calculated using catheterization and is useful in determining if a patient is a candidate for cardiac transplantation.

Reference: Otto C. *Textbook of Clinical Echocardiography, Third Edition.* Philadelphia: Elsevier 2004:231.

123. **Answer = D, None of the above.** All of the given statements are false. Continuous-wave ultrasound cannot produce two-dimensional images. Only pulsed-wave ultrasound can produce two-dimensional images. In the best views for obtaining blood flow velocities with Doppler ultrasound, the blood flow is parallel (*not* perpendicular) to the direction of the ultrasound beam. In the best views for two-dimensional imaging the object of interest is perpendicular (not parallel) to the path of the ultrasound beam.

Reference: Edelman SK. *Understanding Ultrasound Physics.* Woodlands, TX: ESP, Inc. 1994:132.

124. **Answer = B, 1.57 cm² = aortic valve area.** This problem involves the continuity principle: flow through the LVOT is equal to flow through the aortic valve. The 60-degree angle will affect flow through both the left ventricular outflow track and flow through the aortic valve to the same extent. Therefore, the aortic valve calculation should be accurate.

$$Q_{AV} = Q_{LVOT}$$

$$SV_{AV} = SV_{LVOT}$$

$$V_{peak\,AV} * A_{AV} = V_{peak\,LVOT} * A_{LVOT}$$

$$A_{AV} = V_{peak\,LVOT} * A_{LVOT} / V_{peak\,AV}$$

$$A_{AV} = V_{peak\,LVOT} * 2\pi\,(r_{LVOT})^2 / V_{peak\,AV}$$

$$A_{AV} = 1.57\ cm^2$$

- A_{AV} = AVA = aortic valve area
- Q_{AV} = flow through the aortic valve
- Q_{LVOT} = flow through the LVOT
- LVOT = left ventricular outflow tract
- V_{peakAV} = peak instantaneous velocity across the aortic valve
- A_{LVOT} = area of the LVOT
- $V_{peakLVOT}$ = peak instantaneous velocity across the left ventricular outflow tract
- r_{LVOT} = radius of the LVOT
- HR = heart rate
- SV = stroke volume
- CO = cardiac output
- CI = cardiac index

Reference: Sidebotham D, Merry A, Legget M (eds.). *Practical Perioperative Transoesophageal Echocardiography.* Burlington, MA: Butterworth Heinemann 2003:233.

125. **Answer = B, 32 mm Hg = the best estimate of the pressure gradient across the aortic valve.** According to the modified Bernoulli equation: $\Delta P = 4V^2$. Because the angle between the path of the ultrasound beam and the direction of blood flow is 60 degrees this will underestimate the true peak aortic velocity by a factor of cos 60 = 0.5. Therefore, the pressure gradient across the aortic valve is equal to twice the number obtained by the modified Bernoulli equation or $2 * 4 \ (V_{peak\ AV})^2 = 8(2\ m/s)^2 = 32\ mmHg$.

126. **Answer = A, 31.4 cm³ = the best estimate of stroke volume (SV).**

Stroke volume = stroke distance * area =

$TVI_{AV} * A_{AV} = (20\ cm) * 1.57\ cm^2 = \underline{\textbf{31.4cm}^3}$

$Q_{AV} = Q_{LVOT}$

$SV_{AV} = SV_{LVOT}$

$V_{peak\ AV} * A_{AV} = V_{peak\ LVOT} * A_{LVOT}$

$A_{AV} = V_{peak\ LVOT} * A_{LVOT} / V_{peak\ AV}$

$A_{AV} = V_{peak\ LVOT} * 2\pi \ (r_{LVOT})^2 / V_{peak\ AV}$

$A_{AV} = 1.57\ cm^2$

- A_{AV} = AVA = aortic valve area
- Q_{AV} = flow through the aortic valve
- Q_{LVOT} = flow through the LVOT
- LVOT = left ventricular outflow tract
- V_{peakAV} = peak instantaneous velocity across the aortic valve
- A_{LVOT} = area of the LVOT
- $V_{peakLVOT}$ = peak instantaneous velocity across the left ventricular outflow tract
- r_{LVOT} = radius of the LVOT
- HR = heart rate
- SV = stroke volume
- CO = cardiac output
- CI = cardiac index

Reference: Sidebotham D, Merry A, Legget M (eds.). *Practical Perioperative Transoesophageal Echocardiography.* Burlington, MA: Butterworth Heinemann 2003:232.

127. **Answer = A, 3,140 ml/min is the best estimate of the cardiac output (CO).** The calculation is as follows.

$$CO = HR * SV$$

$$CO = (100 \text{ beats/min}) * (31.4 \text{ ml/beat})$$

$$CO = 3140 \text{ ml/min}$$

$$SV = TVI_{AV} * A_{AV} = (20 \text{ cm}) * 1.57 \text{ cm}^2 = 31.4 \text{ cm}^3$$

$$Q_{AV} = Q_{LVOT}$$

$$SV_{AV} = SV_{LVOT}$$

$$V_{peakAV} * A_{AV} = V_{peak\ LVOT} * A_{LVOT}$$

$$A_{AV} = V_{peak\ LVOT} * A_{LVOT} / V_{peakAV}$$

$$A_{AV} = V_{peak\ LVOT} * 2\pi\ (r_{LVOT})^2 / V_{peakAV}$$

$$A_{AV} = 1.57 \text{ cm}^2$$

- A_{AV} = AVA = aortic valve area
- Q_{AV} = flow through the aortic valve
- Q_{LVOT} = flow through the LVOT
- LVOT = left ventricular outflow tract
- V_{peakAV} = peak instantaneous velocity across the aortic valve
- A_{LVOT} = area of the LVOT
- $V_{peakLVOT}$ = peak instantaneous velocity across the left ventricular outflow tract
- r_{LVOT} = radius of the LVOT
- HR = heart rate
- SV = stroke volume
- CO = cardiac output
- CI = cardiac index

Reference: Sidebotham D, Merry A, Legget M (eds.). *Practical Perioperative Transoesophageal Echocardiography.* Burlington, MA: Butterworth Heinemann 2003:232.

128. **Answer = A, 1.57 L/min/m² = the cardiac index (CI).** The calculation is as follows.

$$CI = CO / BSA$$

$$CI = 1,570 \text{ ml/min}$$

$$CO = HR * SV$$

$$CO = (100 \text{ beats/min}) * (31.4 \text{ ml/beat})$$

$$CO = 3,140 \text{ ml/min}$$

- HR = heart rate
- SV = stroke volume
- CO = cardiac output
- CI = cardiac index
- BSA = body surface area

Reference: Sidebotham D, Merry A, Legget M (eds.). *Practical Perioperative Transoesophageal Echocardiography.* Burlington, MA: Butterworth Heinemann 2003:232.

129. **Answer = D, A chiari network is a thin filamentous structure found in the right atrium near the eustachian valve.**

Reference: Sidebotham D, Merry A, Legget M (eds.). *Practical Perioperative Transoesophageal Echocardiography.* Burlington, MA: Butterworth Heinemann 2003:71.

130. **Answer = C, Tricuspid Stenosis. A hepatic venous Doppler flow profile is shown.** This profile consists of four waves: S, V, D, and AR. The AR wave (also known as the A wave) is illustrated. This wave results from right atrial contraction, which causes retrograde flow. In a patient with tricuspid stenosis there is obstruction of flow from the right atrium to the right ventricle, and therefore a prominent AR wave.

Reference: Perrino AC, Reeves S. *A Practical Approach to TEE.* Philadelphia: Lippincott Williams & Wilkins 2003:124.

131. **Answer = E, The midesophageal four-chamber view allows assessment of the tricuspid annulus systolic excursion.**

Reference: Sidebotham D, Merry A, Legget M (eds.). *Practical Perioperative Transoesophageal Echocardiography.* Burlington, MA: Butterworth Heinemann 2003:206.

132. **Answer = A, MVA = 759/deceleration Time = 759/759 = 1cm²**

Reference: Perrino AC, Reeves S. *A Practical Approach to TEE.* Philadelphia: Lippincott Williams & Wilkins 2003:153.

133. **Answer = B, Patient B is most likely to have post operative systolic anterior motion (SAM) of the anterior mitral valve leaflet with left ventricular outflow tract obstruction.** Things that increase the risk of SAM include C-sept distance < 2.5 cm, AL/PL ratio < 1, small ring size, and small TG LVEDd. Techniques to decrease the risk of post repair SAM include use of a partial ring (instead of a complete ring), performance of a sliding leaflet annuloplasty, or shortening of the anterior leaflet such that the anterior leaflet reaches the coaptation point but there is reduced redundant anterior leaflet length.
   - C-sept distance = distance from the coaptation point to the septum
   - AL/PL ratio = anterior leaflet length to post leaflet length
   - TG LVEDd = transgastric mid short axis left ventricular end diastolic dimension

Reference: Perrino AC, Reeves S. *A Practical Approach to TEE.* Philadelphia: Lippincott Williams & Wilkins 2003:124.

134. **Answer = B, 2 to 16% of patients develop systolic anterior motion (SAM) of the anterior mitral valve leaflet with left ventricular outflow tract obstruction after mitral valve repair.** Techniques to decrease the risk of post repair SAM include use of a partial ring (instead of a complete ring), performance of a sliding leaflet annuloplasty, or

shortening of the anterior leaflet such that the anterior leaflet reaches the coaptation point but there is reduced redundant anterior leaflet length.

Reference: Maslow AD, Regan MM, Haering JM, Johnson RG, Levine RA. Echocardiographic predictors of left ventricular outflow tract obstruction and systolic anterior motion of the mitral valve after mitral valve reconstruction for myxomatous valve disease. *J Am Coll Cardiology* 1999:34:2096–2104.

135. **Answer = B, Rheumatic heart disease most often affects the mitral valve.** The valves involved in decreasing order of frequency are:

- Mitral
- Mitral + aortic
- Mitral + aortic + tricuspid

Reference: Otto C. *Textbook of Clinical Echocardiography, Third Edition.* Philadelphia: Elsevier 2004:299.

INDEX

A

Abdominal viscera, 47
Absorption, 250, 290, 352, 395
AC. *See* Attenuation coefficient
Acetone, 271
Acoustic impedance (Z), 32, 40, 40t, 42, 42t, 75, 82, 83, 85, 154, 192, 250, 354t, 396, 461, 501, 502
    material order and, 252, 291
Acoustic interference, 178
Acoustic resonance, 62
Acoustic shadowing, 7, 24, 61, 62, 102, 323, 338
Acoustic speckle, 61
Agitated saline (Echo contrast), 195, 421
AI. *See* Aortic insufficiency
AICD. *See* Automated internal cardiac defibrillator
Akinesis, 344, 386, 415
Albumin, 116, 134
Alcohol toxicity, 277
Aliasing artifact, 157, 158, 194, 195, 505
    decreasing, 63, 374, 409
    eliminating, 465, 504
    Nyquist limit and, 103, 177, 208–209
    pulsed-wave Doppler and, 465, 504–505
Aliasing velocity, 92
AL/PL ratio, 377, 412
American Society of Anesthesiologists (ASA), 350, 392
American Society of Echocardiography
    16-segment model of, 19–20, 32, 33, 129, 142–143, 146, 229–230, 232, 240–242, 327–328, 331, 340–341, 342, 372, 408, 435–436, 449
    wall motion grading scale by, 246, 287, 344, 386, 386t
Amiodarone, 22
Amplitude, 151, 152, 190
    formula for, 249, 290
    intensity and, 459, 500
    tissue thickness and, 353, 396
Amyl nitrate, 487, 523
Amyloidosis, 488
    infiltrative, 14, 167, 171, 202
    restrictive cardiomyopathy caused by, 182, 212, 475, 514
Aneurysm, 164, 201
    aorta, 50, 88, 94, 164, 201, 260, 298, 320, 337, 360, 401, 514
    aortic, 260, 298, 360, 401, 514
    cardiac, 393
    of coronary artery, 226, 239
    interatrial septal, 63, 103, 221, 230, 237, 241, 271, 275, 303, 304, 306
    left ventricular, 216, 234
    pseudo-, 216, 234, 369, 406
    stroke and interatrial septal, 271, 304
    thoracoabdominal, 94
    ventricular septal, 226, 239, 256, 295
Angiography, 52, 165
Angiosarcoma, 270, 303, 370, 407
Angle of incidence, 40, 41, 83, 84, 153, 154, 192, 195, 208, 464, 504
Angular resolution, 42, 85, 145, 156, 194
Annular dilation, 118, 148, 187
Anterior wall, 15, 17, 115, 134, 315, 334, 431, 447
Anteroseptal wall, 15, 17, 130, 231, 241, 431, 447
Anticoagulation, 130, 131
Ao ratio, 425, 444, 473, 513
Aorta, 114, 132, 165, 173, 332, 342, 427, 444
    abdominal, 347, 389
    aneurysm of, 50, 88, 94, 164, 201, 260, 298, 320, 337, 360, 401, 514
    bifurcation in, 164, 360

dissection of, 324, 338
    epiaortic scan of, 201, 232, 233
    overriding, 238
    transesophageal echocardiography and, 165
Aortic abscess cavity, 319, 337
Aortic arch, 165, 382, 416
Aortic cannulation, 165, 201, 474, 514
Aortic clamp, 134
Aortic coarctation, 46, 123, 125, 160, 320, 337, 358t
Aortic dissection, 95, 393, 473, 513
    Marfan's syndrome and, 425, 443
    tests for, 52
Aortic ejection velocity, 308
    Aortic insufficiency (AI), 8, 25, 71, 95, 111, 120, 126, 141, 240, 339, 347, 389, 416
    degree of, 423, 424, 442
    pressure half time method for evaluating, 423, 442
Aortic regurgitation, 10, 119, 228, 240, 318, 326, 335
    fraction of, 260, 298
    indicators for, 423, 424, 442, 443
    volume of, 259, 297
Aortic root, 17, 68, 109, 131, 165
Aortic stenosis (AS), 8, 10, 29, 88, 119, 120, 127, 134, 137–138, 149, 160, 175, 188, 320, 337, 458, 500
    calcific, 348, 389
    degree of, 248, 289
    systolic ejection and, 26
Aortic transvalvular gradient, 119, 137
Aortic valve, 11, 17, 18, 19, 29, 71, 110, 122, 165, 228, 240, 373, 408, 409
    annulus of, 424, 443
    area of, 48, 90, 149, 163, 188, 199, 248, 276, 288, 306, 469, 484, 489, 509, 520, 524
    bicuspid, 19, 20, 46, 88, 125, 279, 309, 319, 337
    clover leaf, 20
    defects in, 88
    evaluating, 323, 338
    function of, 119
    herniated cusp of, 159, 196
    leaflet fluttering in, 180, 211
    leaflets of, 373, 409
    midsystolic closure of, 180, 211, 458, 500
    myxomatous, 19
    papillary fibroelastomas and, 270, 303
    pressure gradient across, 174, 206, 489, 525
    quadracuspid, 20
    sclerosis of, 68, 109, 119
    stroke volume of flow through, 49
    tricuspid, 20
Aortography, 52, 95
Arrhythmia
    myxoma and, 407
    ventricular, 3, 22
Arthritis, cervical, 61, 102
Artifact formation, 62, 102
AS. *See* Aortic stenosis
ASA. *See* American Society of Anesthesiologists
ASD. *See* Atrial septal defect
Assumptions, violation of, 62
Asymmetric septal hypertrophy, 378. *See also* Hypertrophic cardiomyopathy
Asymmetry of pulses, 473, 513
Atherosclerosis, 201, 232, 242, 514
    grading of, 201t
Atrial catheter pressure, 55
Atrial compliance, 34

Atrial contractility, flow velocity profile and, 260, 298
Atrial contraction, 56, 98, 99, 166, 202, 516
Atrial fibrillation, 109, 221
Atrial inversion, 13, 27, 362
Atrial septal defect (ASD), 89, 123, 131, 139, 221
    atrioventricular canal defect and, 257, 295
    coronary sinus, 158, 159, 195, 196
    frequency of, 159, 196, 421
    mitral regurgitation and, 357, 398
    ostium primum, 20, 46, 124, 125, 140, 158, 159, 196, 224, 238, 257, 295, 421, 434, 440, 448
    ostium secundum, 20, 46, 88, 124, 125, 140, 158, 159, 196, 224, 238, 315, 357, 398
    pulmonary veins and, 47
Atrioventricular canal defect, 120, 257, 295, 433, 448
Atrioventricular valves, 399, 409
Atropine, 415
Attenuation, 32, 75, 153, 191, 352, 395, 408
    crystal thickness and, 250, 290
    frequency and, 460, 501
    imaging depth and, 249, 290
    intensity and, 298
    soft tissue and, 250, 290
    tissue thickness and, 191
Attenuation coefficient (AC), 40t, 82, 353, 354t, 395, 460, 501
Audible sound, frequency of, 273, 304
Autocorrelation, 356, 397
Automated internal cardiac defibrillator (AICD), 22
AV. See Aortic valve
Axial resolution, 32, 145, 146, 155, 156, 193, 194, 291, 305, 355, 395, 396, 503.
    See also Longitudinal resolution
    numerical value for, 243, 284
    spatial pulse length and, 463, 503
Azimuthal resolution, 145, 355, 397. See also Lateral resolution
Azygos vein, 233, 242

B

Backing material, 155, 193, 291. See also Damping material
Bacteremia, 271
Bandwidth, 155, 193, 253, 289, 293
Beam alignment, 150
Beam diameter, 156, 194, 502
    lateral resolution and, 355, 397
Beam divergence, 52, 85
Beam focusing, 255, 293
Beam intensity, tissue thickness and, 152, 153, 191
Beam steering, 255, 293
Beam thickness, 146, 186
Beam velocity, 39
Beam width, 337
    lateral resolution and, 274, 305
Beam width artifacts, 61, 62
Benzocaine, 271
Bernoulli equation, modified, 160, 196
Bernoulli's physiology, 160
Beta blockers, 325, 339, 473, 513
Beta-myosin heavy chain gene, 412
Bezold-Jarisch reflex, 415
Bicuspid aortic valve, 19, 20, 46, 88, 125
    in neonates, 279, 309
Blalock-Taussig shunt, 358, 399
Blood flow, 45, 88, 157, 164, 194, 195, 200
    diastolic, 161, 197
    direction of, 280, 310
    pulsed-wave Doppler measurement of, 375
    turbulent, 125, 140
    velocity of, 177, 208, 352, 395, 484, 521
    ventricular inversion and, 358, 399
Blood pressure, arterial, 116
Body surface area (BSA), 468, 508
Bradycardia, paradoxical, 381, 415
Bradykinin, 110, 311

Bronchus, left main, 427, 444
BSA. See Body surface area

C

CABG. See Coronary artery bypass graft
Calcific mitral stenosis, 220, 236
Calcium chloride, 115, 116
Carcinoid syndrome, 14, 71, 72, 110, 220, 221, 236, 274, 281, 310, 311, 348, 389
Cardiac aneurysm, 393
Cardiac apex, 47
Cardiac arrhythmia, 271
Cardiac defibrillator, 394
Cardiac index, 48, 90, 181, 452, 456, 468, 469, 490, 496, 499, 508, 510, 526
Cardiac myxoma, 269, 302
Cardiac output, 48, 89, 174, 206, 456, 469, 484, 490, 509, 518, 520, 526
    calculating, 314, 334
    left ventricular output tract and, 48
    mitral valve and, 499
    right ventricular, 467, 507
Cardiomyopathy, 394
    dilated, 175, 181, 207, 211, 277–279, 308, 309, 377, 412, 487, 488, 522, 524
    hypertrophic, 52, 175, 180–182, 211–212, 232, 241, 278, 279, 308, 309, 378, 413, 487, 523
    hypertrophic obstructive, 8, 346, 377, 378, 388, 393, 412, 458, 500
    postpartum, 277
    restrictive, 12, 68, 109, 175, 182, 212, 475, 488, 514, 523
Cardioplegia, 386–387, 393
Cardioplegia catheter, 121
Cardioplegia, retrograde, 195
Cardiopulmonary bypass (CPB), 114, 317, 474, 514
Carotid arteries, 134
Carpentier classification, 18, 29, 119, 137, 137t, 181, 211, 212t, 219, 229, 236, 319, 336, 336t
Catheter(s), retrograde coronary sinus, 131
Cavity dilation, 70
Celiac trunk, 50
Central venous line, 121
Central venous pressure (CVP), 100
Cerebrovascular accident, 221, 237, 304. See also Stroke
Cervical arthritis, 61, 102
Cervical spine instability, 176, 208
Chagas disease, 181, 211
Chemotherapy, 130, 131
Chiari network, 11, 62, 103, 121, 122, 124, 130, 179, 221, 222, 273, 304, 438, 450, 490, 527
    treatment of, 223, 237
Chirp-Z transforms, 356, 397
Chordae tendinae, 34, 76, 147, 187, 246, 287, 346, 388
Christa terminalis, 11, 321, 338
Chronic coronary artery disease, 66
Chronic hypertension, 68, 109, 379, 413
Clover leaf aortic valve, 20
Coagulopathy, 102, 176
Coanda effect, 218, 235
Coaption line, 347, 389
Coaption point, 23, 389
Cobalt toxicity, 277, 279, 309
Color flow Doppler, 23, 45, 52, 88, 157, 178, 194, 224, 256, 420, 440, 487, 523
    autocorrelation and, 397
    jet area in, 412
    jet height in, 339
    mitral regurgitation and, 35, 383, 388, 416
    Nyquist limit and, 383, 416
Color flow map, 124, 125, 140
Color M-mode Doppler flow propagation velocity, 53, 55, 68, 97, 151, 190, 365, 404
    transmitral, 13
Comet tail artifact, 329, 330, 341, 342, 371f, 372, 407
Compression, 374, 409
Computed tomography (CT), 52, 95
Conal ventricular septal defect, 357, 398
Conductivity, 153
Congenital heart defects, 46, 88, 393

Congenital heart disease, 197
Congestive heart failure, 166, 202
Constrictive pericarditis, 12, 14, 52, 60, 95, 102, 171, 176, 207, 369, 406, 475, 514, 515
    flow waves and, 268, 302
    spontaneous inspiration and, 60
Constrictive systolic dysfunction, 14
Continuity equation, 71, 90, 120, 138, 188
Continuity principle, 499, 500
Continuous wave Doppler, 34, 43, 76, 93, 103, 156, 157, 172f, 193, 194, 205, 284, 382, 384, 416, 487, 523
    aliasing and, 465, 504
    disadvantages of, 284
    flow velocity profile from, 217, 454, 497
    frequency of, 252, 292
    mitral inflow profile from, 347, 389
    modified Bernoulli equation and, 160, 196
    processing for, 343, 386
    pulmonary artery systolic pressure and, 432, 447
    pulsed-wave v., 177, 208
Continuous wave ultrasound
    advantages of, 464, 503
    beam for, 43
    intensity for, 460, 501
Cor triatriatum, 62, 63, 72, 124, 140, 160, 382, 416
Coronary artery, 17, 134, 221, 453, 496
    aneurysm of, 226, 239
    circumflex, 17, 28, 32, 33, 70, 75, 115, 146, 147, 187, 247, 287, 346, 381, 382, 388, 415
    ischemia of, 70, 110, 115
    left, 33
    left anterior descending, 17, 32, 33, 70, 75, 76, 115, 146, 147, 187, 315, 334, 346, 382, 388, 415
    left main, 70, 131, 143
    obtuse marginal branches of, 147
    occlusion of, 180, 211
    posterior descending, 146, 147, 186, 187
    right, 17, 32, 33, 70, 75, 115, 131, 146, 147, 187, 247, 287, 382, 415
Coronary artery bypass graft (CABG), 53, 107, 115, 161, 165, 473, 513
Coronary artery disease, 69, 415
    left main, 183, 212
Coronary blood supply, 32, 146, 147, 186, 187
    papillary muscles and, 188
Coronary cusp, 126, 141
    left, 422, 441
    right, 223, 237, 422, 441, 457, 500
Coronary ostia, 386–387
Coronary reserve, 66
Coronary revascularization, 12
Coronary sinus, 17, 20, 30, 46, 122, 124, 125, 131, 132, 221, 237, 317, 335
    atrial septal defect of, 158, 159, 195, 196
    cannulation of, 179, 210
    dilated, 179, 210, 274, 305, 433, 448
Coumadin ridge, 62, 63, 124, 428, 444
CPB. See Cardiopulmonary bypass
Crawford classification system, 50, 94, 94t, 164, 201, 260, 298, 360, 401, 512t
Crista terminalis, 62, 63, 103, 130, 179
Critical temperature, 153, 154, 193
C-sept distance, 377, 412
CT. See Computed tomography
Curie temperature, 193
CVP. See Central venous pressure

D
Damping material, 155, 193, 251, 273, 291, 305
    depth resolution and, 355, 396
DeBakey classification, 51, 94, 94t, 339t, 472, 512t, 513t
Deceleration time (DT), 54, 60, 71, 97, 98, 167, 173, 299, 492, 527
    peak E-wave, 151
Density, 153, 154, 192
Depth resolution, 146, 355, 397
    damping material and, 355, 396

Depth-dependent amplification, 274
Dextrocardia, 47, 161, 197
Dextroinversus, 47, 161
Dextrotransposition, 47, 161
Dextroversion, 47, 161
Diaphragm, 165
Diastasis, 56, 98, 99, 166, 202
Diastole, 416
    paradoxical septal motion in, 60
    phases of, 56, 58, 166, 202
Diastolic blood flow, 161, 197
Diastolic dimension, 23
Diastolic dysfunction, 55, 95–98, 101, 167, 474, 514
    congestive heart failure and, 166, 202
    pseudonormal, 265, 300, 362, 403, 516
    restrictive, 300, 360, 364, 402, 403, 488, 523
Diastolic flow reversal, 423, 442
Diastolic function, 27, 53, 55, 57, 98, 170, 172, 261, 264, 299, 363, 366, 403, 404, 476, 515
    aging and, 54, 361, 402
    constrictive, 53
    impaired relaxation, 53
    mitral regurgitation and, 175, 207
    pseudonormal, 53
    restrictive, 53, 267, 301, 361, 402
Diastolic inflow, 76
Diastolic pressure, 123
    pulmonary artery, 349, 390, 466, 506
Diastolic transmitral inflow velocity, 168, 203
Dilated cardiomyopathy, 175, 181, 207, 211, 279, 309, 377, 412, 488, 524
    fractional area change and, 487, 522
    mitral regurgitation and, 278, 308
    potential causes of, 277, 308
Diplopia, 230
Dobutamine stress echocardiography (DSE), 67, 69, 107, 110, 179, 180
    left main coronary artery disease and, 183, 212
    sensitivity of, 183, 213
    side effects of infusion for, 381, 415
Doppler flashing, 178
Doppler shift, 44, 86, 140
    angle and, 310
    highest measurable, 375, 410
    maximum measurable, 177, 209
Doppler ultrasound, 43–45
Down's syndrome, 88, 159, 196, 448
    dp/dt, 217, 218, 234
Dressler's syndrome, 176, 207, 342
DT. See Deceleration time
Duchenne's muscular dystrophy, 181
Ductus arteriosus, 36, 78
    patent, 123, 124, 139, 160, 183, 213
Duty factor, 249, 289, 351–394
Dynamic range, 66, 106–107, 178, 209
Dyskinesis, 3, 344, 386, 428, 445. See also Akinesis; Hypokinesis
    inferior wall, 330, 342
    septal, 453, 496
Dysphagia, 61, 102, 176, 370

E
E/A ratio, 53, 95, 96t, 97, 109, 151, 167, 168, 190, 202–204, 262, 299–300
Early filling, 56, 98, 99, 166, 202
    velocity of, 97
Early filling velocity, 99
Ebstein's anomaly, 71, 72, 220, 236, 281, 311, 358t
ECG. See Electrocardiogram
Echo contrast media, 195, 421
Echo dropout. See Acoustic shadowing
Echocardiography machine, operating frequencies of, 31, 74
E/E$_M$ ratio, 55
Eisenmenger's physiology, 160, 197
Ejection fraction, 67, 68, 218, 452, 495
    qualitative estimate of, 217, 234

Ejection time, 173
Electrocardiogram (ECG), 216
Elevational resolution, 146, 186
Embolism, 22, 374, 409
    papillary fibroelastoma and, 270, 303
    segmental wall motion abnormalities and, 344, 386–387
Endocardial cushion defect, 315, 334
Endocardial thickening, 245, 286
Endocarditis, 71, 110, 128, 142, 393, 394
    tricuspid valve, 522
Enhancement artifact, 373, 408
Ephedrine, 116
Epiaortic ultrasound scan, 165, 201, 232, 233
Epicardium, 115, 134
Epinephrine, 115, 127, 142
E-point to septal separation (EPSS), 277, 308
Esmolol, 318, 336
Esophageal diverticulum, 102
Esophageal strictures, 371, 407
Esophageal trauma, 167
Esophageal varices, 102
Esophagus, 201
Eustachian valve, 11, 62, 102, 121, 122, 130, 131, 179, 241, 320, 421, 440, 527
Euvolemia, 16, 28
E-wave peak pressure, 60
E-wave peak velocity, 60, 97

F

FAC. See Fractional area change
False lumen (FL), 52, 95
Fast Fourier transform, 343, 356, 386, 397
Femoral artery, 114
Femoral vein, 114, 421, 441
Fibroma, 130, 269, 302
Fibrotic leaflets, 110
Filling pressure, 166, 167, 202, 361, 402
Filling velocities, 97
FL. See False lumen
Flow velocity, 160, 196
    preload reduction and, 300t
Flow velocity profile, 57f, 95, 96t, 260, 298, 475, 515
Flow volume loops, 8, 9
Flow waves, 267, 268, 301, 474, 514
Focal depth, 85, 464
    frequency and, 462, 502
Focal length, 153, 191, 254, 293, 462, 502
Focal zones, 69, 109
    multiple, 464, 503
Focus, 66, 145, 178, 186
    location of, 255, 293
Focused beam, 186
Foramen ovale, 241, 440
    patent, 20, 62, 103, 225, 230, 239, 241, 271, 275, 303, 304, 306, 348, 389, 390
Fossa ovalis, 46, 88
Fractional area change (FAC), 3, 22, 60, 174, 206, 217–218, 451, 453, 495–497
    dilated cardiomyopathy and, 487, 522
Fractional shortening (FS), 4, 22–23, 59, 101, 174, 205, 217–218, 451, 453, 487, 495–497, 523
Frame rate, 43, 69, 86, 109, 182, 194, 212, 309, 397
Free wall thickness, 68, 379, 413
FS. See Fractional shortening (FS)

G

Gain, 66, 178
Gastric trauma, 167, 202
Genetics
    dynamic LVOT obstruction and, 412
    hypertrophic cardiomyopathy and, 279, 309
Ghosting, 178, 209
Glenn shunt, 358, 399
Glutaraldehyde, 175, 207, 304
Glycogen storage diseases, 488

H

Half power distance, 153, 191
Half-value layer thickness, 250, 290
Halothane, 225, 238
Heart block, complete, 478, 516
Heart disease, hypertensive, 175
Heart rate (HR), 43, 47t, 156, 168, 203
    flow velocity profile and, 260, 298
Heart transplantation, 12, 60, 101, 393, 524
Hemochromatosis, 488
Hepatic vein, 15, 16, 28, 60, 68, 102, 109
    flow profile for, 168f, 169, 203, 479f
    flow reversal in, 428, 445
    flow wave in, 262, 299, 491, 491f, 527
    holosystolic flow reversal in, 486, 522
Hetastarch, 123, 127
Hiatal hernia, 102
Hibernating myocardium, 66, 107, 344, 381, 387, 415
    in inferior wall, 179, 210, 280, 310
Histamine, 110, 311
Hodgkin's disease, 14, 28
Holodiastolic flow reversal, 183, 213, 347, 389
HR. See Heart rate
Hydrophilicity, 153
Hypereosinophilic syndrome, 488, 523
Hypertension
    chronic, 68, 109, 379, 413
    pulmonary, 14, 160, 197
Hypertensive heart disease, 175
Hypertrophic cardiomyopathy, 52, 175, 180–182, 211–212, 232, 241, 278, 308, 487, 523
    genetics of, 279, 309
    left ventricular outflow obstruction and, 279, 309, 378, 413
Hypertrophic obstructive cardiomyopathy, 8, 346, 377, 378, 388, 393, 412, 458, 500
Hypertrophy
    of left ventricle, 52, 67, 68, 108, 108t, 109, 134, 228, 231, 240, 241, 241t, 278, 308, 344, 386, 430, 447, 523t
    of right ventricle, 238
Hypertrophy, severity of, 231, 241, 241t, 278, 308
Hypokinesis, 3, 245, 246, 286, 287, 334
Hypotension, 127, 142
Hypovolemia, 4, 16, 28, 227, 239, 245, 286, 344, 345, 387

I

Idiopathic hypertrophic subaortic stenosis (IHSS), 238, 378. See also Hypertrophic cardiomyopathy
IHSS. See Idiopathic hypertrophic subaortic stenosis
Ileal cancer, 281, 311
Ileum, 281, 311
Image quality, spatial pulse length and, 352, 395
Imaging depth, 43, 69, 86, 152, 156, 182, 191, 212, 374, 409
    attenuation and, 249, 290
    decreasing, 375, 409
    pulse repetition frequency and, 310
    temporal resolution and, 255, 294
Impaired relaxation, 95, 96, 109, 167, 170, 172, 182, 204, 212
    diastolic function and, 53
    left ventricle and, 261, 298–300
Incidence, 41
    angle of, 40, 41, 83, 84, 153, 154, 192, 195, 208, 464, 504
    intensity of, 250
    oblique, 84, 85
Incident angle, 40, 41, 83, 84, 153, 154, 192, 195, 208, 464, 504
Incident intensity, 154
Infarcted myocardium, 108
Inferior vena cava (IVC), 11, 63, 102, 103, 132, 241, 322, 338, 406, 441, 445
    restrictive cardiomyopathy and, 109
Inferior wall, 15, 115, 280, 310, 315, 334
    dyskinesis of, 330, 342
    hibernating myocardium in, 179, 210, 280, 310
Infiltrative amyloidosis, 14, 167, 171, 202

Inhibited myocardium, 66
Inlet ventricular septal defect, 257, 295, 433, 434, 448
Inotropes, 318, 336
Intensity
    amplitude and, 459, 500
    continuous-wave ultrasound and, 460, 501
    probes and, 460, 501
    ultrasound, 353, 395–396, 459, 500
Intensity reflection coefficient, 154, 192, 250, 291
Intensity transmission coefficient, 154, 192
Interatrial septum, 88, 124, 150
    aneurysm of, 63, 103, 221, 230, 237, 241, 271, 275, 303, 304, 306
    lipomatous, 13, 27, 62, 321, 337
    myxoma and, 407
    stroke and aneurysm of, 271, 304
    thrombus in, 241
Interventricular septum, 7, 275, 306, 517
    lipomatous, 14
    right ventricular volume overload and, 382, 416
Intra-aortic balloon pump, 121, 142, 394
Intracardiac shunt, 160, 224, 225, 238, 239, 420, 440
Intracardiac thrombectomy, 393
Intracardiac thrombus, 230, 241
Intrathoracic pressure, 27, 102, 402, 517
Intraventricular septum, 24, 402
Ischemia, 95, 107, 210
    anterior wall, 134
    circumflex coronary artery, 70
    coronary artery, 70, 110, 115
    fixed irreversible, 281, 310
    left anterior descending, 70
    left main coronary artery, 70
    mitral regurgitation and, 118
    myocardial, 52, 66, 67, 69, 70, 110, 167, 171, 202, 204, 344, 386–387, 393, 415
    right coronary artery, 70
    TEE sensitivity for, 141–142
Ischemic myocardium, 66, 67, 107
Ischemic period, 53
Isovolumic left ventricular contraction, 217, 452, 495
Isovolumic relaxation, 13, 56, 98, 99, 101, 166, 202
Isovolumic relaxation time (IVRT), 54, 60, 97, 101, 151, 167, 173, 202, 205, 369, 406
    diastolic dysfunction and, 260, 298
IVC. See Inferior vena cava
IVRT. See Isovolumic relaxation time

K
Kartagener's syndrome, 10, 123
Kidney transplantation, 2

L
Lambls' excrescences, 373, 408, 409
Laminar flow, 52, 124, 140, 294
LAP. See Left atrial pressure
Late ventricular filling, 56
Lateral mitral annular tissue Doppler E_M, 13, 27, 53, 54, 55, 60, 97, 98, 102, 145, 151, 186, 204, 475, 514, 515
    chronic hypertension and, 379, 413
    restrictive diastolic dysfunction and, 360, 402
Lateral resolution, 32, 42, 85, 109, 156, 177, 194, 208, 254, 284, 293, 320, 337, 355, 356, 396–397, 397, 463, 502
    beam diameter and, 355, 397
    improving, 274, 305
    pulses per scan line and, 380, 381, 415
Lateral wall, 15, 17, 115, 130, 227, 239, 431, 447
    dyskinetic, 428, 445
Leaflet fluttering, 180, 211, 458, 500
Leaflet prolapse, 72, 111, 148
Leakage current, 371, 407
Left anterior descending artery, 53
Left atrial appendage, 178, 179, 210
    inverted, 275, 305

Left atrial pressure (LAP), 49, 91, 97, 483, 519
    chronically elevated, 101
Left atrium, 11, 12, 13, 14, 27, 28, 102, 223, 237, 325, 339, 426, 437, 440, 444, 449, 458, 500, 516
    cor triatrium and, 382, 416
    diameter of, 377, 412
    dilation of, 60, 101, 379, 413, 485, 521
    enlargement of, 109
    mitral regurgitation and, 497
    myxoma in, 269, 302
Left ventricle, 11, 13, 14, 28, 134
    aneurism of, 216, 234
    blood supply to, 131, 143
    cavity dilation of, 70
    compliance of, 98, 244, 260, 285, 298, 364, 403
    dilation of, 4, 23
    ejection fraction of, 141
    hyperdynamic, 70, 110
    hypertrophy of, 52, 67, 68, 108, 108t, 109, 134, 228, 231, 240, 241, 241t, 278, 308, 344, 386, 430, 447, 523t
    impaired relaxation of, 261, 298–300
    isovolumetric contraction of, 217, 452, 495
    nondilated thick, 182, 212
    pseudoaneurysm of, 369, 406
    remodeling of, 67
    stroke volume of, 163, 199, 207, 276, 307, 467, 484, 507, 517, 520
    thrombus in, 275, 306
    wall of, 70, 127, 181
    wall stress in, 379, 380, 413, 414
    wall tension in, 380, 414
    wall thickness in, 487, 523
Left ventricular band, 437, 449
Left ventricular diastolic dysfunction, 119
Left ventricular ejection fraction (LVEF), 68, 116, 127, 134, 141, 142
Left ventricular end diastolic diameter (LVEDd), 101
Left ventricular end diastolic pressure (LVEDP), 58, 99, 258, 259, 296, 297, 380, 414
Left ventricular end systolic diameter (LVEDp), 101
Left ventricular outflow tract (LVOT), 12, 23–24, 25–26, 35t, 117, 131, 149, 150, 157, 173, 188, 189, 211, 239, 339, 523
    aortic insufficiency and, 423, 442
    bacterial vegetation in, 486, 522
    cardiac output through, 48
    continuity equation and, 120, 138
    diameter of, 314, 334
    flow through, 524
    hypertrophic cardiomyopathy and obstruction of, 279, 309, 378, 413
    obstruction of, 71, 279, 309, 318, 335, 336, 377, 378, 407, 412, 492, 527
    stroke volume of, 48, 117, 136, 161, 197, 247, 259, 288, 297
Left ventricular pressure, 26
Ligamentum arteriosum, 114
Line density, 43, 69, 86, 109, 182, 212, 309, 503
Listening time, 86, 255, 294
Lodine, 271
Longitudinal resolution, 42, 85, 146, 156, 194, 254, 293, 355, 397
Low-frequency transducer, 32, 75
Lung transplantation, 35, 393
LVEDd. See Left ventricular end diastolic diameter
LVEDP. See Left ventricular end diastolic pressure; Left ventricular end systolic diameter
LVEF. See Left ventricular ejection fraction
LVOT. See Left ventricular outflow tract

M
Magnetic resonance imaging (MRI), 52, 95
Marfan's syndrome, 71, 325, 339, 425, 443, 473, 513
Matching layer, 145, 186, 461, 502
    reflection and, 502
Mediastinal mass, 28
Mediastinal radiation treatment, 61, 102
Medtronic Hall single tilting disc prosthesis, 322, 338
Midsystolic closure, 458, 500
Miller's physiology, 160

Milrinone, 123, 127, 139, 142
Mineral oil, 271
Mirror image artifact, 272, 304
Mirroring, 61, 62
Mitral annular, 76, 149
  dilation of, 118, 148, 187, 454, 497
  tissue Doppler velocities of, 363, 403, 404
Mitral annular calcification, 68, 102, 109, 110
Mitral insufficiency, 36, 120
Mitral regurgitation (MR), 6, 8, 14, 24, 34, 35, 48, 70, 71, 72, 111, 119, 124, 137, 148, 181, 187, 211, 318, 405, 487, 523
  atrial septal defect and, 357, 398
  causes of, 224, 238
  cleft valve leaflet and, 433, 448
  color flow Doppler evaluation of, 35, 383, 388, 416
  continuity equation and, 138
  degree of, 37, 150, 190, 457, 471, 500, 512
  diastolic function and, 175, 207
  dilated cardiomyopathy and, 278, 308
  flow profile of, 454, 497
  flow rate of, 376, 410
  flow velocities and, 168, 203, 217
  fraction of, 37, 50, 81, 94, 162, 198, 471, 512
  hypereosinophilic syndrome and, 523
  hypertrophic obstructive cardiomyopathy and, 346, 388
  ischemic, 118
  jet area of, 7, 377, 412
  jet velocity and, 346, 388–389, 497
  leaflet motion and, 219, 220, 236
  left atrium and, 497
  measurements of, 7
  mechanism for, 118, 137, 318, 335
  orifice area of, 37, 49, 80, 91, 92, 118, 136, 150, 162, 189, 198, 376, 410, 471, 511
  severity of, 162, 198, 218, 219, 235, 236, 317, 319, 335, 336, 377, 411, 454, 474, 497, 514
  systolic function and, 217, 234
  vena contracta, 454, 497
  volume of, 36, 50, 76, 79, 92, 93, 118, 136, 150, 162, 189, 198, 376, 411, 470, 511
Mitral stenosis (MS), 5, 8, 25, 26, 37, 71, 81, 111, 127, 160, 516
  atrial reversal wave and, 475, 514
  calcific, 220, 236
  causes of, 72
  degenerative calcific, 72
  degree of, 248, 289, 471, 512
  rheumatic heart disease and, 348, 389
  segmental wall motion abnormalities and, 344, 345, 387–388
Mitral valve, 11, 13, 47t, 71, 121, 128, 142
  annulus of, 34
  area of, 7, 25, 36, 71, 77, 111, 221, 237, 383, 416–417, 455, 468, 470, 492, 498, 509, 510, 527
  assessing, 346, 388
  cardiac output of, 499
  chordae tendinae of, 34, 76, 147, 187, 246, 287
  cleft, 46, 125, 140
  commissure of, 116, 135, 219, 235
  complications for, 71
  disease of, 220, 236, 260, 298
  leaflets of, 4, 5, 7, 18, 23, 29, 34, 72, 76, 88, 117, 118, 119, 127, 128, 135, 137, 137t, 148, 187, 219, 220, 236, 246, 318, 320, 335, 336, 337, 412, 523, 527
  myxomatous, 118
  myxomatous degeneration of, 148, 187
  prolapse of, 224, 238, 357, 398
  reduction of leaflet length in repairing, 347, 389
  repair of, 71, 72, 110, 275, 318, 335, 347, 389, 492
  replacement of, 316, 335
  rheumatic disease of, 220, 236, 493, 528
  scallops of, 6, 24, 72, 116, 128, 134, 142, 148, 187, 220, 236–237, 246, 287, 345, 383, 388, 416
  St. Jude prosthetic, 316, 326–327, 335, 339–340
  stroke volume of, 36, 50, 78, 93, 117, 135, 149, 161, 188, 197, 259, 296, 455, 470, 498, 510
  systolic anterior motion and, 318, 335, 336, 347, 389
Mixed venous oxygen saturation, 181, 211
Moderator band, 62, 63, 122, 130, 139, 143, 275, 306, 383, 416

Monoamine oxidases, 110, 311, 389
MR. See Mitral regurgitation
MRI. See Magnetic resonance imaging
MS. See Mitral stenosis
Myocardial contrast echocardiography, 67, 107
Myocardial dysfunction, 66
Myocardial infarction, 12, 69, 175, 176, 275, 306
  segmental wall motion abnormalities and, 386–387
Myocardial ischemia, 52, 66, 67, 69, 70, 110, 167, 171, 202, 204, 344, 386–387, 393, 415
Myocardial oxygen, 142
Myocardial performance, 54
  index of, 96, 218
Myocardial segment, 32
Myocardial segments (16-segment model), 19–20, 32, 33
Myocardial viability, 67, 107–108
Myocardium
  hibernating, 66, 107, 179, 210, 280, 310, 344, 381, 387, 415
  infarcted, 108
  inhibited, 66
  ischemic, 66, 67, 107
  nonviable, 310
  perfusion to, 373, 408
  somnolent, 66
  stunned, 66, 67, 107, 344, 387
  thinned, 234
  viability of, 180, 210
Myxoma, 303, 370, 467, 487, 522
  arrhythmia and, 407
  interatrial septum and, 407
  left atrium and, 269, 302
Myxomatous aortic valve, 19
Myxomatous degeneration, 148, 187, 347, 389
Myxomatous mitral valve, 118
Myxomatous valve disease, 71, 128

N
Natriuretic peptide, 127
Near field length. See Focal length
Near-zone length, 156, 194
Nitric oxide, 12
Nitroglycerin, 57, 98, 265, 300, 362, 403
Nodules of Arantius, 373, 409
Noncoronary cusp, 422, 442
Noonan's physiology, 160
Noonan's syndrome, 348, 389–390
Norepinephrine, 123
Normal incidence, 153, 154, 192
Nyquist limit, 24, 63, 103, 177, 194, 374, 409, 410, 464, 504
  aliasing and, 208–209
  color flow Doppler map and, 383, 416
  pulse repetition frequency and, 356, 398

O
Oblique incidence, 84–85, 153, 192, 251, 291
Obtuse incidence, 153, 192
Octopus. See Stabilizing device
Odynophagia, 61, 102, 176, 370
Oral pharynx, 61, 102
Oropharyngeal trauma, 167, 202
Orthogonal incidence, 153
Ostium primum atrial septal defect, 20, 46, 124, 125, 140, 158, 159, 196, 224, 238, 257, 295, 421, 434, 440, 448
Ostium secundum atrial septal defect, 20, 46, 88, 124, 125, 140, 158, 159, 196, 224, 238, 315, 357, 398
  rate of occurrence of, 224, 238

P
P$_2$ prolapse, 72, 111
Papillary fibroelastoma, 270, 303, 374, 409, 482, 519
  complications of, 270, 303
Papillary muscle, 15, 28, 76, 110, 122, 187, 246, 275, 287, 306, 346, 388
  anterolateral, 130, 329, 341, 346, 388, 437, 449

anteromedial, 388
    perfusion of, 247, 287
    posteromedial, 130, 143, 330, 331, 341, 342, 345, 388
    rupture of, 148, 188
Paradoxical septal motion, 60, 101, 160, 196, 453, 496
PASP. *See* Pulmonary artery systolic pressure
Patent ductus arteriosus, 123, 124, 139, 160, 183, 213
Patent foramen ovale, 62, 103, 225, 230, 239, 241, 271, 275, 303, 304, 306
    occurrence of, 348, 390
Peak E-wave deceleration time, 151
Peak mitral diastolic inflow velocity, 92, 93
Peak temporal average intensity
    maximum spatial, 243, 284
    spatial, 146, 186
Peak transvalvular velocity, 120, 137
Pectinate muscles, 178, 179
Pericardectomy, 393
Pericardial drainage, 12, 27
Pericardial effusion, 12, 13, 14, 27, 122, 171, 176, 207, 268, 301, 301f, 331, 332, 362, 368, 393, 402, 405, 480, 516–517
    Dressler's syndrome and, 342
    hemodynamically significant, 14
    severity of, 369, 406
Pericardial tamponade, 12, 27, 368, 369, 405, 480, 516
Pericarditis, 394
    causes of, 175, 207
    constrictive, 12, 14, 52, 60, 95, 102, 171, 176, 207, 268, 302, 369, 406, 475, 514, 515
Perimembranous ventricular septal defect, 46, 226, 239, 256, 295, 357, 398
Perioperative transesophageal echocardiography, 67
PET scanning. *See* Positron emission tomography
Phenylephrine, 115, 123, 127, 134, 318, 336
Piezoelectric crystal (PZT), 42, 42t, 43, 85
    attenuation and, 250, 290
    composition of, 154, 155, 193
    damping material and, 305
    focal length and, 293
    frequency and, 153, 191
    matching layer and, 461, 502
    resonant frequency of, 155, 193, 253, 292
    size of, 156, 194
    thickness of, 154, 193, 252, 291
    wavelength and, 252, 291
PISA. *See* Proximal isovelocity surface area method
Pleural effusion, 331
Pleuropulmonary diseases, 394
Positive pressure inspiration, 481, 517
Positive pressure ventilation, 482, 518
Positron emission tomography (PET scanning), 67, 108, 108t
Posterior wall, 15, 17, 115, 130, 415
    thickness of, 278, 308
Posteromedial commissure, 434, 448
Postpartum cardiomyopathy, 277
Power, 38, 66, 81, 82, 178
    tissue thickness and, 461, 501
P-R interval, 71
Preload, 95, 96t, 97, 300, 403
    decrease in, 53
Pressure
    change with respect to time in, 217, 218, 234, 452, 495
    formulas for, 152, 191
    left atrial, 483, 519
    mean pulmonary artery, 350, 359, 392, 399, 466, 505
Pressure gradient, 160
    across aortic valve, 174, 206, 489, 525
    diastolic transmitral, 347, 389
    peak instantaneous, 382, 416, 430, 446, 469, 509
Pressure half time, 120, 173, 383, 384, 416–417, 510
    aortic insufficiency and, 423, 442
Pressure overload, 60, 101
Pressure tracing, 68
PRF. *See* Pulse repetition frequency
Probes, 154, 167, 175, 193, 202, 207. *See also* Transducers
    attenuation and, 460, 501

cleaning, 175, 207
    damage to, 271, 304
    intensity and, 460, 501
    phased-array, 463, 503
Propagation speed artifact, 272, 304
Propagation velocity, 69, 74, 109
Prostaglandins, 110, 311
Proximal isovelocity surface area method (PISA), 25, 35t, 71, 77, 78, 79, 80, 92, 93, 111, 120
PRP. *See* Pulse repetition period
Pseudoaneurysm, 216, 234, 369, 406
Pulmonary artery, 12, 78, 122, 131, 143, 178, 181, 221
    bifurcation in, 64, 103
    catheter in, 394
    diastolic pressure in, 349, 359, 390, 400, 466, 506
    left, 426, 427, 444
    mean pressure in, 350, 359, 392, 399, 466, 505
    right, 132, 322, 324, 326, 338, 339
    stroke volume through, 349, 391, 456, 500
    systolic pressure, 123, 124, 140
Pulmonary artery catheter, 121, 138, 426, 429, 444, 445
Pulmonary artery systolic pressure (PASP), 164, 181, 200, 258, 277, 296, 307, 360, 375, 401, 410, 429, 432, 446, 447, 467, 506
Pulmonary embolectomy, 393
Pulmonary flow
    systemic flow and, 164, 200, 277, 307, 420, 440, 468, 508
    systolic reversal of, 514
Pulmonary flow velocity, 123
Pulmonary hypertension, 14, 160, 197
Pulmonary insufficiency, 457
Pulmonary vascular resistance, 488, 524
Pulmonary veins (PV), 55, 57, 131, 132, 143, 171, 204
    atrial reversal wave in, 96, 478, 478f, 516
    atrial septal defects and, 47
    flow reversal in, 475, 514
    flow velocity profile of, 265f, 266, 476f, 477, 478f, 515
    left upper, 8, 179, 333, 342
    pulsed-wave Doppler flow velocities in, 367, 367f, 404
    right lower, 438, 450
    right upper, 332, 342, 437, 438, 450
Pulmonary venous return, anomalous, 125, 274, 334, 421, 440
Pulmonic insufficiency, 36
    regurgitant volume, 349, 391
Pulmonic regurgitation, 10, 26, 124, 183, 213
    orifice area for, 350, 391
Pulmonic stenosis, 10, 26, 78, 124, 140, 429, 446, 447
Pulmonic valve, 11, 26, 71, 76, 110, 121, 122, 139, 223, 237, 322, 324, 338
    area of, 123
    cusps of, 33
    Noonan's syndrome and, 389–390
    pressure gradient across, 430, 446
    sclerosis of, 281
    stroke volume of flow through, 65, 104
Pulse duration, 152, 289
    wavelength and, 459, 500
Pulse length, 500
Pulse repetition frequency (PRF), 63, 152, 156, 191, 194, 255, 274, 280, 290, 294, 305, 309–310, 355, 374, 397, 409
    aliasing and, 465, 504–505
    duty factor and, 351, 394
    imaging depth and, 310
    Nyquist limit and, 356, 398
    sample volume and, 343, 386
    temporal resolution and, 274, 305
Pulse repetition period (PRP), 38, 81, 152, 156, 191, 194, 249, 255, 289, 294
Pulsed-wave Doppler, 52, 53, 57, 63, 68, 95, 96, 97, 98, 99, 102, 109, 157, 158, 160, 166, 170, 194, 195, 203, 260, 263, 298, 363, 396, 397
    aliasing and, 465, 504–505
    continuous wave v., 177, 208
    flow velocities from, 169f, 170–171, 170f, 171f, 266f, 267, 267f, 301, 362, 365, 404, 476, 515
    frequency of, 252, 253, 292
    optimum conditions for, 375, 409
    processing for, 343, 386

Pulsed-wave Doppler, *cont'd*
   range resolution and, 396–397, 464, 503–504
   spectral analysis for, 356, 397
   transducers and, 158, 195, 253, 292
   velocity profiles from, 265
   wavelength of, 252, 291
PV. *See* Pulmonary veins
PZT. *See* Piezoelectric crystal

Q

Q waves, 216, 234, 330, 342
Quadracuspid aortic valve, 20
Quality factor (Q factor), 155, 193, 253, 254, 291, 292, 293, 355, 396, 502

R

Radial arterial line, 115
Radial resolution, 145, 146, 284
Radiation therapy, 102, 130, 131
   mediastinal, 61
Range ambiguity, 273, 305, 505
Range resolution, 177, 208–209, 355, 396, 397, 503
definitions of, 397
Rarefaction, 374, 409
Rayleigh scattering, 352, 395
Reciprocal changes, 405
Recurrent laryngeal nerve, 473, 513
Red blood cells, Doppler shift and, 44–45
Reflection, 40, 41, 83, 84, 85, 145, 186, 192, 251, 352, 354, 395, 396
   depth of, 154, 192
   matching layer and, 502
   oblique incidence and, 291
Reflection coefficients, 352, 395
Refraction, 39, 40, 82, 154, 192, 251, 291, 354, 396
   Snell's law and, 84
Refraction artifact, 272, 304
Regional wall motion abnormality (RWMA), 70, 108, 315
Regurgitant fraction, 65, 118, 136, 162, 198, 471, 512
   aortic, 260, 298
Regurgitant orifice, 66
   area of, 471, 512
Regurgitant volume, 36, 50, 65, 76, 79, 92, 93, 105, 118, 136, 150, 162, 189, 198
   pulmonic valve, 349, 391
Regurgitation
   aortic, 240, 297, 298, 335, 442, 443
   mitral, 7, 14
Renal arteries, 94, 347, 389, 401
Renal cell carcinoma, 486, 522
Renal perfusion, 3, 22
Reperfusion, 66, 107
Resonant frequency, 155, 156, 193, 289, 292, 293, 396
Respiratory filling patterns, 102
Restrictive cardiomyopathy, 12, 68, 175
   amyloidosis and, 182, 212, 475, 514
   causes of, 488, 523
   systolic function and, 109
Restrictive diastolic dysfunction, 53, 98, 267, 300, 301, 360, 361, 364, 402, 403, 488, 523
Retrograde flow, 299
Revascularization, 107, 180, 210
Reverberation artifact, 7, 61, 62, 102, 178, 342, 371f, 372, 407. *See also* Comet tail artifact
Rhabdomyoma, 130, 269, 302–303, 482, 486, 518, 519, 522
Rhabdomyosarcoma, 128
Rheumatic heart disease, 71, 72, 111, 128, 160, 220, 236, 493, 528
   mitral stenosis and, 348, 389
   tricuspid stenosis and, 281, 310
Rheumatic mitral disease, 118
Right atrial inversion, 368, 405
Right atrial pressure, 123, 140, 448
Right atrial pressure tracing, 68
Right atrium, 11, 12, 13, 14, 122, 179, 441, 490, 517
   angiosarcomas in, 270, 303

trabeculated portion of, 63, 103
   tumor in, 321, 338
Right ventricle, 11, 12, 13, 14, 27, 458, 500
   cardiac output of, 467, 507
   dilation of, 160, 196
   hypertrophy of, 238
   stroke volume of, 64, 103, 163, 199, 276, 306, 368, 405, 467, 485, 507, 521
   systolic function of, 122, 139
   systolic pressure, 59, 466, 505
   volume overload of, 382, 416
Right ventricular collapse, 362
Right ventricular inflow, 27
Right ventricular outflow tract (RVOT), 160, 173, 196
   obstruction of, 238
Right ventricular pressure overload, 60, 282, 311
Right ventricular systolic pressure (RVSP), 36, 59, 100, 258, 295, 329, 341, 359, 400, 401, 429, 445, 455, 466, 497, 505
Ring-down artifact. *See* Comet tail artifact
Ringing, 145
Risk/benefit ratio, 392
R-R interval, 314, 334
Ruptured chord, 118, 137
RVOT. *See* Right ventricular outflow tract
RVSP. *See* Right ventricular systolic pressure
RWMA. *See* Regional wall motion abnormality

S

St. Jude mitral valve prosthesis, 316, 326, 335
   cleansing jets in, 327, 339, 340
Sample depth, 63, 103
Sample gate, 63, 464, 503
Sample volume, 63, 343, 386, 464, 503
Sarcoidosis, 488
SCA. *See* Society of Cardiovascular Anesthesiologists
Scan lines, 43, 109, 156, 503
   focal zones per, 69
   pulses per, 380, 381, 415
   time to image, 255, 294
Scar tissue, 180, 210
Scattering, 153, 191, 395
Segmental wall motion, 3
   abnormal, 344, 386–387
   normal, 245, 286
Segmental wall motion abnormalities (SWMA), 141–142, 316
Septal dyskinesis, 453, 496
Septal motion, paradoxical, 60, 101, 160, 196, 453, 496
Septal wall, 17, 228, 240, 430, 447
   systolic thickening of, 453, 496
   thickness of, 278, 308
Serotonin, 110, 311
Side lobe artifact, 428, 445
Simpson's method of discs, 217
Single photon emission computerized tomography (SPECT), 67
Sinotubular ridge, 17, 18, 29, 47t, 325, 339, 424, 443
Sinus of Valsalva, 17, 18, 29, 47t, 131, 165, 179, 325, 339, 424, 443, 513
   dilation of, 425, 444
Sinus venarum, 63, 103
Sinus venosus, 20, 46, 89, 124, 125, 131, 158, 159, 334, 398
   embryologic remnants of, 62, 102, 273, 304
Sinus venosus defect, 421, 440
Situs inversus, 47, 89, 161
Sliding valvuloplasty, 347, 389
Snake bite toxicity, 277
Snell's law, 83, 84
Society of Cardiovascular Anesthesiologists (SCA), 350, 392
Somnolent myocardium, 66
Sound
   propagation of, 374, 409
   speed of, 31, 74
Spatial pulse length, 145, 155, 193, 273, 284, 291, 305, 351, 394, 395, 502
   axial resolution and, 463, 503
   image quality and, 358, 395

Spatial resolution, 32, 145, 177, 208
Specific heat, 153
SPECT imaging. *See* Single photon emission computerized tomography
Splenic injury, 271
Spontaneous expiration, 481, 518
Spontaneous inspiration, 13, 27, 102, 176, 207, 402, 405, 516–517
   constrictive pericarditis and, 60
ST segment elevation, 216
Stabilizing device (octopus), 115, 134, 334
Stanford type A dissection, 51, 94, 325, 338, 339, 473, 513, 514
Stanford type B dissection, 51, 94, 324, 325, 338, 339, 473, 513
Stroke, 22
   interatrial septal aneurysm and, 271, 304
Stroke volume, 36, 48, 49, 50, 64, 65, 78, 90, 92, 93, 102, 117, 135, 136, 161, 197, 206, 455, 456, 489, 498, 500, 525
   left ventricular, 163, 199, 207, 276, 307, 467, 484, 507, 517, 520
   left ventricular outflow tract, 48, 117, 136, 161, 197, 247, 259, 288, 297
   mitral valve, 36, 50, 78, 93, 117, 135, 149, 161, 188, 197, 259, 296, 455, 470, 498, 510
   in pulmonary artery, 349, 391, 456, 500
   pulmonic valve, 65, 104
   right ventricular, 64, 103, 163, 199, 276, 306, 368, 405, 467, 485, 507, 521
   tricuspid valve, 65, 104
ST-segment analysis, 67
Stunned myocardium, 66, 67, 107, 344, 387
Subclavian artery, 50, 51f, 94, 134, 201, 260, 338
Superior vena cava (SVC), 63, 64, 68, 103, 104, 131, 132, 143, 222, 237, 323, 332, 338, 342, 427, 441, 444
   persistent left, 158, 178, 195, 210, 274, 315, 334, 422, 433, 441, 448
Supraventricular membrane, 124
SVC. *See* Superior vena cava
SVR. *See* Systemic vascular resistance
Sweep speed, 168
SWMA. *See* Segmental wall motion abnormalities
Systemic flow, pulmonary flow and, 164, 200, 277, 307, 420, 440, 468, 508
Systemic vascular resistance (SVR), 238, 244, 285
Systole, 52, 95, 101, 405
   paradoxical septal motion in, 60
   right ventricular pressure overload during, 282, 311
Systolic anterior motion (SAM), 5, 23–24, 412, 492, 527
   of mitral valve leaflet, 318, 335, 336
   mitral valve repair and, 347, 389
Systolic dimension, 23
Systolic dysfunction, 138, 139
Systolic ejection, aortic stenosis and, 26
Systolic flow reversal, 428, 445
Systolic function, 2, 3, 14, 22, 114, 116, 134, 227, 239, 452, 496
   decreased, 244, 284
   determining, 217, 234
   estimates of, 218, 234
   globally decreased, 70
   mitral regurgitation and, 217, 234
   restrictive cardiomyopathy and, 109
   right ventricular, 122, 139
Systolic pressure, 78, 123, 181, 200, 258, 277, 296, 307, 360, 375, 401, 410, 429, 432, 446, 447, 467, 506. *See also* Pulmonary artery systolic pressure; Right ventricular systolic pressure
   gradient of, 360, 400–401, 469, 509

T
Tachycardia, 381
Technetium-99m sestamibi assessment, 67
TEE. *See* Transesophageal echocardiography
Temporal resolution, 32, 43, 69, 86, 145, 156, 177, 191, 194, 208, 243, 254, 284, 293, 310, 337, 355, 397
   imaging depth and, 255, 294
   neonatal bicuspid aortic valve and, 279, 309
   pulse repetition frequency and, 274, 305
   pulses per scan line and, 381, 415
Tetralogy of fallot, 225, 238, 357, 398
Thallium scintigraphy, 67
Thebesian valve, 179, 210

Thermal injury, 271
Thiamine deficiency, 181
Thoracic viscera, 47
Thoracoabdominal aneurysm, 94
Thromboembolic events, 374, 409
Thrombus, 3, 5, 14, 22, 128, 130, 178, 210, 523
   detecting, 485, 521
   intracardiac, 230, 241
   in left ventricle, 275, 306
   St. Jude valve prosthesis and, 339, 340
   surgical excision of, 230, 241
Time gain compensation, 66, 178, 274, 305
Time velocity integral (TVI), 35t, 47t, 79, 80, 89, 117, 135, 136, 137, 149, 161, 188, 197, 308
   AV, 137, 138
   LVOT, 136, 137, 138
   proximal to aortic valve, 314, 334
Tissue thickness, 152, 191, 353, 396
   beam attenuation and, 153
   power and, 461, 501
TL. *See* True lumen
TR. *See* Tricuspid regurgitation
Trabecular ventricular septal defect, 257, 295
Trachea, 201, 370, 427, 444
Transducers, 45, 69, 86, 109, 157–158
   aliasing artifact and, 158, 195
   bandwidth of, 253, 293
   continuous-wave, 156, 193
   Doppler shift and, 45, 87, 88
   5-MHz, 243
   focal length and, 254, 293
   linear phased-array, 255, 293
   matching layer in, 145, 186
   phased-array, 381, 415, 463, 503
   pulsed-wave Doppler and, 158, 195, 253, 292
Transesophageal echocardiography (TEE), 52, 95
   aorta and, 165, 201
   complications of intraoperative, 271, 304, 370, 407
   contraindications to, 61, 102, 176, 208, 371, 407, 483, 519
   indications for, 350, 392–394
   leakage current from, 371, 407
   limitations of, 453, 496
   perioperative, 67
   probes for, 154, 167, 175, 193, 202, 207, 371, 407, 460, 463, 501, 503
   TTE v., 150
Transmission, 40, 41, 83, 354, 396
   angle of, 41, 83
Transmitral early filling, 97, 98
Transmitral flow peak velocities, 55
Transmitral flow velocity, 12, 13, 182, 212, 261, 261f, 262, 266f, 267, 299, 301
Transmitral regurgitant jet, 34, 76
Transplant rejection, 60, 101
Transthoracic echocardiography (TTE), 150, 485, 496, 521
Transtricuspid flow peak early filling velocity, 13, 27
Transvalvular regurgitation, 316, 446
Transverse resolution, 42, 85, 156, 194
Transverse sinus, 62, 63, 178
Tricuspid annular plane systolic excursion, 123, 139, 348, 390, 491, 527
Tricuspid aortic valve, 20
Tricuspid atresia, 358t
Tricuspid regurgitation (TR), 15, 28, 35, 124, 140, 274, 310, 428, 445, 447, 522
   degree of, 329, 341
   intensity of signal from, 184, 213
Tricuspid regurgitation (TR), *cont'd*
   jet area of, 77, 148, 188, 247, 287
   severity of, 247, 287, 431, 447
Tricuspid stenosis, 124, 131, 249, 262, 274, 289, 299, 491, 527
   rheumatic heart disease and, 281, 310
Tricuspid valve (TV), 11, 13, 27, 65, 71, 110, 121, 122, 138, 160, 173
   area of, 248, 288, 456, 499
   endocarditis in, 522
   leaflets of, 10, 26, 281, 311, 345, 388

Tricuspid valve (TV), *cont'd*
    regurgitant fraction of, 65, 105
    regurgitant orifice area of, 66, 106
    regurgitant volume through, 65, 105
    sclerosis of, 281
    stroke volume through, 65, 104
    ventricular inversion and, 357, 398–399
Trisomy 21, 434, 448
Troponin, 127, 141
True lumen (TL), 52, 95
TTE. *See* Transthoracic echocardiography
Tuberculosis, 176
Tuberous sclerosis, 303
Turbulent flow, 256, 294
TV. *See* Tricuspid valve
TVI. *See* Time velocity integral

U

Ultrasound beam
    blood flow direction and, 280, 310
    continuous wave, 43, 460, 464, 501, 503
    Doppler, 43–45
    epiaortic scan with, 165, 201, 232, 233
    frequency of, 374, 409
    intensity of, 353, 395–396, 459, 500
    near-zone length of, 156, 194
    velocity of, 39, 82, 154, 192, 253, 292
Ultrasound gel, 42
Ultrasound probe, 43
Ultrasound propagation velocity, 31
Ultrasound system
    dynamic range and, 106–107
    multifocus, 381, 415
output power of, 38, 39
    power of, 38, 81, 82
Uremia, 175, 176

V

V. *See* Velocity
Variance color flow Doppler map, 18
Vascular accident, 3, 22
Vasoconstriction, 142, 318, 336
Vasodepressor, 415
Vasodilation, 12
Vasopressin, 127, 134, 318, 336
Vegetation, 128, 142
    bacterial, 486, 522
Velocity (V), 39, 40t, 193, 354t
    aliasing, 92
    aortic ejection, 308
    beam, 39
    of blood flow, 177, 208, 352, 395, 484, 521
    of circumferential shortening, 218, 235
    diastolic transmitral inflow, 168, 203
    early filling, 97
    E-wave peak, 60
    flow, 160, 196, 300t
    maximum measurable, 177, 209
    measuring high, 464, 503
    MR jet, 346, 388–389, 497
    peak, 92
    peak mitral diastolic inflow, 92, 93
    peak transvalvular, 120, 137
    propagation, 69, 74, 109
    pulmonary flow, 123
    transmitral flow, 12, 13, 182, 212, 261, 261f, 262, 266f, 267, 299, 301
    of ultrasound beam, 39, 82, 154, 192, 253, 292

Vena cava, 30
    inferior, 11, 63, 102, 103, 109, 132, 241, 322, 338, 406, 441, 445
    persistent left superior, 125, 158, 178, 195, 210, 274, 315, 334, 422, 433, 441, 448
    superior, 63, 64, 68, 103, 104, 131, 132, 143, 222, 237, 323, 332, 338, 342, 427, 441, 444
Vena contracta, 7, 24, 454, 497
Venous cannula, 115, 134, 222, 237
Ventricular arrhythmia, 22
Ventricular dilation, 4, 23
Ventricular dysfunction, 66
Ventricular fibrillation, 5
Ventricular filling, 14, 56, 207
Ventricular hypertrophy, 4, 14, 181, 211, 211t
    left, 52, 67, 68, 108, 108t, 109, 134, 228, 231, 240, 241, 241t, 278, 308, 344, 386, 430, 447, 523t
    right, 238
Ventricular inversion, 357, 358, 358t, 398
Ventricular mass, 13, 14, 27, 28
Ventricular rupture, 71, 110
Ventricular septal aneurysm, 226, 239
    defects and, 256, 295
Ventricular septal defect (VSD), 20, 88, 123, 139, 159, 160, 196, 238, 320, 337, 356, 358t, 398
    aneurysms and, 226, 239, 256, 295
    atrioventricular canal defect and, 257, 295
    conal, 357, 398
    inlet, 257, 295, 433, 448
    perimembranous, 46, 226, 239, 256, 295, 357, 398
    tetralogy of fallot and, 357, 398
    trabecular, 257, 295
    types of, 257, 295
Ventricular wall, 14, 76, 146, 186, 187
    chordae tendinae and, 187
    hyperdynamic, 70
    restrictive cardiomyopathy and, 109
    stress on, 100
Vocal cord paralysis, 370
Volume overload, 101, 196
    interventricular septum displacement and, 382, 416
    right ventricular, 382, 416
Volume status, 16, 28, 227, 239, 453, 497. *See also* Hypovolemia
    decreased, 245, 286
VSD. *See* Ventricular septal defect

W

Wake Forest grading system, 201t
Wall motion
    abnormal, 70
    American Society of Echocardiography grading scale for, 246, 287, 344, 386, 386t
    dyskinetic, 330, 342
    hibernating myocardium and, 310
    impaired, 107
Wall stress, 59
    left ventricular, 379, 380, 413, 414
Wall tension, 59, 99, 100
    left ventricular, 380, 414
Wall thickness, 101, 102, 109, 175, 181, 207, 211, 228, 240, 278, 308, 523t
    free, 68, 379, 413
    left ventricular, 487, 523
    posterior, 278, 308
    septal, 278, 308
Wavelength, pulse length and, 459, 500

Z

Z. *See* Acoustic impedance
Zero crossing detection, 356, 397
Zvara's physiology, 160